THE NUTRITION DESK REFERENCE

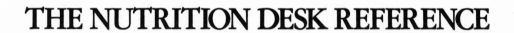

Keats Titles of Relevant Interest

Brain Allergies by William H. Philpott, M.D. and Dwight K. Kalita, Ph.D.

Diet and Disease by E. Cheraskin, M.D., D.M.D.,
  W.M. Ringsdorf, D.M.D., and J.W. Clark, D.D.S.

Diverticular Disease of the Colon by Neil Painter, M.D.

Mental and Elemental Nutrients by Carl C. Pfeiffer, Ph.D., M.D.

Minerals and Your Health by Len Mervyn, Ph.D.

1984: The Yearbook of Nutritional Medicine,
  edited by Jeffrey Bland, Ph.D.

Nourishing Your Child by Ray C. Wunderlich, Jr., M.D. and
  Dwight K. Kalita, Ph.D.

Nutrients to Age Without Senility by Abram Hoffer, Ph.D., M.D. and
  Morton Walker, D.P.M.

Orthomolecular Nutrition by Abram Hoffer, Ph.D., M.D. and
  Morton Walker, D.P.M.

Physician's Handbook on Orthomolecular Medicine, edited by
  Roger J. Williams, Ph.D. and Dwight K. Kalita, Ph.D.

The Poisons Around Us by Henry A. Schroeder, M.D.

Predictive Medicine by E. Cheraskin, M.D. and W.M. Ringsdorf, D.M.D.

The Saccharine Disease by T.L. Cleave, M.D.

Selenium as Food and Medicine by Richard A. Passwater, Ph.D.

Solved: The Riddle of Illness by Stephen E. Langer, M.D.
  with James F. Scheer

Trace Elements, Hair Analysis and Nutrition by Richard A. Passwater, Ph.D.
  and Elmer M. Cranton, M.D.

Victory Over Diabetes: A Bio-Ecologic Triumph by
  William H. Philpott, M.D., and Dwight K. Kalita, Ph.D.

THE NUTRITION DESK REFERENCE

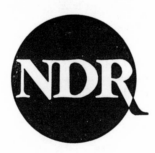

Robert H. Garrison, Jr., M.A., R.Ph.
and
Elizabeth Somer, M.A.

Keats Publishing, Inc. New Canaan, Connecticut

Library of Congress Cataloging in Publication Data

Garrison, Robert H., Jr.
  The nutrition desk reference.

  Includes bibliographies and index.
  1. Nutrition—Handbooks, manuals, etc.   2. Drug-
nutrient interactions—Handbooks, manuals, etc.
3. Cardiovascular system—Diseases—Nutritional aspects—
Handbooks, manuals, etc.   4. Cancer—Nutritional
aspects—Handbooks, manuals, etc.   I. Somer, Elizabeth.
II. Title. [DNLM: 1. Cardiovascular Diseases—handbooks.
2. Medical Oncology—handbooks.   3. Nutrition—handbooks.
QU 39 G242n]
QP141.G33   1985   613.2   84-26098
ISBN 0-87983-328-9

THE NUTRITION DESK REFERENCE

Printed in the United States of America

Keats Publishing, Inc.
27 Pine Street (Box 876)
New Canaan, Connecticut 06840

TABLE OF CONTENTS

.........FIGURES.........

•••••••••••••••••••••••••••••••TABLES•••••••••••••••••••••••••••••••

··············ACKNOWLEDGMENTS·················

We would like to express our sincere appreciation to the staff at Health Media of America—Therese Argoud, Timothy Holsather, Sharisse Parker and Kristi Paulson—for their role in developing the *Nutrition Desk Reference*. We are especially grateful to Lisa Garrison Moye for her superb research assistance.

Ellen Kapustka's editorial support in shepherding this book from manuscript through to finished pages deserves more than our gratitude. We both believe it is accurate to say that there would be no *Nutrition Desk Reference* without her.

Robert H. Garrison, Jr.
Elizabeth Somer

$\bullet$ P R E F A C E $\bullet$

THE NUTRITION DESK REFERENCE provides health professionals and the interested general reader with basic nutrition information as well as the latest findings in nutrition research. The fundamentals of nutrition are included to give the reader a foundation, as well as a synopsis of verified research findings on the individual roles of the nutrients. More recent, and often more controversial, research findings on vitamins and minerals and their role in the prevention and treatment of disease are included as well. Some sections, such as those covering cardiovascular disease and cancer, present a comprehensive accumulation of the research, old and new.

The *Nutrition Desk Reference* is unique. No other book combines nutrition basics and current research in a documented format for the health professional and the general public. It is hoped that no matter what a person's connection to nutrition—whether as a dietitian, pharmacist, physician, beginner or advanced student in the health sciences, or general reader interested in diet and health—the book will make a contribution to increased knowledge and the ability to make informed decisions. The authors have sought to avoid the over-simplification and ultimately the vagueness of introductory nutrition books designed for the general public while refraining from in-depth biochemical explanations for nutrient roles in health and disease. In addition, the *Nutrition Desk Reference* provides accurate, up-to-date information which can stand alone or supplement a basic nutrition text.

Interest in nutrition and diet has proliferated since the dawn of man. Nutrition as a science, however, is relatively new and this novelty breeds popular interest as well as faddism. The role of nutrition in the prevention and treatment of degenerative conditions and diseases has been extensively researched. Health pro-

fessionals attempt to sort fact from fiction to determine the relationship of nutrition to cancer, heart disease, diabetes, obesity, arthritis, depression, aging and numerous other conditions. Qualified health professionals are not the only ones preaching their views on nutrition. Nutrition is a popular topic, and many less qualified individuals jump aboard the band wagon to prescribe and recommend. Every magazine designed for the general reader includes articles on nutrition and the latest claims for vitamins, minerals and other nutrients. This deluge of printed material is eagerly received by individuals seeking information about foods, supplements and health habits that may cure an ailment or provide guidelines for optimal health and longevity. At this time, the science of nutrition does not have definitive answers to many health and disease questions, and consumers are forced to choose among conflicting reports, beliefs and opinions.

The individual must take responsibility for gathering information in order to make informed choices, while health professionals must stay abreast of current information and translate the research into practical terms for all to understand. In spite of the lack of consistency, the data on health and nutrition continue to accumulate. Unfortunately, this accumulation of information is often presented to the consumer and the health professional in a fragmented and incomplete fashion, further complicating the decision-making process. The *Nutrition Desk Reference* seeks to alleviate this problem by bringing together important topics in nutrition research in a concise, readable style.

From 1960 to 1982, the cost of health care in the United States escalated from $27 billion to $290 billion, an increase of over 900 percent. Of every Federal dollar spent, eleven cents went to health care. Unless the health care system is dramatically altered, this figure will continue to rise. A large proportion of health care costs has been devoted to treating diseases which are in fact a product of faulty lifestyle habits. This after-the-fact treatment approach to disease has not resulted in substantial improvements in the nation's health. A preventive approach which includes individual responsibility for changing life-threatening habits must be encouraged.

Because 75 percent of the deaths in this country are due to lifestyle-related degenerative diseases such as cardiovascular disease and cancer, the *Nutrition Desk Reference* includes extensive coverage of these topics and the verified as well as controversial nutrition research relating to their development and treatment. The dietary recommendations section, based on the *Dietary Goals for the United States*, provides the rationale and tools to assist health professionals and the general public in designing an eating pattern that includes shopping, preparing foods and dining out.

The final section of the book addresses the relationship between drugs and nutrition. The chapter on drug-nutrient interactions provides health professionals and pharmacists with information on drug-induced nutrient deficiencies which can help them in making dietary recommendations to clients and patients. This section provides the general public with information about the relationship between prescription or over-the-counter drugs and nutritional status. The reader should use this information in conjunction with a consultation with a pharmacist regarding appropriate diet and supplement changes to counteract drug influences. The chapter on nutrition and alcohol and drug abuse shows the critical role diet and nutritional status play in the perpetuation of these conditions. This section is designed for use by all those affected by alcoholism and drug abuse. For health professionals, this section provides useful information for improving compliance in rehabilitation programs.

Part I
DIETARY FACTORS

1
······························INTRODUCTION TO DIETARY FACTORS··········

IN THE FOLLOWING CHAPTERS, you will be presented with succinct information on the macronutrients and the micronutrients, including noteworthy recent research findings. Space limitations do not allow the inclusion of all relevant research in the literature, so the summaries will reflect the most promising areas for continuing investigation.

For the benefit of the general reader, an overview of nutritional constituents is offered. Detailed information on research for specific nutrients is provided in subsequent chapters. If one nutrient or aspect of therapeutic application is of specific interest, consult the table of contents and the index for quick reference.

Nutrition is the study of foods and their constituents—their ingestion, digestion, absorption, transport and utilization. The term nutrition includes the action, interaction and balance of food constituents as they pertain to human health and disease. The functions of normal nutrition are to sustain life, provide energy, promote growth, and replace loss. Therapeutic nutrition is the manipulation of dietary factors to prevent or treat disease, or to influence non-nutritional regimens of therapy.

SHORT SUMMARY OF NUTRITIONAL BREAKTHROUGHS

The oldest extant records of human nutritional awareness are 7,000-year-old Egyptian pictographs. Circa B.C. 1500, Egyptian medical writings on papyrus offered dietary cures for various afflictions and diseases. The Old Testament contains numerous records of "laws" for the selection, preparation and storage of foods.

The Father of Medicine, Hippocrates (born B.C.

460), emphasized the role of diet in the control of disease. Although most of his aphorisms were without scientific foundation, they set a medical precedent in considering nutritional factors.

René de Réaumur (b. 1683) is credited with pioneering investigations into the chemical nature of digestion. Antoine Laurent Lavoisier (b. 1743) established the basis for the scientific study of energy metabolism in laboratory animals.

In the mid-1700s, Dr. James Lind showed the effect of consuming citrus fruits on the treatment and prevention of scurvy. The mechanism was not understood, but the effect was that British sailors—thereafter called "limeys"—could sail around the world without fear of contracting scurvy.

In 1862, the first experimental chamber large enough to allow the study of human heat production and oxygen/carbon dioxide exchange was constructed in Germany. Using chambers of this type, scientists were able to prove the law of the conservation of energy for higher animals.

Justus von Liebig (b. 1803) developed analytical methods for determining the composition of foods, body tissue, and excrement. One of Liebig's students, Carl von Voit, studied the influence of nitrogen on protein metabolism.

Researchers in Switzerland and France determined in the early 1800s the dietary importance of calcium in dental and bone growth and health. In Sweden in 1838, the chemist Berzelius determined the role of iron in hemoglobin formation and opened the field of dietary therapy for anemia. At approximately the same time, J. B. Boussingault proposed that iodine could be used to prevent goiter, based on an observed relationship between diet and the incidence of the disease in South America.

In 1897, P. Eijkmann of the Netherlands demonstrated that beriberi could be induced or cured by dietary substitution of processed or unmilled rice, respectively. In the first decade of this century, the Englishman J. G. Hopkins determined that laboratory animals required more than proteins, carbohydrates, fats, and salts to sustain life. The missing nutritional factors were labeled ''vitamines'' in 1911 by Casimir Funk.

Researchers at Yale University and the University of Wisconsin isolated vitamin A in the second decade of the twentieth century, using controlled diets for laboratory animals.

In the mid-1930s, Rudolf Schoenheimer of Columbia University demonstrated the use of hydrogen isotopes in tracing metabolic reactions.

In 1953, the field of genetics was revolutionized by the discovery of DNA structure and function. By explaining DNA's double-helix structure and the process of its replication, Francis H. C. Crick and James D. Watson greatly advanced nutritional studies.

THE THOUSANDFOLD INCREASE IN NUTRITIONAL RESEARCH

The number and importance of nutritional discoveries per month in the 1980s correspond to advances in research equal to entire centuries of previous collective discovery. Nutrition research today involves tools and techniques that were unknown even a decade ago.

According to some authorities, the total set of human knowledge is currently estimated to double every two years. The challenge to individuals interested in nutrition is to sort through the sheer volume of research findings, and view each research contribution in a broader context.

The science of nutrition is no longer a single field. Nutritional research is a co-mingling of the findings of geneticists, molecular biologists, psychobiologists, immunologists, pharmacologists, biochemists, neuroscientists, and researchers in an incredible range of other scientific fields.

Only seventy years have passed since the first vitamin was identified. Today the rate of laboratory and clinical findings is so accelerated that if an individual is not abreast of the findings published in the last few years, he or she may be light-years away from the current state of nutritional understanding.

WATER: THE MEDIUM FOR LIFE

The body's need for water is second in importance only to its need for oxygen. Adult body weight is approximately 55 to 65 percent water, with infants' body weight comprising as much as 70 percent. A 10 percent loss of body water poses significant health risks, and a 20 percent loss may result in death.

The importance of water in the body should be considered in terms of osmotic pressure relationships, as an acid-base balance, as a mechanism for the movement of nutrients into cells (and the removal of wastes from cells) and as the solution holding the electrolytes. Briefly, electrolytes are salts that allow the conveyance of electrical currents. Sodium and chloride are found primarily in blood and the extracellular body fluids. Potassium is the major intracellular electrolyte.

Water is the medium for all body fluids including blood, lymph, the digestive juices, urine and perspiration.

AN INTRODUCTION TO THE MACRONUTRIENTS

The macronutrients are so named because they comprise the greatest portion of human diet. They supply fuel for work and they help to regulate body heat. The macronutrients are carbohydrates, lipids and protein. Their consumption as a percentage of the average American diet is depicted in Figure 1.

The fuel potential of the macronutrients is expressed in kilocalories (or ''calories'' in the vernacular). The term calorie is derived from the Latin *calor*, which means heat. A calorie is the amount of energy needed to raise the temperature of one gram of water by one degree centigrade (from an accepted standard temperature), at one atmospheric pressure. A gram of water is approximately two or three raindrops; one degree centigrade is approximately 1.8 degrees Fahrenheit; and one atmospheric pressure is that existing at sea level.

Food is usually defined quantitatively in terms of calories as a convenient basis for comparing relative energy value. For example, lipids (fats) contain 9 calories per gram, while protein and carbohydrates contain 4 calories per gram.

Carbohydrates: Sugars and starch serve as the body's chief source of energy, and help regulate the metabolism of protein and lipids. Fiber is another component of carbohydrates that serves to facilitate digestion.

Proteins: Protein is the most plentiful substance in the

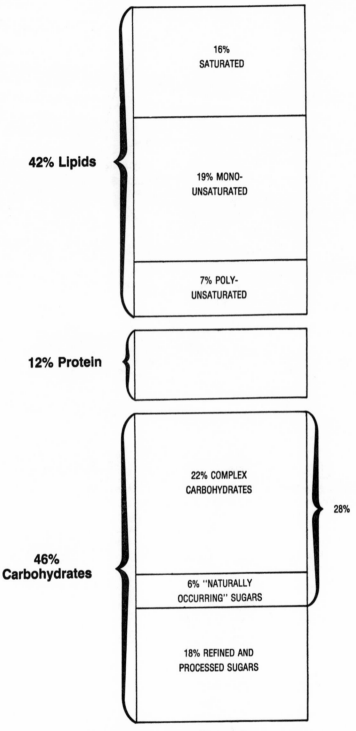

Figure 1

*The lipid, protein and carbohydrate components of a
typical American's diet (excluding alcoholic beverages)*

Adapted from *Dietary Goals for the United States*, 2nd ed. Select
Committee on Nutrition and Human Needs, United States Senate.
Washington, D.C.: U.S. Government Printing Office, 1977, p. 5.

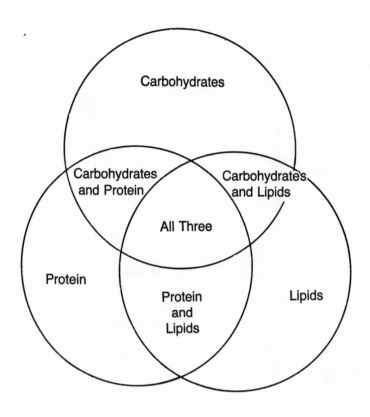

Carbohydrates:
    carrots
    oranges
    sugar
    bananas

Carbohydrates
and Protein:
    beans (dry)
    bread
    corn
    macaroni
    oatmeal
    potato

Protein only:
    (none naturally)

All Three:
    cookies (chocolate
        chip)
    crackers (saltine)

    ice cream
    milk (whole)
    peanut butter

Protein and Lipids:
    cheese (cheddar)
    eggs
    hamburgers
    hot dogs (all-meat)
    roasts
    tuna fish

Carbohydrates
and Lipids:
    pie (apple)
    salad dressing
        (mayonnaise
        type)

Lipids Only:
    margarine

Figure 2

How some common foods can be classified as carbohydrates and/or lipids and/or protein.

Adapted from Travis, S. and Fry, B. *Energy: Our Food and Our Needs*. Ithaca, N.Y.: Division of Nutritional Sciences, Cornell University.

body after water. Protein consists of large molecules that are broken down into amino acids during digestion. Amino acids are necessary for the construction of body proteins, which are vital for the growth and maintenance of muscles, blood, internal organs, skin, hair and nails. In addition, protein is vital to the formation of hormones, enzymes and antibodies.

Lipids: The most concentrated energy source in our diet is lipids, which are found in foods derived from animal and plant sources. Lipids are the carriers for fat-soluble vitamins (A, D, E and K), and serve to control the rate of digestion in the stomach. Lipids are designated as saturated, unsaturated, or polyunsaturated on the basis of their physical and functional properties.

Figure 2 shows how some common foods can be classified as predominantly composed of one or more of the macronutrients. Eaten in excess, protein can be fattening, just like carbohydrates or lipids. "Fattening" is a function of the consumption of more calories than are expended, with the unused energy stored as reserves for future needs.

AN INTRODUCTION TO THE MICRONUTRIENTS

Vitamins and minerals are the micronutrients. They have no caloric or energy value, but are absolutely necessary for good health. With very few exceptions, essential micronutrients are not manufactured within the human body and must be obtained from food or supplements.

Vitamins: These complex organic molecules are essential for biochemical transformations; they sometimes fulfill hormone-like functions and aid in the protection of cell membranes.

Minerals: These naturally occurring inorganic elements perform structural and catalytic roles, including the activation of enzymes and hormones. Unlike vitamins, minerals are not destroyed during cooking. Certain minerals (such as silicon and fluoride) are nutritionally essential, but too little is known about their biochemical functions to establish daily requirements.

Accessory Nutrients: There are two types of accessory nutrients. The first group is considered nonessential although it plays a critical metabolic role; this group includes choline, inositol, carnitine, taurine, lipoic acid, etc. The second group (including PABA and bioflavonoids) are food compounds that have been clinically demonstrated to serve preventive or therapeutic purposes, even though they do not provide any proven role in metabolism.

ESSENTIAL VS. NONESSENTIAL

A distinction is made between "essential" and "nonessential" nutrients on the basis of bioavailability. Essential nutrients are absolutely indispensable to human life and cannot be manufactured by the body itself. The essential nutrients include water, carbohydrates, linoleic acid (a lipid), eight amino acids (plus an additional one for infants), at least thirteen vitamins, and at least fifteen minerals.

Nonessential nutrients are manufactured within our bodies, synthesized from essential nutrients. For example, niacin can be produced from a particular amino acid. The term "nonessential" should not be construed to imply a lack of importance to human health. Quite the contrary, "nonessential" is merely a label for identifying relative dependence on external sources.

FOOD ADDITIVES

Considerable controversy has been associated with the potential threats and possible benefits of food additives. Additives serve to preserve foods for extended shelf life, to establish and prolong a desired appearance or flavor, and to impart certain qualities to the foodstuff.

Most of the additives on the FDA list (see Table I) are derived from natural flavors and oils, and have been used for at least twenty-five years. Occasionally, substances are removed from the FDA list in response to clinical evidence of threat. Saccharin and the cyclamate sweeteners are examples of such substances.

DIGESTION AND ABSORPTION

The nutritional value of food must be unlocked physically and chemically to yield nutrients that are digestible and absorbable.

THE DIGESTIVE TRACT

Digestion begins with mastication. As the teeth are grinding and crushing the food, saliva softens and lubricates the mass. The three salivary glands are identified in Figure 3. Saliva serves to lubricate the food for ease in swallowing, and the enzyme ptyalin breaks up dextrins and maltose.

TABLE 1
Food Additive Groups on the FDA's List of "Generally Recognized As Safe"

Anticaking Agents
Aluminum calcium silicate
Calcium silicate
Magnesium silicate
Sodium aluminosilicate
Sodium calcium aluminosilicate
Tricalcium silicate

Chemical Preservatives
Ascorbic acid
Ascorbyl palmitate
Benzoic acid
Butylated hydroxyanisole
Butylated hydroxytoluene
Calcium ascorbate
Calcium propionate
Calcium sorbate
Caprylic acid
Dilauryl thiodipropionate
Erythorbic acid
Gum guaiac
Methylparaben
Potassium bisulfite
Potassium metabisulfite
Potassium sorbate
Propionic acid
Propyl gallate
Propylparaben
Sodium ascorbate
Sodium benzoate
Sodium bisulfite
Sodium metabisulfite
Sodium propionate
Sodium sorbate
Sodium sulfite
Sorbic acid
Stannous chloride
Sulfur dioxide
Thiodipropionic acid
Tocopherols

Emulsifying Agents
Cholic acid
Desoxycholic acid
Diacetyl tartaric acid esters of mono- and diglycerides
Glycocholic acid
Mono- and diglycerides
Monosodium phosphate derivatives of above
Propylene glycol
Ox bile extract
Taurocholic acid

Nutrients and Dietary Supplements
Alanine
Arginine
Ascorbic acid
Aspartic acid
Biotin
Calcium carbonate
Calcium citrate
Calcium glycerophosphate
Calcium oxide
Calcium pantothenate
Calcium phosphate
Calcium pyrophosphate
Calcium sulfate
Carotene
Choline bitartrate
Choline chloride
Copper gluconate
Cuprous iodide
Cysteine

Cystine
Ferric phosphate
Ferric pyrophosphate
Ferric sodium pyrophosphate
Ferrous gluconate
Ferrous lactate
Ferrous sulfate
Glycine
Histidine
Inositol
Iron, reduced
Isoleucine
Leucine
Linoleic acid
Lysine
Magnesium oxide
Magnesium phosphate
Magnesium sulfate
Manganese chloride
Manganese citrate
Manganese gluconate
Manganese glycerophosphate
Manganese hypophosphite
Manganese sulfate
Manganous oxide
Mannitol
Methionine
Methionine hydroxy analogue
Niacin
Niacinamide
D-pantothenyl alcohol
Phenylalanine
Potassium chloride
Potassium glycerophosphate
Potassium iodide
Proline
Pyridoxine hydrochloride
Riboflavin
Riboflavin-5-phosphate
Serine
Sodium pantothenate
Sodium phosphate
Sorbitol
Thiamine hydrochloride
Thiamine mononitrate
Threonine
Tocopherols
Tocopherol acetate
Tryptophane
Tyrosine
Valine
Vitamin A
Vitamin A acetate
Vitamin A palmitate
Vitamin B12
Vitamin D2
Vitamin D3
Zinc sulfate
Zinc gluconate
Zinc chloride
Zinc oxide
Zinc stearate

Sequestrants
Calcium acetate
Calcium chloride
Calcium citrate
Calcium diacetate
Calcium gluconate
Calcium hexametaphosphate
Calcium phosphate, monobasic
Calcium phytate
Citric acid
Dipotassium phosphate

Disodium phosphate
Isopropyl citrate
Monoisopropyl citrate
Potassium citrate
Sodium acid phosphate
Sodium citrate
Sodium diacetate
Sodium gluconate
Sodium hexametaphosphate
Sodium metaphosphate
Sodium phosphate
Sodium potassium tartrate
Sodium pyrophosphate
Sodium pyrophosphate, tetra
Sodium tartrate
Sodium thiosulfate
Sodium tripolyphosphate
Stearyl citrate
Tartaric acid

Stabilizers
Acacia (gum arabic)
Agar-agar
Ammonium alginate
Calcium alginate
Carob bean gum
Chondrus extract
Ghatti gum
Guar gum
Potassium alginate
Sodium alginate
Sterculia (or karaya) gum
Tragacanth

Miscellaneous Additives
Acetic acid
Adipic acid
Aluminum ammonium sulfate
Aluminum potassium sulfate
Aluminum sodium sulfate
Aluminum sulfate
Ammonium bicarbonate
Ammonium carbonate
Ammonium hydroxide
Ammonium phosphate
Ammonium sulfate
Beeswax
Bentonite
Butane
Caffeine
Calcium carbonate
Calcium chloride
Calcium citrate
Calcium gluconate
Calcium hydroxide
Calcium lactate
Calcium oxide
Calcium phosphate
Caramel
Carbon dioxide
Carnauba wax
Citric acid
Dextrans
Ethyl formate
Glutamic acid
Glutamic acid hydrochloride
Glycerin
Glyceryl monostearate
Helium
Hydrochloric acid
Hydrogen peroxide
Lactic acid
Lecithin
Magnesium carbonate

Magnesium hydroxide
Magnesium oxide
Magnesium stearate
Malic acid
Methylcellulose
Monoammonium glutamate
Monopotassium glutamate
Nitrogen
Nitrous oxide
Papain
Phosphoric acid
Potassium acid tartrate
Potassium bicarbonate
Potassium carbonate
Potassium citrate
Potassium hydroxide
Potassium sulfate
Propane
Propylene glycol
Rennet
Silica aerogel
Sodium acetate
Sodium acid pyrophosphate
Sodium aluminum phosphate
Sodium bicarbonate
Sodium carbonate
Sodium citrate
Sodium carboxy-methylcellulose
Sodium caseinate
Sodium citrate
Sodium hydroxide
Sodium pectinate
Sodium phosphate
Sodium potassium tartrate
Sodium sesquicarbonate
Sodium tripolyphosphate
Succinic acid
Sulfuric acid
Tartaric acid
Triacetin
Triethyl citrate

Synthetic Flavoring Substances
Acetaldehyde
Acetoin
Aconitic acid
Anethole
Benzaldehyde
N-butyric acid
d- or l-carvone
Cinnamaldehyde
Citral
Decanal
Diacetyl
Ethyl acetate
Ethyl butyrate
Ethyl vanillin
Eugenol
Geraniol
Geranyl acetate
Glycerol tributyrate
Limonene
Linalool
Linalyl acetate
1-malic acid
Methyl anthranilate
3-Methyl-3-phenyl glycidic acid ethyl ester
Piperonal
Vanillin

Source: Kermode, G.O., *Food Additives in Human Nutrition: Readings from Scientific American.* San Francisco: W. H. Freeman and Co., 1978.

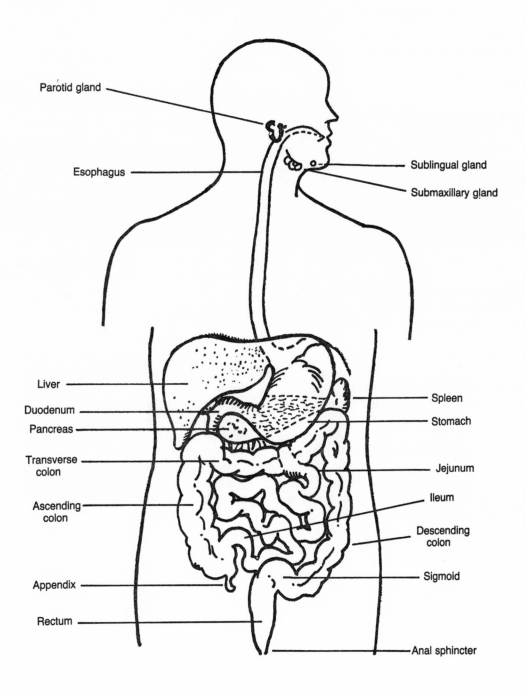

Parotid gland

Esophagus

Sublingual gland

Submaxillary gland

Liver

Duodenum

Pancreas

Transverse colon

Ascending colon

Appendix

Rectum

Spleen

Stomach

Jejunum

Ileum

Descending colon

Sigmoid

Anal sphincter

Figure 3
The digestive tract

As food enters the mouth, the senses should be positively stimulated, inducing further eating. As the food bolus is formed and positioned on the back of the tongue, reflexive swallowing moves the materials through the pharynx to the esophagus. Passage down the esophagus is accomplished by involuntary deglutition through waves of contraction. The cardiac sphincter is the circular muscle that controls the bolus's entry into the stomach.

In the pouch-like fundus of the stomach, the semi-solid food aggregates are manipulated by tonic contractions. Digestion is advanced by gastric hydrochloric acid (with a pH of 1.5 to 2.5), and enzymatic action (particularly pepsin, milk-curdling rennin, and gastric lipase). During this process, pepsinogen is converted to pepsin; ferric iron is reduced to ferrous iron; emulsified lipids are broken into fatty acids and glycerol; casein becomes paracasein; and proteins are converted to proteoses, peptones and polypeptides.

The gastric mucosa also secrete water and mucin, which act as a protective lubricant. The bactericidal and bacteriostatic actions of the stomach secretions provide protection against bacteria-related food poisoning, while at the same time controlling the levels of intestinal flora.

After an average of 3 to 4.5 hours (for a mixed solid meal) the pyloric sphincter at the base of the stomach opens to admit the chyme (the thick, semifluid mass of partially digested food) into the duodenum. Liquid ingesta remain in the stomach only briefly. Of the solids, lipids pass through the stomach most slowly and have an inhibitory action on gastric function. Thus the consumption of even small amounts of lipids may offer a prolonged sense of satiation. Proteins pass through the stomach somewhat more quickly than lipids, but not as rapidly as carbohydrates.

Emotions can profoundly effect gastric digestion. Hostility, for example, produces hyperfunction, while fear or depression slows the gastric rate. The gastric glands are also controlled by the senses (for example, the sight and smell of appetizing food) and humoral action originating in the duodenum (gastric secretion is increased when protein products interact with the duodenal mucosa and are decreased by lipid interaction).

In the small intestine, chyme is controlled by short-surge and lengthy-contraction peristaltic waves. This action mixes the chyme with the intestinal mucosa, and facilitates the surface exposure to enzymatic action. The pancreatic juices are stimulated by hormones. These juices are alkaline and help to neutralize acidic chyme. The pancreas also secretes enzymes called pancreozymins. These include: amylase, which hydrolyzes starch to maltose and dextrins; chymotrypsinogen, the inactive precursor of chymotrypsin, which splits proteins into proteoses, peptones and polypeptides; trypsinogen, the inactive precursor of trypsin, which splits specific links in the peptide chain; peptidase, which further breaks down the polypeptides into amino acids and smaller peptides; and lipase, which splits lipids into monoglycerides, fatty acids and glycerol.

The succus entericus (intestinal juice) is stimulated by a hormone (enterocrinin) and by mechanical action of the passing materials. The alkaline intestinal juice contains several digestive enzymes. Peptidases free single amino acids; phosphatases separate certain compounds into absorbable phosphate; carbohydrases (sucrase, maltase and lactase) split disaccharides into monosaccharide components; and intestinal lipase further splits lipids. Nucleinase converts nucleic acid into nucleotides, which are converted into nucleosides and phosphoric acid by nucleotidase.

The hepatic cells secrete bile, which is released into the duodenum by gallbladder contraction initiated by the hormone cholecystokinin. The constituents of bile— salts, acids, pigments, cholesterol and mucin—serve to neutralize acid chyme, emulsify fats and facilitate the absorption of fat-soluble vitamins. As the macro-nutrients—protein, carbohydrate and fats—are broken down into their constituents, vitamins and minerals entrapped in the complex molecules are released.

The large intestine absorbs the remaining food constituents as well as excess fluid. In the reservoir of the large intestine, bacterial action degrades some previously undigested materials.

The microbial population of the large intestine is dominated by the genera Streptococcus, Lactobacillus and Diplococcus. These intestinal flora vary according to the type of foods consumed; a high-carbohydrate diet results in increased gram-positive fermentative flora, while a predominately protein diet increases the gram-negative putrefactive flora. The intestinal flora synthesize essential and non-essential nutrients.

The fecal material that evacuates the large intestine includes bacteria, cellular material from the gastrointestinal tract and intestinal secretions/excretions. The remainder of the fecal material is the undigested plant fiber ("bulk" or "roughage"), which, although it has no nutritional value, is important for ease and frequency of fecal discharge and the prevention of a number of disease conditions.

ABSORPTION OF NUTRIENTS

The process of assimilating nutrients from the digestive tract into the bloodstream is called absorption. The human body is remarkably efficient in absorbing the macronutrients. For example, an estimated 95 percent of dietary fat is absorbed.

Almost all absorption of nutrients occurs in the intestines. Only alcohol is absorbed in the stomach, while everything else (water included) is passed on. In the intestines, complex molecules are broken into absorbable constituents which are diffused into the intestinal capillaries and lymphatics via semipermeable mucosal barriers. Intestinal absorption of nutrients is influenced by numerous factors, including membrane permeability, solute diffusibility, solute concentration, membrane surface tension, temperature, electrical membrane potentials and the forces of the living properties of the intestinal mucosa.

Carbohydrate is absorbed into the bloodstream in the form of glucose, galactose and fructose. In the liver, fructose and galactose are converted to glucose, which can then be used as fuel or converted to glycogen for storage.

Lipid digestion produces water-soluble triglyceride products that are easily absorbed in the bloodstream. The remaining monoglycerides, diglycerides and long-chain fatty acids need a wetting agent (bile salts) because they are less water soluble. The final fat products (fatty acids, phospholipids, free cholesterol, cholesterol esters and triglycerides) are formed through the metabolic action of the intestinal mucosa.

Amino acids, the water-soluble end-products of protein digestion, are rapidly absorbed from the small intestine directly into the bloodstream. The micronutrients, vitamins and minerals, are absorbed at specific sites along the small intestine. Fiber and non-digestive components of food travel to the large intestine and are eventually excreted.

AFTER ABSORPTION: TRANSPORTATION AND METABOLISM

After nutrients enter the bloodstream, the portal vein conveys them to the liver, then to the various tissues. When the nutrients are carried by the blood to the cells requiring the nutrients, an osmotic exchange occurs on the capillary, interstitial fluid, and cellular levels. The nutrients move from areas of higher concentration (in the blood) through the endothelial cells,

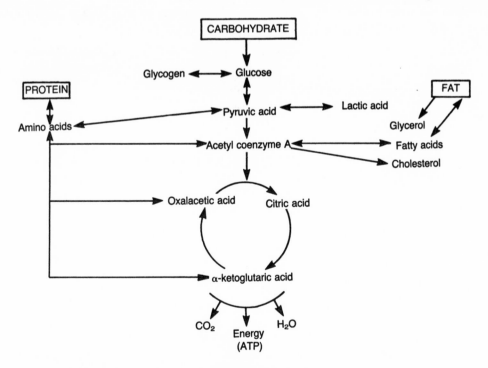

Figure 4
Simplified metabolic pathways of the macronutrients

dissolve in the extracellular fluid bathing the cell proper and finally into the cell. Some nutrients must be actively transported or "pumped" across membranes against a concentration gradient.

Basically, nutrients follow the same course (although the process is simpler) as oxygen does in its transport from the blood to the cells. It should be noted that although oxygen is derived through capillary action in the lungs (rather than ingestion), it should properly be considered a "nutrient" at the cellular level.

Within the cells, the nutrients are chemically transformed through the metabolic processes of oxidation, reduction, interconversion, transformation, energy release, synthesis and storage. Metabolic homeostasis, the normal balance of cellular metabolism, is dependent on nutrient availability, enzymatic action and hormone secretion rates.

Carbohydrate, lipids, and protein are metabolized interdependently through catabolic and anabolic reacations, as depicted in simple fashion in Figure 4. Glucose, fatty acids and amino acids enter through common pathways that produce energy (ATP). Glucose can be metabolized to form cholesterol, fatty acids and oxidative products that form amino acids when combined with amino groups. Amino acids can also serve as potential sources for the formation of fatty acids or glucose. The macronutrients are mutually dependent on the presence and activity of vitamins, as well as on correct concentrations of the electrolytes and other minerals.

REFERENCES

1. Hamilton, E. M. N., and Whitney, E. N. *Nutrition: Concepts and Controversies*. St. Paul, Minn.: West Publishing Co., 1982.

2. Eagles, J. A., and Randall, M. N. *Handbook of Normal and Therapeutic Nutrition*. New York: Raven Press, 1980.

3. Kirschmann, J. D. *Nutrition Almanac*. New York: McGraw-Hill Book Company, 1979.

4. Friend, B. Changes in nutrients in the U.S. diet caused by alternations in food intake patterns. U.S. Department of Agriculture, 1974.

5. Robinson, C. H. *Fundamentals of Normal Nutrition*. New York: The Macmillan Company, 1973.

6. Kermode, G. O. *Food Additives in Human Nutrition: Readings from Scientific American*. San Francisco: W. H. Freeman and Company, 1978.

7. Burton, T. B. *The Heinz Handbook of Nutrition*. New York: McGraw-Hill Book Company, 1965.

8. Williams, S. R. *Nutrition and Diet Therapy*. St. Louis: The C. V. Mosby Company, 1977.

9. Robinson, C. H. *Normal and Therapeutic Nutrition*. New York: The Macmillan Company, 1972.

2

···············THE MACRONUTRIENTS: ································
Carbohydrates, Proteins, Lipids

CARBOHYDRATES

DEFINITION

BRIEFLY STATED, dietary carbohydrates are 1) sugars or simple carbohydrates found in table sugar, honey, natural fruit sugars and molasses; 2) starches or complex carbohydrates found in legumes, grains, vegetables and fruits; and 3) fiber, such as cellulose, hemicellulose and pectin found in whole grains, legumes, vegetables and fruits. Carbohydrates are formed by green plants as a product of photosynthesis and are the most abundant compounds found on earth.

Literally speaking, carbohydrates are organically derived compounds composed of carbon atoms coupled to "hydrates" (such as water, H_2O). All carbohydrates follow the empirical formula of $C_n H_{2n} O_n$. Biochemically, carbohydrates are polyhydroxy alcohols with aldehyde or ketone groups that are potentially active.

Dietary carbohydrates are the principal source of energy for all body functions, including the digestion and absorption of other foods. Although proteins and lipids can be converted into energy, carbohydrates are the body's preferred source of energy.

Overindulgence in simple carbohydrates may cause nutritional deficiencies, obesity and dental decay. Inadequate intake of dietary carbohydrates may result in nutritional deficiencies, ketosis, energy loss, depression and loss of essential body protein.

CLASSIFICATIONS

Carbohydrates are classified according to their structure. Monosaccharides are single (or simple) sugars; oligosaccharides are multiple sugars; and polysaccharides are complex molecules made of simple sugars.

Monosaccharides are naturally occurring simple sugars containing 3 to 7 carbon atoms each. The hexoses ($C_6 H_{12} O_6$), so named because of the 6 carbon atoms, are of the greatest importance dietarily. The empiric formula of the hexoses is the same; the differences among the various sugars (identified below) are in their arrangements of atoms about the carbon chains.

GLUCOSE (also called dextrose, corn sugar, grape sugar) is the form of carbohydrate circulating in the blood (blood sugar) and is the carbohydrate used by cells for energy. Dietary glucose is soluble in hot or cold water, crystallizes easily and is somewhat less sweet than cane sugar.

FRUCTOSE (levulose, fruit sugar) is found in honey, ripe fruits and some vegetables. Much sweeter than cane sugar, fructose is highly soluble, does not crystallize and is not absorbed directly into the bloodstream. Fructose is also produced as a product of the hydrolysis of sucrose.

GALACTOSE is a monosaccharide that is produced during the digestion of lactose (milk sugar).

MANNOSE is a minor hexose carbohydrate. Similarly, XYLOSE and ARABINOSE are pentose carbohydrates that are produced during the digestion of certain fruits and meats. RIBOSE is another pentose produced during digestion; it is also synthesized by the human body. Ribose is a constituent of riboflavin (a B complex vitamin), ribonucleic acid (RNA) and deoxyribonucleic acid (DNA).

Oligosaccharides are two or more hexoses combined with the loss of a water molecule ($C_{12} H_{22} O_{11}$). They are of varying sweetness, but are all water soluble and can crystallize.

SUCROSE (common table sugar) is derived from sugar cane, sugar beets, sorghum, molasses, or maple sugar. Sucrose is a disaccharide of one molecule of fructose and one molecule of glucose. Some vegetables and many fruits contain at least some sucrose.

LACTOSE (milk sugar) is the only nutritionally significant carbohydrate of animal origin. Depending on the species of mammal, lactose may account for 2 to 8 percent of the milk by volume. Lactose is a disaccharide containing one molecule of glucose and one molecule of galactose.

MALTOSE (malt sugar) is consumed in malted beers, malted snacks, and some breakfast cereals. Maltose, a short chain of glucose molecules, is also an intermediate product in the digestive hydrolysis of starch.

Polysaccharides are complex compounds that represent the starches. Following the empirical formula $C_6 H_{10} O_5$, the polysaccharides have several characteristics in common: they are not sweet, do not crystallize and are not water soluble.

STARCH is a polysaccharide composed of long chains of glucose units. The amorphous starch granules are encased in cell walls and burst free when cooked because the granules absorb water and expand. If the polysaccharide chains structurally comprise long, straight lines of glucose, the starch is labelled AMYLOSE. If the glucose chains are short and branched, the starch is AMYLOPECTIN.[13]

DEXTRINS are shorter chains of glucose units that are the intermediate products of the hydrolysis of starch.

GLYCOGEN (also called the "animal starch") is synthesized in the human liver and muscle from glucose. Structurally, glycogen is similar to amylopectin starch, but with more branches.

Indigestible polysaccharides is a categorical grouping for the various forms of fiber. In addition to cellulose, hemicellulose and lignin, the indigestible polysaccharides include agar, alginate and carrageen. Agar and alginate are derived from seaweed and are useful for the physical properties they bring to certain foods and cosmetics. Carrageenin is derived from carrageen (Irish moss) and is used to enhance the smoothness of some dairy products.

Carbohydrate derivatives are produced when sugars chemically react to produce amino sugars, uronic acids, sugar alcohols, glycosides, etc. For example, SORBITOL is a sweet sugar alcohol that is found in ripe cherries and berries. ASCORBIC ACID (vitamin C) is a hexose derivative synthesized by plants and most animals.

DIETARY REQUIREMENTS

The dietary requirements for carbohydrates have not been agreed upon by the government and the scientific and nutrition communities.

The wide range of dietary consumption includes both Oriental diets (principally rice) of very high levels of carbohydrates, and the practically carbohydrate-free diet of certain Eskimo tribes. Carbohydrates are recognized as an important component in the contemporary American's diet—a diet generally characterized by too much animal protein, with its attendant health problems. Many nutritionists recommend increased dietary intake of the complex carbohydrates to promote good health and for therapeutic manipulation of specific conditions.

SOURCES

In the United States, the average person obtains approximately 46 percent of his dietary calories from carbohydrates.[1] In the Caribbean, carbohydrates constitute 65 percent of the dietary calories; in Africa, that amount is nearly 80 percent.[2]

The appeal of carbohydrate as a dominant contributor to the human diet is a result of its ready accessibility from a variety of palatable plant sources, its low cost and its ability to be stored for future consumption. In a world in which starvation is commonplace, it should be noted that carbohydrate-producing food crops yield far more food energy per acre than would be produced if the same land were used for herding animals.

The most common crop source of dietary carbohydrates is wheat (360 million metric tons harvested worldwide per year), followed by rice (320 million metric tons). Corn (maize) and potatoes are tied (300 million tons), followed by barley (170 million tons), sweet potatoes (130 million) and cassava (100 million). In descending order of harvest tonnage, dietary carbohydrates are derived from grapes, soybeans, oats, sorghum, sugar cane, millet, bananas, tomatoes, sugar beets, rye, oranges, coconut, cottonseed oil, apples, yams, peanuts, watermelons, cabbage, onions, beans, peas, sunflower seeds and mangoes.[3]

TABLE 2
**The Carbohydrate Content of Common American Foods, Including Grams
and Percentages for Specific Servings**

Food Type	Sample Portion	Grams per Serving	Grams of Carbohydrate	Percent Carbohydrate by Weight
Complex Carbohydrates				
Bread, all kinds	1 slice	25	13	50–56
Cereals, breakfast, dry	1 cup wheat flakes	30	24	68–84
Crackers, all kinds	4 saltines	11	8	67–73
Flour, all kinds	2 tablespoons	14	11	71–80
Legumes, dry	½ cup navy beans, cooked	95	20	60–63
Macaroni, spaghetti, dry	½ cup cooked	70	16	75
Nuts	¼ cup peanuts	36	7	15–20
Pie crust, baked	⅙ shell	30	13	44
Potatoes, white, raw	1 boiled	122	18	17
Rice, dry	½ cup cooked	105	25	80
Complex and Simple Carbohydrates				
Cake, plain and iced	1 piece layer, iced	75	45	52–68
Cookies	1 chocolate chip	10	6	51–80
Simple Carbohydrates				
Beverages, carbonated	8 ounces cola	246	24	8–12
Candy (without nuts)	1 ounce milk chocolate	28	16	75–95
Fruit, dried	4 prunes	32	18	59–69
Fruit, fresh	1 apple	150	18	6–22
Fruit, sweetened, canned or frozen	½ cup peaches	128	26	16–28
Ice cream	½ cup	67	14	18–21
Milk	1 cup	244	12	5
Pudding	½ cup vanilla	128	21	16–26
Sugar, all kinds	1 tablespoon white	11	11	96–100
Syrups, molasses, honey	1 tablespoon molasses	20	13	65–82
Vegetables	½ cup green beans	63	4	4–18

After carbohydrate-rich crops are harvested, the food-stuff is processed and refined. In the course of food processing (milling, bleaching, and refining), much of the nutritional value of the food is lost, especially the vitamins. "Fortified" and "enriched" flours contain some nutrients as partial replacements for those lost during the processing. Unfortunately, the nutrients that are added almost never match the losses, qualitatively or quantitatively. The result often is "convenience" food containing low-nutrient, high-calorie starches and sugars.

Of the starches and sugars consumed by Americans, one-third are from refined and processed sugars; that constitutes approximately one-fifth of all calories consumed daily. "Refined" sugars are derived from cane and beet sources; "processed" sugars include corn sugar, syrups, molasses and honey. The typical American diet contains approximately one calorie derived from "naturally occurring" sugars for every three calories derived from refined and processed sugars. "Naturally occurring" sugars are indigenous in fruits, fruit juices and vegetables. When "natural" and "manufactured" sugars are considered together, they constitute approximately one-fourth of the calories in the typical American diet.[1]

Complex carbohydrates (starches) represent another one-fourth of the caloric intake of the average American diet. Food sources for starches include beans, bread, cake, cereals, corn, crackers, flour, fruits (canned, dried and fresh), macaroni, noodles, peas, rice and pasta.

Although most Americans have discovered that eating more calories from carbohydrates (as well as fats and protein) than they burn off through exercise leads to weight-gain problems, athletes (especially those engaged in endurance sports such as long-distance running, swimming or cycling) take a different view of carbohydrates. Dietary carbohydrates are the body's preferred source of energy, are easily digested and produce glycogen reserves in the muscle and liver. (Glycogen, the storage form of glucose, is a complex starch molecule that animals can synthesize from glucose.) Athletes engaged in endurance sports have found that eating very-high-carbohydrate diets (up to 90 percent of caloric intake) for several days before competition may give them a physical endurance advantage.[4]

Table 2 identifies the carbohydrate content of some typical foods. In this table, the identification of simple carbohydrates (monosaccharides) and complex carbohydrates (oligosaccharides and polysaccharides) is a reflection of the predominating type of carbohydrate present in the food.

FIBER

Dietary fiber comprises all palatable foods that are consumed by single-stomach animals (including humans) and that remain essentially undigested by the time they reach the large intestine. Many fibers, such as cellulose, hemicellulose and pectin, are carbohydrates and thus are composed of carbon, hydrogen and oxygen. Humans do not produce the enzyme necessary for breaking down the bonds linking the individual fiber units. The monogastric ("single-stomach") distinction is important because cows and other animals with ruminant stomachs can digest grasses and other fiber-rich plants.

In America and other industrialized nations, there has been a prevailing trend in the past century to eat less fiber-rich food, in favor of more processed packaged food. There has been a parallel increase in the incidence of constipation, diverticulosis, colon cancer and gastrointestinal disorders. In recent years, there has been much interest in the health community and general population in the vital role of fiber in nutrition. Table 3 identifies the fiber content of some foods.

Because fiber is essentially not digested, it provides no caloric contribution. But fiber increases the ability

TABLE 3
Fiber Content of Major Food Groups, Identified by Soluble and Insoluble Components

BREADS, CEREALS	Serving Size (•½ cup cooked (unless otherwise indicated	Total Fiber (gms)	Soluble Fiber (gms)	Insoluble Fiber (gms)
Bran (100%) cereal	•	10.0	0.3	9.7
Popcorn	3 cups	2.8	0.8	2.0
Rye bread	1 slice	2.7	0.8	1.9
Whole grain bread	1 slice	2.7	0.08	2.8
Rye wafers	3	2.3	0.06	2.2
Corn grits	•	1.9	0.6	1.3
Oats, whole	•	1.6	0.5	1.1
Graham crackers	2	1.4	0.04	1.4
Brown rice	•	1.3	0	1.3
French bread	1 slice	1.0	0.4	0.6
Dinner roll	1	0.8	0.03	0.8
Egg noodles	•	0.8	0.3	0.8
Spaghetti	•	0.8	.02	0.8
White bread	1 slice	0.8	0.03	0.8
White rice	•	0.5	0	0.5

FRUITS	Serving Size (raw)	Total Fiber (gms)	Soluble Fiber (gms)	Insoluble Fiber (gms)
Apple	1 small	3.9	2.3	1.6
Blackberries	½ cup	3.7	0.7	3.0
Pear	1 small	2.5	0.6	1.9
Strawberries	¾ cup	2.4	0.9	1.5
Plums	2 med	2.3	1.3	1.0
Tangerine	1 med	1.6	1.4	0.4
Apricots	2 med	1.3	0.9	0.4
Banana	1 small	1.3	0.6	0.7
Grapefruit	½	1.3	0.9	0.4
Peaches	1 med	1.0	0.5	0.5
Cherries	10	0.9	0.3	0.6
Pineapple	½ cup	0.8	0.2	0.6
Grapes	10	0.4	0.1	0.3

LEGUMES	Serving Size (•½ cup cooked unless otherwise marked)	Total Fiber (gms)	Soluble Fiber (gms)	Insoluble Fiber (gms)
Kidney beans	•	4.5	0.5	4.0
White beans	•	4.2	0.4	3.8
Pinto beans	•	3.0	0.3	2.7
Lima beans	•	1.4	0.2	1.2

NUTS				
Almonds	10	1.0		
Peanuts	10	1.0		
Walnuts, black	1 tsp. chopped	0.6		
Pecans	2	0.5		

VEGETABLES				
Peas	•	5.2	2.0	3.2
Parsnips	•	4.4	.04	4.0
Potatoes	1 small	3.8	2.2	1.6
Broccoli	•	2.6	1.6	1.0
Zucchini	•	2.5	1.1	1.4
Squash, summer	•	2.3	1.1	1.2
Lettuce	½ cup raw	0.5	0.2	0.3

of fecal stools to bind large amounts of water, making their passage easier and more rapid. A single gram of fiber can bind up to 15 grams of water.[4]

Dietary fiber is the fiber that remains in the colon after digestion. Crude fiber is the fiber that withstands laboratory analysis with dilute acids and alkalis. For every gram of crude fiber, there are about two to three grams of dietary fiber. Crude fiber is composed of cellulose, which is a starch-like complex molecule of glucose molecules. Cellulose is the nondigestible plant structure commonly found in the skins of fruits and vegetables. The white tissue of an orange is a good example of cellulose. When the orange industry began in Florida a half century or more ago, the growers were burdened with small mountains of cellulose waste (discarded orange rinds after dejuicing). After a few years, they discovered that the citrus cellulose could be used as a noncaloric flour substitute for "diet" bread and baked goods, thus spawning the "diet" bread industry.

Related to cellulose is hemicellulose, the carbohydrate gums that are found in the cell walls of plants. Hemicelluloses are primarily of importance for their ability to absorb water. Bacteria can break down hemicellulose to allow some absorption by the human body as an energy source. One type of hemicellulose is pectin (used commercially in making jelly and in certain pharmaceuticals). Pectin in the human digestive tract can lower the amount of fat the body absorbs (a high priority in any good weight-reduction program). Another hemicellulose is psyllium, which absorbs water and speeds bowel transit time. Psyllium seed is a popular fiber supplement, currently added to many foods (bread, peanut butter, etc.). Uncooked pure pectin, the type used in making jam and jelly, can cause gastrointestinal discomfort, bloating and cramping. It should not be used as a dietary source of fiber. Pectin can be safely added to the diet in the form of apples and oranges.

Lignin is the principal component of the woody structure of plants. Although not a carbohydrate, lignin is of plant origin and is indigestible; hence its inclusion in crude fiber estimates on food packages.

In Japan, the konjac root (also called glucomannan or konjac mannan) is an important dietary carbohydrate used in the preparation of konnyaku. In the United States, konjac root powder or flour is gaining popularity as a dietary supplement for use in weight reduction and diabetes control. It may also help in lowering cholesterol levels.[5,6] Also in the mannan family is guar gum, which prevents the rapid uptake of glucose in the small intestine,[7,8] slows gastric emptying,[9] has been used to treat patients with diabetes mellitus[10] and has proven effective in the treatment of hypercholesterolemia.[11]

Chitosan, another fiber product, belongs to a group of carbohydrates called aminopolysaccharides. Derived from oyster shells and certain insects, chitosan has been used to reduce cholesterol levels.

FUNCTIONS

Dietary carbohydrates are primarily an energy source, but they also serve a function in the metabolism of fat and in forming body compounds. Dietary hydrocarbons can be stored in almost unlimited amounts as body fat or in small quantities as glycogen in the liver and muscles.

As an energy source, 1 gram of carbohydrate yields 4 calories of energy. By way of comparison, 1 gram of protein has 4 calories; 1 gram of alcohol has 7 calories; and 1 gram of lipids has 9 calories.

In combination with proteins, carbohydrates form substances that are essential to fighting infection, lubricating the joints and maintaining the health and growth of bones, skin, nails, cartilage and tendons.

The fiber component of carbohydrates functions to regulate gastrointestinal transit time and facilitate efficient elimination. Proper elimination reduces abdominal pressures which can cause hemorrhoids and certain types of hernia. When elimination is difficult, because of lack of bulk or fiber in the diet, diverticulosis may occur. This condition, in which "outpouchings" develop in weak areas of the intestinal wall, often requires surgery. Appendicitis is another condition that may be associated with inadequate fiber content in the diet.

A high-fiber diet has been shown to reduce the rate of colon and rectal cancers by allowing carcinogens in the food to move more quickly through the intestinal tract. According to Seymour Handler, M.D., of the North Memorial Medical Center in Minneapolis:

> Most of the serious organic diseases of the colon are etiologically linked to the high-saturated-fat and low-fiber Western diet. Benign but common conditions such as appendicitis and diverticular disease of the colon appear to be due to deficiency of fiber and attendant low-bulk stools. Colon cancer appears to be due to carcinogens created in the colon itself. Contributing to carcinogen produc-

tions are cocarcinogens in bile and an increase in anaerobic bacteria, both directly related to high levels of saturated fat in the diet. If these common disorders of the colon are to be controlled, our diet will require major modification. Changes will have to include reduction of saturated fats of animal origin and increase in cereal grains.[12]

See Chapter 8, Fat, Fiber and Cancer, and Chapter 13, Fat, Fiber and the Cardiovascular Connection, for a detailed account of the role of fiber in health.

DIGESTION AND ABSORPTION

The first step in the digestion of carbohydrates is their chemical decomposition by reaction with water (hydrolysis). In various parts of the gastrointestinal tract, the complex carbohydrates are broken down into basic monosaccharide subunits. Figure 5 identifies the major carbohydrases, which are digestive enzymes that convert polysaccharides and oligosaccharides into monosaccharide components.

Saliva begins the process of converting starches and glycogen into dextrins and maltose. The pancreatic α-amylase further digests the dextrins into maltose, isomaltose and glucose. The final steps in digestion occur in the intestinal mucosal lining. Enzymes hydrolyze the partially digested carbohydrates to produce glucose, fructose and galactose. These three endproducts are readily absorbed into the bloodstream through the intestinal mucosal cells.

Glucose and galactose have comparable rates of absorption. The rate for fructose is approximately half that of glucose. Mannose and xylose are poorly absorbed, because of preferential selectivity at the absorption sites.

Carbohydrates can be used to meet the body's energy needs directly (as glucose) or indirectly (after conversion to fat). If a person consumes more carbohydrates than the body can readily use, the excess is stored in the muscle cells and in the liver. The stored form is called glycogen, a highly branched polysaccharide. The muscle glycogen can be used by the muscles, while the glycogen in the liver can be released as glucose for transport by the bloodstream. If the carbohydrate intake surpasses usable glucose levels or the storage capacity of the liver and muscles, the excess glucose is converted by the liver into body fat (lipogenesis).

In normal, healthy individuals, there can be an efficiency factor as great as 98 percent in the digestion and absorption of usable carbohydrates.[14] The ability to digest certain carbohydrates may be influenced by race. Caucasians tend to produce adequate lactase, the intestinal enzyme responsible for breaking lactose down into its components, glucose and galactose. Consequently, few cases of lactose intolerance are reported. Other races, however, are more prone to diminished or absent levels of this enzyme, resulting in undigested lactose. The resulting increased concentration of sugar in the intestinal tract causes bloating from pooling of excess fluids and excessive gas production, as well as cramping and diarrhea, typical symptoms of lactose intolerance.

CARBOHYDRATE METABOLISM

Whether derived by absorption from the diet or from synthesis by the liver, glucose is the most important carbohydrate available to the human body. Glucose metabolism is an interrelated series of enzyme-regulated biochemical reactions that are closely tied to the metabolism of lipids and protein. A full discussion of carbohydrate metabolism is beyond the scope of this work, but the following paragraphs are provided as an overview to lay readers and a refresher to health professionals.

Monosaccharides are transported from the bloodstream to the liver after absorption from the small intestine. The liver controls the pathways of the glucose, regulating blood sugar levels and synthesizing essential compounds from glucose. Influencing the carbohydrate-related activities of the liver are the pancreas, adrenal, pituitary and thyroid glands.

The renal threshold for glucose is the liver-controlled upper limit for glucose concentrations in the blood. For most individuals this limit is 160 to 180 mg of glucose per 100 ml blood. By way of comparison, the glucose level is commonly 70 to 90 mg per 100 ml during a fasting state, and 140 to 150 mg during the few hours immediately after ingesting carbohydrate-rich foods.

The sources of blood glucose are absorbed sugars from the diet, breakdown of liver glycogen (glycogenolysis), conversion of glucogenic amino acids and the glycerol of fats (gluconeogenesis), and the reconversion of pyruvic and lactic acids formed in the glycolytic pathway shown in Figure 6.[13]

The hormones affecting increased supplies of blood glucose include the thyroid hormone (increasing absorp-

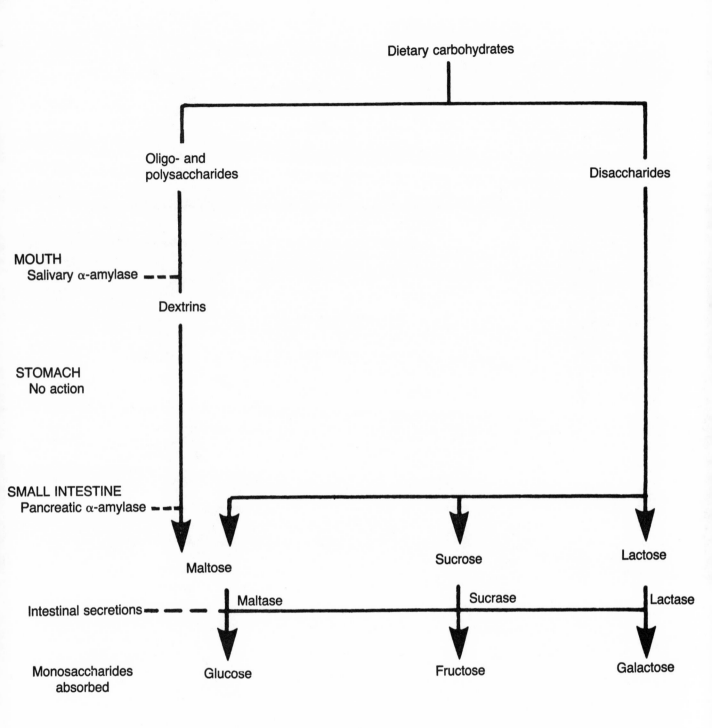

Figure 5

Digestive organs and action of the
carbohydrate-digesting enzymes

Adapted from Orten, J. M. and Neuhaus, O. W. *Human Biochemistry,*
10th ed. St. Louis: The C. V. Mosby Co., 1982, p. 224.

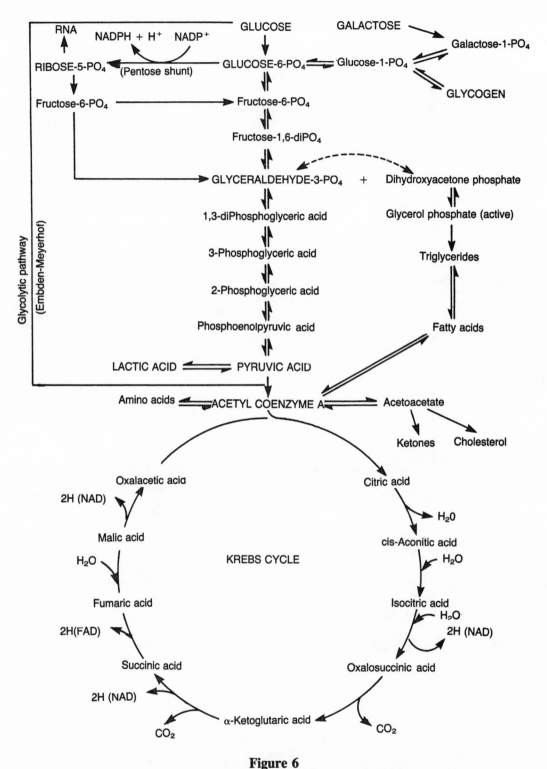

Figure 6

Metabolic pathways for the oxidation and energy-release of carbohydrates, via the anaerobic Embden-Meyerhof mechanism, the aerobic "pentose" shunt, and the CO_2-releasing Krebs cycle.

tion rates), glucagon (pancreatic activator of phosphorylase), epinephrine (adrenal hormone that hastens glycogen breakdown), steroids (which induce gluconeogenesis), and adrenocorticotropic hormone (anti-insulin agent).

The pathways for the reduction of blood glucose levels are oxidation for energy by the cells, glycogenesis, lipogenesis, and synthesis of glucuronic acid, hyaluronic acid, heparin, chondroitin sulfates, immunopolysaccharides, DNA, RNA, galactolipins, glycosides, and other carbohydrate derivatives and urinary excretion when the renal threshold is exceeded.[13]

The only hormone known to lower blood glucose levels is insulin. This pancreatic hormone, produced by the beta cells of the islets of Langerhans, is released when concentrations of blood glucose increase. Insulin serves to facilitate the liver's synthesis of glycogen, increase cell membrane transport activity and convert glucose to fatty acids.

Figure 6 summarizes the complex process whereby glucose is oxidized by enzymic action for the gradual release of energy. The catabolism includes glycolysis (the anaerobic phase yielding pyruvic and lactic acids) and the Krebs cycle (aerobic phase releasing carbon dioxide and water).

CARBOHYDRATES: A SUMMARY

The primary dietary carbohydrates are starch, sugar and fiber. Monosaccharides are the simplest form of carbohydrate; they consist of one sugar unit—glucose, galactose or fructose. The disaccharides—sucrose (table sugar), lactose (milk sugar) and maltose—are compounds of two monosaccharides linked together. Mono- and disaccharides are the sugars or simple carbohydrates.

Glucose, also called dextrose, is the primary source of energy used by the central nervous system. It is also called blood sugar. Glucose, when strung into long chains, forms starch (complex carbohydrate or polysaccharides). Glycogen, the storage form of carbohydrate in the body, is a highly branched chain of glucose units.

Cellulose is composed of many glucose units linked together in such a way that the human body can not break it down to individual units. It is the undigestible fiber, or bulk, in plant foods. All forms of carbohydrates, except fibers, provide four calories per gram.

Carbohydrate's prime function is as a source of energy. It is also important in normal metabolism of fat, in forming mucopolysaccharides and other body lubricants, and in sparing protein for use in building and repairing tissue. Fiber regulates bowel activity, and some forms of fiber, such as pectin, lower serum cholesterol levels.

Carbohydrate digestion begins in the mouth. Here, salivary amylase breaks large molecules down into dextrins. No further digestion of carbohydrate occurs until the food reaches the small intestine, where sucrases, amylases, lactases and maltases, in the alkaline environment, break carbohydrate down into monosaccharides. Once absorbed, all monosaccharides are converted to glucose. If present in excess of immediate energy needs, glucose is converted to glycogen or fat.

Dietary sources of sugars include the naturally occurring sugars in fruits, vegetables and milk and the added or refined sugars in such foods as pastries, candies, cakes and convenience foods. Starches and fibers are obtained from fruits, vegetables, legumes and whole grains. In a 2000-calorie diet, at least 1000 to 1200 calories should come from complex carbohydrates.

PROTEINS AND AMINO ACIDS

DEFINITION

Protein is the second most plentiful substance in our bodies (after water) and constitutes roughly one-fifth of our weight. Muscles, skin, hair, nails, eyes and enzymes are mostly protein. Protein is essential to forming infection-fighting antibodies; it is also essential to growth and maintenance of all tissues.

Protein is composed of carbon, hydrogen, oxygen and nitrogen, and is responsible for building and repairing body tissues. Protein molecules are composed of a class of organic compounds known as amino acids. These amino acids are linked end to end to form long chains, helixes, spheres and branched structures. The characteristics of each protein are determined by the number, variety and order of amino acids in the structural chains.

Twenty amino acids are required to build protein, but half of these are synthesized by the human body. The essential amino acids are: isoleucine, leucine, lysine, methionine, phenylalanine, threonine, tryptophan and valine. Arginine and histidine are considered semiessential.

The most common dietary sources of protein are meat (beef, pork, fowl, etc.), fish and seafood, eggs, dairy products, grain products, and legumes (beans and peas). Americans eat far more meat than their bodies require. This excessive protein consumption taxes the kidneys and can contribute to obesity. Since meat is also an excellent source of fat, eating large quantities is associated with heart disease and cancer. See Part IV: Nutrition and Cardiovascular Disease for a detailed account of the role of meat consumption in heart disease and how to reduce the risk.

CLASSIFICATIONS

All amino acids are compounds consisting of an amine group (NH_2) and a carboxyl group (COOH) linked to the same terminal carbon of the molecule. Unlike carbohydrates or lipids (which are composed of carbon, hydrogen and oxygen), protein contains nitrogen atoms in the form of an amine group.

In a protein molecule, hundreds to thousands of amino acids are linked together by peptide bonds and secondary nonpeptide bonds. The result is a multiplicity of protein structural forms: helixes, spheres, branched units, etc. Fibrous proteins are long polypeptide chains arranged in parallel, as in muscle fibers. Globular proteins (as in hemoglobin and insulin) are spherical to ellipsoidal. In extreme heat, proteins coagulate; in the presence of heavy metal salts, they precipitate. Proteins are amphoteric—they may act as bases or acids. Proteins form true salts, as well as combining with metals in nonionic complexes.

The properties of specific proteins vary depending on the number and type of individual amino acids and their arrangement and structure in the molecule. On the basis of physical and chemical properties, proteins may be classified as simple (yielding amino acids or their derivatives upon hydrolysis), conjugated (simple proteins plus nonprotein substances) or derived (resulting from the decomposition of simple or conjugated proteins).

Proteins are classified nutritionally as being complete or incomplete. Complete proteins (such as egg-derived) are capable of promoting growth and health. Partially complete protein (such as gliadin in wheat) can maintain life, but lacks certain amino acids necessary to promote growth. Totally incomplete proteins (such as zein in corn) are incapable, when consumed alone, of sustaining life processes.

Amino acids are also classified as being essential or nonessential. The nonessential amino acids, which are manufactured within the body, include: alanine, aspartic acid, cysteine, cystine, glutamic acid, glycine, hydroxyproline, hydroxylysine, proline, serine, and tyrosine.

The following paragraphs identify the nutritionally essential amino acids.

ARGININE and HISTIDINE: These two amino acids do not fall clearly into the categories of essential or nonessential. Arginine is synthesized in the body at a rate that is sufficient for maintenance in the adult. During growth periods, however, arginine synthesis may not be rapid enough. Therefore, arginine is essential for growth but nonessential for maintenance. Histidine, like arginine, is a semiessential amino acid. It must be obtained from the diet during growth periods and is therefore essential for children. But apparently histidine is adequately synthesized in adults and therefore nonessential for this age group.

ISOLEUCINE: α-amino-β methylvaleric acid, $C_6H_{13}NO_2$. Isoleucine follows metabolic pathways similar to those of leucine and valine, and is used to manufacture other biochemical components, some of which are used for energy production. Isoleucine is normally metabolized through a series of steps to produce simple acids.

LEUCINE: α-aminoisocaproic acid, $C_6H_{13}NO_2$. Obtainable from the hydrolysis of such foods as milk, this growth-essential amino acid is found throughout the body. Pediatrically, leucine is perhaps best known for the metabolic anomaly known as leucine-induced hypoglycemia. At about the fourth month, an infant with this disease may show growth retardation, symptoms such as those of Cushing's syndrome, and convulsions. Because all protein foods contain leucine, these infants cannot be treated with leucine-free diets. But by careful dietary manipulation, the child can survive until the disease has run its course, usually within five or six years.

LYSINE: α, ϵ-diaminocaproic acid, $C_6H_{14}N_2O_2$. The hydrochloride salt of lysine is used to produce systemic acidosis and increase responsiveness to mercurial diuretics.[19] One important function of lysine is to regulate absorption of calcium. Lysine is also important in the formation of collagen (the protein that forms the matrix of bone, cartilage and connective tissue). The conversion of lysine into a collagen constituent is controlled by vitamin C. Lysine has found recent questionable notoriety in the treatment of herpes simplex.

METHIONINE: DL-2-amino-4(methylthio)butyric acid, $C_5H_{11}NO_2S$. This amino acid is necessary for normal metabolism and growth in that it furnishes both labile methyl groups and sulfur. Methionine's role in sulfur supply prevents disorders of the skin and nails. Methionine is a member of the lipotropic team, which includes choline, inositol and betaine. Its primary lipotropic function is to prevent excessive fat accumulation in the liver by increasing lecithin production. Methionine is used in the prevention and treatment of certain types of liver damage.[20] Methionine is a methyl donor that is included in nutritional supplements used as anti-fatigue agents.

PHENYLALANINE: α-amino-β-phenyl-propionic acid, $C_9H_{11}NO_2$. Among its other important functions, phenylalanine is used by the brain to manufacture norepinephrine, which is a neurotransmitter involved in learning and memory. When experimental animals are given drugs for the specific purpose of decreasing norepinephrine in the brain, scientists find that the animal's capacity for learning is temporarily limited. With an injection of norepinephrine, their learning ability returns. Phenylalanine is used experimentally to improve learning and as an antidepressant. When combined with aspartic acid, it forms aspartame, the new synthetic sweetener recently added to diet drinks and foods.

THREONINE: α-amino-β-hydroxybutyric acid, $C_4H_9NO_3$. Threonine is an important constituent of collagen, elastin and enamel protein. In the absence of adequate choline levels, threonine assumes the role of a lipotrope in controlling fatty buildup in the liver.

TRYPTOPHAN: l-α-aminoindole-3-propionic acid, $C_{11}H_{12}N_2O_2$. This amino acid is a component of casein and other proteins. Vitamin B6 is required for the proper metabolism of tryptophan; dietary tryptophan can be used by the body to manufacture niacin. Tryptophan supplements are used therapeutically to manipulate levels of serotonin, a neurotransmitter in the brain that influences sleep and moods. Tryptophan supplements are being used clinically as antidepressants with effects comparable to those of the commonly prescribed drugs imipramine and amitriptyline, but without unwanted side effects. Similarly, tryptophan is effective and safe in controlling some sleep disorders and migraine headaches, and in promoting immunity (through enhancement of antibody effectiveness).[20]

VALINE: α-aminoisovaleric acid, $C_5H_{11}NO_2$. Valine is a constituent of many proteins and is essential to man and many animals. Valine follows metabolic pathways similar to those of leucine and isoleucine, and, with these two amino acids, is involved in a disease known as "maple syrup urine." In this disease, the three amino acids are not metabolized and are eliminated via the urine which has an odor of maple syrup. Infants with this disease appear normal at birth, but are unable to suck or swallow properly within a few days. If they survive the seizures, the risk of severe mental retardation is great.

SOURCES

Adequate amounts of the essential amino acids should be consumed daily. High-quality protein foods from the meat and dairy categories of the "four food groups" are the most common sources in the United States and other industrialized countries. These much-advertised "protein-rich" foods include all types of palatable meats (from the land, air and waters), milk products and eggs.

Although there is a relative deficiency of lysine, tryptophan and methionine in plant sources of protein, an excellent balance can be achieved by mixing complementary vegetarian fare. For example, a dietary mix of grain products and beans can fully satisfy the body's needs for amino acids. Similarly, beans and milk, or rice and sunflower seeds (to name but two pairs) represent complementary protein sources from the plant kingdom.

Because protein synthesis is hindered by the deficiency of specific amino acids in the diet, the "limiting" amino acids are important to vegetarians seeking adequate protein sources.

Plant Source	Amino Acid Deficiency
Corn	Tryptophan, threonine
Grain cereals	Lysine
Legumes	Methionine, tryptophan
Peanuts	Methionine, lysine
Rice	Tryptophan, threonine
Soybeans	Methionine

The body will synthesize protein only until the point at which it runs out of adequate supplies of a vital amino acid. The remainder of the amino acids at that point will be burned as energy or converted to fat.

The "biological value" of foods is the degree to which the amino acid distribution in specific dietary sources matches the body's qualitative and quantitative requirements. The Net Protein Utilization (NPU) is the measure of biological value and protein digestibility of

TABLE 4
Protein Content of Foods, Based on Averages for Food Types

Food	Average Serving	Protein g
Milk Group		
Milk, whole or skim	1 cup	9
Nonfat dry milk	⅞ ounce (3–5 tablespoons)	9
Cottage cheese	2 ounces	10
American cheese	1 ounce	7
Ice cream	⅛ quart	3
Meat Group		
Meat, fish, poultry	3 ounces, cooked	15–25
Egg	1 whole	6
Dried beans or peas	½ cup cooked	7–8
Peanut butter	1 tablespoon	4
Vegetable-Fruit Group		
Vegetables	½ cup	1–3
Fruits	½ cup	1–2
Bread-Cereals Group		
Breakfast cereals, wheat	½ cup cooked	2–3
	¾ cup dry	2–3
Bread, wheat	1 slice	2–3
Macaroni, noodles, spaghetti	½ cup cooked	2
Rice	½ cup cooked	2
Cornmeal and cereals	½ cup cooked	2

TABLE 5
Recommended Daily Allowances for Dietary Intake of Protein Reflecting Average Health and a Variety of Common Foods

	Age (years)	Weight (kg)	Weight (lb)	Height (cm)	Height (in)	Protein (g)
Infants	0.0–0.5	6	13	60	24	kg × 2.2
	0.5–1.0	9	20	71	28	kg × 2.0
Children	1–3	13	29	90	35	23
	4–6	20	44	112	44	30
	7–10	28	62	132	52	34
Males	11–14	45	99	157	62	45
	15–18	66	145	176	69	56
	19–22	70	154	177	70	56
	23–50	70	154	178	70	56
	51+	70	154	178	70	56
Females	11–14	46	101	157	62	46
	15–18	55	120	163	64	46
	19–22	55	120	163	64	44
	23–50	55	120	163	64	44
	51+	55	120	163	64	44
Pregnant						+30
Lactating						+20

Source: Recommended Dietary Allowance, 9th ed. Committee on Dietary Allowances, Food and Nutrition Board, National Research Council. Washington, D.C.: National Academy of Sciences, 1980.

specific foods. Although there is no "perfect" protein source, eggs most nearly reflect the mix of amino acids required by healthy human bodies. Thus, the chicken egg is the standard by which other protein sources are measured. The common foods with the highest NPU are, in descending order, eggs, fish, cheese, brown rice, red meat and poultry. Table 4 summarizes the average protein content of foods according to the four food groups.

In the last fifty years, Americans have doubled their dietary consumption of beef and veal, and increased their consumption of poultry two-and-a-half-fold. The reasons for these dietary trends are advertising, availability, improved refrigeration (commercial and residential), relative cost reductions and the social aspects of meats as "status" foods. Although North Americans constitute only 7 percent of the world's population, they consume roughly 30 percent of the of the world's supply of animal protein. Americans consume thirty times as much meat as the Japanese and sixty-six times as much meat as the average Asian.[17]

Worldwide, pork is the most common meat from domesticated stock, followed closely by beef, then poultry (chicken, duck and turkey), lamb, goat, buffalo and horse.[18]

FUNCTIONS

The functions of protein are maintenance and growth, regulation of the body processes and provision of energy.

Proteins are the major constituents of every living cell and body fluid except bile and urine. Thus, the continuous cell-building and regeneration that is the basis for life requires continuous supplies of proteins. As shown in Table 5, protein requirements are greatest during the years of most rapid growth.

Enzymes and some hormones are proteins as well. In a single cell, there may be a thousand enzymes, each one enabling the union or disunion of substances. Hormones composed of protein include insulin and thyroxin. These substances regulate blood glucose levels and the body's metabolic rate.

Hemoglobin, an iron-bearing protein, carries blood, nutrients and oxygen to the tissues via red blood cells.

The plasma proteins regulate osmotic pressure and water balance. Blood proteins maintain alkaline balance. Antibodies are proteins that fight infection and disease.

As an energy source, protein yields 4 calories per gram. If the dietary intake of carbohydrates and lipids is inadequate to meet energy needs, the body will use protein for energy. If the diet fails to meet energy needs, the body will break down tissue protein. Amino acids cannot be stored the way body fat is, but they can provide immediate energy through the destruction of body protein.

Protein deficiency may result in abnormalities of growth and tissue development. A child lacking adequate dietary protein may be physically small and even mentally impaired. Kwashiorkor is a sometimes fatal disease affecting young children; its symptoms are growth failure, edema, skin lesion and changes in hair color. Marasmus is an even more severe disease caused by combined deficiencies of protein and calories. Pregnant women who do not obtain adequate protein have a tendency to miscarry, give birth prematurely and suffer anemia. Worldwide, an estimated 700 million people suffer from harmful deficiencies of dietary protein.[14]

DIETARY REQUIREMENTS

There are no universally accepted dietary requirements for protein from vegetable or animal sources. However, a decade ago, the World Health Organization (WHO) reported that 0.45 grams of protein were needed daily for each kilogram of body weight to meet the needs of almost all members of the general world population.[15] This figure used eggs as the reference protein source.

The need for protein must be considered in light of such factors as usable protein within the diet, protein needs as a function of the age of the individual (infants have higher requirements for growth, the elderly have lower needs), the degree of stress, and energy requirements to accomplish specific types of work.

Considering all these factors, according to one source, the recommended protein allowance for health maintenance following the current average American diet should be 0.8 grams per kilogram of body weight per day.[16] Pregnant and lactating women have additional protein requirements.

Table 5 presents the dietary protein recommendations of the Food and Nutrition Board of the U.S. National Academy of Sciences. These allowances are intended as averages and should be amended to reflect personal health factors and environmental conditions.

Table 6 provides minimum daily requirements of essential amino acids. Note that methionine requirements are given for varying levels of cystine, and phenylalanine requirements are given for varying levels of tyrosine. Cystine and tyrosine are classified as nonessential amino acids because the body synthesizes them. If the levels of these two nonessential nutrients are great enough, the requirements decrease for dietary sources of methionine and phenylalanine, respectively.

DIGESTION AND ABSORPTION

Digestion of proteins begins when the food is in the stomach, where hydrochloric acid, pepsin and protease (an enzyme) assault specific linkages in the protein chains. Proteins are usually composed of more than one amino acid, and the acids are coupled together by peptide links. Amino acid chains are called peptides; the combination of two amino acids is a dipeptide; three amino acids may be joined to form a tripeptide; and the union of several acids is a polypeptide.

The first step in chemical digestion is attacking these linkages, beginning on the end of the protein chains. The precursor of pepsin is pepsinogen, which is activated as a proteolytic (protein-splitting) gastric juice by the action of the hydrocholoric acid. Figure 7 shows a summary of the digestive breakdown of dietary proteins to constituent amino acids.[21]

In the duodenum, the food is converted from an acid to a slightly basic state. The pancreatic juice containing the enzyme trypsin breaks the carboxyl groups' bonds, thereby converting polypeptides to dipeptides and tripeptides.

Farther down the small intestine, the remaining polypeptides and tripeptides are reduced to dipeptides, and the dipeptides are subdivided into single amino acids. Carboxypeptidases further attack the bonds at the carboxyl ends of the peptide linkages. Aminopeptidases attack the amino groups on the peptide linkages. Dipeptidases, acting either inside or outside the lumen of the small intestine, break the remaining linkages of the paired amino acids.

The single amino acids are absorbed by active transport or simple diffusion across the intestinal wall into the bloodstream. The portal vein carries the absorbed amino acids to the liver. From there, the amino acids are carried by the bloodstream to cells throughout the body.

TABLE 6
Minimum Essential Amino Acid Requirements for the Average American Infant, Adult Male and Adult Female

Essential Amino Acid	Minimal Requirements		
	Infants mg/kg/day	Men g per day	Women g per day
Histidine	32		
Isoleucine	90	0.70	0.45
Leucine	120	1.10	0.62
Lysine	90	0.80	0.50
Methionine			
In absence of cystine		1.10	
In presence of 15 mg cystine per kg	85		
In presence of 50 mg cystine per kg	65		
In presence of 200 mg cystine			0.35
In presence of 810 mg cystine		0.20	
Phenylalanine			
In absence of tyrosine		1.10	
In presence of 175 mg tyrosine per kg	90		
In presence of 1100 mg tyrosine		0.30	
In presence of 900 mg tyrosine			0.22
Threonine	60	0.50	0.30
Tryptophan	30	0.25	0.16
Valine	93	0.80	0.65

Source: Robinson, C. *Fundamentals of Normal Nutrition*. New York: Macmillan, 1983.

PROTEIN METABOLISM

Protein metabolism is one facet of the synthetic (anabolic) and degradative (catabolic) process of animals for the utilization of nutrients via biochemical reactions. The mechanisms of protein and amino acid metabolism are integrated into the metabolism of carbohydrates, lipids and the micronutrients. Figure 8 summarizes the metabolic pathways common to the three macronutrients.[13]

The overall metabolism of protein is reflected in the body's nitrogen balance.[2] Nitrogen enters the body from dietary protein sources, and the end-products of nitrogen metabolism are excreted primarily in the urine (and secondarily through fecal and dermal losses). It is the sum total of nitrogen in versus nitrogen out that indicates tissue growth, degradation or maintenance.

The liver is the primary site of amino acid metabolism and serves as the principal storage site for the labile amino acid metabolic pool. Exogenous amino acids are those derived from the diet. Endogenous amino acids (accounting for two-thirds of the pool) are "recycled" from worn-out tissue proteins.

Approximately 75 percent of the amino acids in the normal human adult are metabolized for the purpose of creating proteins (tissue proteins, enzymes and protein hormones).[19] The creation of these new proteins is required because of the constant destruction of body proteins. As a point of reference, approximately one-half of the muscle proteins at a given time will have been catabolized after 180 days. By way of comparison, the "half-life" of liver proteins is 10 days. The half-life of insulin is estimated at 6.5 to 9 minutes.[14]

Most of the amino acids not used to create proteins are converted to essential nonprotein nitrogenous tissue constituents. These include purines, pyrimidines, choline, creatine, niacin, porphyrins, epinephrine, thyroxine, bile acids, melanin and detoxication products.

Within cells, amino acids are combined to make

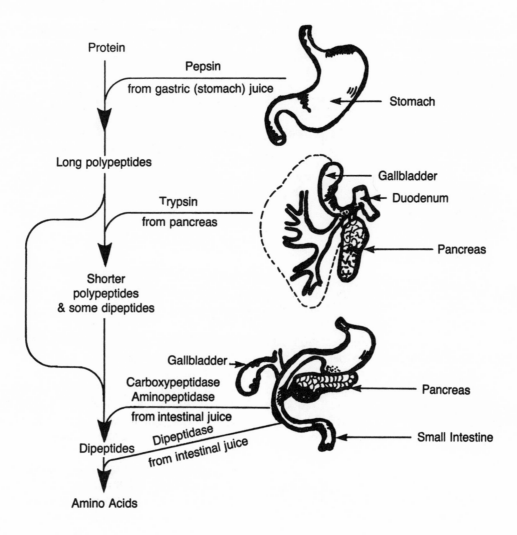

Figure 7
Digestive organs and action of the
protein-digesting enzymes

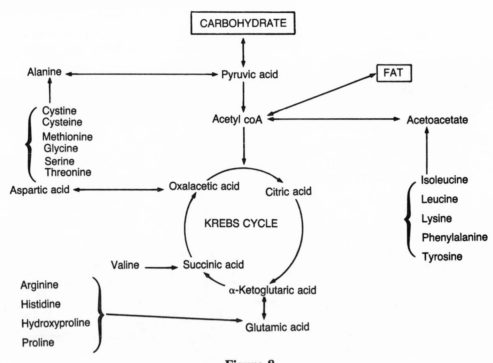

Figure 8

*Metabolic pathways of amino acids as elements in
the metabolism of carbohydrates and lipids*

proteins for use by those cells or for secretion into lymph or blood. Protein synthesis, the making of protein from amino acids, is controlled by deoxyribonucleic acid (DNA). The DNA in the nucleus of each cell in the human body is identical, with specialized cells using only that part of the genetically defined "blueprint" which pertains to replicating that type of specialized cell.

When a new body protein is required, the DNA molecule divides to form an identical copy of itself. The messenger ribonucleic acid (RNA)—the copy—passes through the nuclear membrane and attaches itself to a ribosome, which is a protein-making structure that itself is composed of protein and RNA. The messenger RNA then "supervises" to insure that the blueprint is followed exactly. Thousands of transfer RNAs collect the various amino acids from the cell fluid and add them to the ribosome in the required sequence. The transfer RNAs act as delivery vehicles, unloading their materials at the molecular construction site. Specific proteins are created from the sequencing of exact quantities of the endogenous and exogenous amino acids, which are linked by enzymatic action. In a cell, a hundred amino acids can be added to a growing protein strand in a second or less.[22] What is

more amazing, each human cell contains enough DNA to code approximately 7 million different protein molecules.[14]

An adult male is estimated to manufacture approximately 300 grams of new protein daily.[23] The synthesis of most protein occurs at the site where the protein will be incorporated into the tissue. In the synthesis of nonprotein nitrogenous tissue constituents, the metabolic pathways may involve cooperation among tissues in several organs. For example, creatine synthesis commences in the kidney with arginine and glycine forming guanidoacetic acid. The reaction product is transferred to the liver where creatine is formed through methylation. From the liver the creatine is transported by the bloodstream to muscle tissue, where it is concentrated.

PROTEIN: A SUMMARY

Protein is distinct from the other macronutrients in that it contains nitrogen, as an amine group, as well as carbon, oxygen and hydrogen. Amino acids are the building blocks of protein. Of the over twenty amino acids, eight are not synthesized by the body and must be obtained from the diet, hence the term "essential."

Depending on the sequencing of the individual amino acids in the protein chain, proteins can be helical, spherical or branched. They can vary from four to hundreds of amino acids in length.

Proteins function as enzymes, hormones, hemoglobin and antibodies. They are important in regulating fluid and salt balance between compartments of the body and as buffers in maintaining the normal acid-base balance. Proteins are the major constituents of every cell and body fluid except urine and bile. They are necessary for growth, maintenance and repair of all tissue. Amino acids can also be used for energy.

Digestion of protein begins in the stomach when hydrocholoric acid denatures the large molecules and enzymes begin systematic hydrolysis of the peptide bonds. In the small intestine, peptides and tripeptides are broken down to individual amino acids. Once absorbed, amino acids are taken up by cells to be incorporated directly into proteins, converted to non-essential amino acids, broken down to glucose or converted to fats. DNA dictates the code for cellular anabolism. If an essential amino acid is lacking, the protein cannot be built and the other amino acids are wasted or used elsewhere.

The daily requirement for protein depends on age, the quality and digestibility of the dietary source, the energy supply and the individual's nutritional status, degree of stress and health. The RDA for protein is 0.8 grams per kilogram of ideal body weight. Pregnant and lactating women require an additional 30 and 20 grams, respectively.

Foods which supply all the essential amino acids and therefore are considered high-quality protein sources include meat, chicken, fish, milk and milk products and eggs. Plant foods such as grains and legumes provide excellent protein but must be combined to provide all of the essential amino acids. Americans consume ample, even excessive, quantities of protein. In third-world countries however, protein deficiencies, such as are seen in the diseases kwashiorkor and marasmus, are not uncommon.

THE LIPIDS

DEFINITION

Lipids are a group of fats and fatlike substances that share the common property of insolubility in water and solubility in the fat solvents. This group includes fats, fatty acids, fatty oils, waxes, sterols, and esters of fatty acids.

Like carbohydrates, lipids are composed of carbon, hydrogen and oxygen. Dietary lipids serve as a source of energy, can be converted to other essential tissue constituents, or are transformed into stored energy as reserve fat in adipose tissue.

Lipids (not to be confused with just "body fat") account for over 10 percent of the body weight of normal adults.[14] Although fats in the diet have received much bad press because of their implication in heart disease, dietary lipids are a good source of nutrition when consumed in moderation. In addition to serving as a high-energy food, lipids facilitate the digestion and metabolism of some other nutrients. Lipids play an important role in the absorption and transport of the fat-soluble vitamins (A, D, E and K).

If lipids are eliminated from the diet, the body will synthesize some fatty acids from other macronutrients to meet the body's needs. One fatty acid, linoleic acid, is "essential," meaning that it cannot be synthesized from other macronutrients and must be obtained from food or supplements. Linoleic acid is important as a precursor to a series of hormone-like substances called prostaglandins.

At the cellular level, lipids are vital structural and functional materials.

CLASSIFICATION

Triglycerides are the primary form of fat. They comprise the bulk of fat in foods, the storage form of fat in the body and a primary form of fat in the blood. Only triglycerides provide calories or energy to the body. Triglycerides come in all shapes and sizes, but they all exhibit a similar structure—a glycerol molecule with three fatty acids attached. It is the length and degree of saturation of these fatty acids that determines the physical characteristics of a given fat. Fatty acids are composed of carbon atoms—usually sixteen to eighteen in number, but ranging from two to twenty—linked together. If each carbon atom is also bound to its maximum number of hydrogens, it is said to be saturated. If two adjoining carbon atoms are linked in a double bond and could bind to additional hydrogens, the fat is said to be monounsaturated. If more than one spot on the carbon chain could accept more hydrogen atoms, the fat is polyunsaturated. Linoleic acid is a polyunsaturated fatty acid; oleic acid is a monounsaturated fatty acid.

An unsaturated fat is more fluid at room temperature than a saturated fat. For example, safflower oil, high in polyunsaturated fatty acids, is liquid at room temperature, while lard, high in saturated fats, is solid. This is due to the molecular shape of the respective acids. If a fatty acid is saturated with hydrogen atoms, it is regular in shape and the fatty acids fit uniformly and closely together like stacked spoons. Unsaturated fatty acids are kinked and do not lie in a compact fashion. Consequently, the former is more dense and solid; the latter is less dense and fluid.

For a detailed review of trans fatty acids and hydrogenated fats and their role in disease, see pp. 168–169.

HYDROGENATION refers to the process of adding hydrogen atoms at the double bonds of unsaturated fatty acids. Hydrogenation is used to prolong the storage time (shelf life) of fats, and serve to change liquid unsaturated fats to firm, semisolid form. Hydrogenation solidifies liquid oil, as in the conversion of corn oil to margarine. The process of hydrogenation converts the structured form of some unsaturated fatty acids from their natural cis configuration to the trans configuration. Trans fatty acids are under investigation for their potential carcinogenic properties and ability to impair prostaglandin synthesis. (See pp. 168–169.)

CHOLESTEROL is a white crystalline substance, $C_{27}H_{45}OH$, that is a constituent of egg yolk, all animal fats and oils, bile, gallstones, nervous tissue and blood. Cholesterol is found in practically all body tissues, but is particularly concentrated in the liver, blood and brain. Only animals synthesize cholesterol, the most commonly known type of sterol (an alcohol). ERGOSTEROL and SITOSTEROL are the most common sterols produced by plants. Cholesterol and its role in health and disease are reviewed in detail on pp. 159–163.

LINOLEIC ACID and linolenic acid are the essential polyunsaturated fatty acids that must be obtained from dietary sources. Rich sources include vegetable oils, nuts and seeds. ARACHIDONIC acid is a "nonessential" lipid synthesized within the body when adequate linoleic acid is supplied.

DIETARY REQUIREMENTS

Americans eat an average of 155 grams (approximately one-third pound) of fat each day. During the lifetime of a single generation, today's senior citizens, the eating habits of Americans have changed so that we now consume a third more of our calories as fat than was the case around the time of World War I.[24] Increased lipid consumption results from the greater use of salad and cooking oils, hydrogenated cooking fats, vegetable shortening and meat.

There is no Recommended Daily Allowance (RDA) for fat. Although fats are one of the three macronutrients, there is no need for dietary fats per se. Some nutritionists suggest that the essential fatty acid, linoleic acid, should supply 1 to 2 percent of the total calories in the daily diet.[24]

The RDA for dietary fat suggested by the National Academy of Sciences, to ensure adequate intake of essential fatty acids and to act as a carrier for fat-soluble vitamins, is 15 to 25 grams of dietary fat.[25] The fat-soluble vitamins and essential fatty acids could be obtained through supplementation. But the elimination of all lipids from the diet is both unwarranted and practically impossible (because of their co-presence with proteins and carbohydrates in almost all foods).

SOURCES

Lipids occur in meats, dairy products and plant-derived foods. Vegetables that are rich in lipids include olives, avocado, nuts, peanuts and soybeans. But meats (red meat, fish, poultry and lard) and dairy products (butter, cream and cheese) are the most visible and well-known sources.

Cholesterol, a highly publicized form of dietary lipids, is found in concentration in egg yolks and almost all animal fats, particularly in liver.

Saturated fats are metabolized differently from unsaturated fats and are generally associated with an increased risk of heart disease, cancer and other disorders. On the other hand, unsaturated fats, unless adequately protected by nutrients (such as vitamin E), can be transformed into reactive substances which may play a role in diseases such as cancer and arthritis.

Sources of saturated and unsaturated fatty acids[14]

SATURATED FATTY ACIDS

Animal sources	pork, beef, poultry, fish, egg yolks, dairy products
Plant sources	coconut and palm

UNSATURATED FATTY ACIDS

Monounsaturated (plant)	olive
Polyunsaturated (plant)	corn, safflower, cottonseed, soybean, peanut

Foods usually contain a mixture of saturated and unsaturated fatty acids. As a rule, animal-derived fats have a higher concentration of saturated fatty acids than vegetable-derived fats. Poultry and fish have higher proportions of unsaturated fats than other meats. As shown below, most vegetable oils (except palm and coconut) are composed chiefly of unsaturated fatty acids.

A relationship exists between the consumption by affluent cultures of fatty foods and their high incidence of coronary disease, diabetes and cancer. By way of comparison, Americans derive 40 to 45 percent of total dietary calories from lipids, while the average person in the Orient (eating mostly grains and vegetables) obtains 10 percent of total calories from lipids.[21] Americans lead the world in incidence of cardiovascular disease, whereas this degenerative disease is relatively rare in Oriental cultures.

Because lipids are the most calorie-rich macronutrient (with 9 calories per gram), there may be a temptation to restrict intake severely or eliminate them from the diet altogether. The problem with lipid-free diets is that they tend to be boring (with no meat, no eggs, no butter or margarine, no salad dressings, no milk, or cheese, no fried foods, no baked goods, no gravies, few sauces and limited vegetables). Lipids are present in almost every protein source, so the key element in dieting is moderation.

Lipids, even in small amounts, have a remarkable ability to reduce or negate the sense of hunger. Physiologically, this is accomplished because lipids in the stomach increase the levels of enterogastrone, a hormone that serves to inhibit gastric function and retard food discharge. Because lipids linger in the stomach, the person has an ''unfounded'' sense of not being hungry for several hours. Lipids also stimulate the release of cholecystokinin from the intestinal wall, and cholecystokinin seems to have an appetite-suppressing effect via the central nervous system. Lipids thus are said to have a high satiety value.

Most of the lipids consumed by Americans are hidden in foods the consumer may not consider to be lipid-rich. Examples include coffee creamers, whipped toppings, potato chips and pastries.

In ''pure'' form, all lipids have the same caloric content, which is 252 calories per ounce.[21] When measured by volume, however, the liquid oils weigh slightly more than solid fats because the oils are denser, thus offering more calories per tablespoon. Similarly,

''whipped'' butter and margarine have fewer calories by weight and volume, because air and water are included in the product. The high-fat diet consumed by the average American is associated with the major killers in this country—cardiovascular disease, obesity, diabetes and cancer. Fat intake in all forms must be reduced if these diseases are to be prevented, treated or regressed. For a detailed look at the role of fat in disease, see Parts III and IV.

FUNCTIONS

The principal function of lipids is to serve as a ready source of energy. Lipids supply over half the energy used in basal metabolism.[14] Dietary fats, or triglycerides, yield 9 calories per gram; this is more than twice the energy value of either carbohydrates or protein (4 calories each).

The second function of lipids is that of a thermal blanket. Subcutaneous tissue (that is, just beneath the skin) insulates the body against heat loss. In times of distress (famine or severe disease), the body fat in the thermal blanket can be converted from stored energy to ready-to-use energy.

The third function of lipids is as a component of cell membranes. Lipids also serve as a protective cushion for many tissues and organs. Finally, lipids constitute a structure for secondary sex characteristics.

DIGESTION AND ABSORPTION

The lipid digestive process is initiated in the mouth as foods are chewed and partially separated. In the esophagus, body heat softens the solid fats.

In the stomach, gastric lipase (a lipid-splitting enzyme) initiates fat breakdown. More important, the proteolytic enzymes acting on proteins and the amylases acting on carbohydrates serve to free the lipid constituents of the food.

The small intestine is the principal site of lipid digestion. Lipids enter the upper small intestine (duodenum) in small amounts. Bile emulsifies the fats, permitting intestinal and pancreatic lipases (steapsin) to split the triglycerides into diglycerides and monoglycerides, and finally into free fatty acids and glycerol. Unsaturated fatty acids are hydrolyzed more readily than saturated fatty acids.

As fat enters the duodenum, it stimulates the intestinal wall to secrete secretin, pancreozymin and cholecystokinin. Secretin increases the electrolyte and fluid components of the pancreatic juice. Pancreozymin stimulates secretion of the pancreatic enzymes. When the hormone cholecystokinin is carried by the bloodstream to the gallbladder, the gallbladder contracts, forcing bile into the small intestine.

The bile salts function to make the lipids water-soluble. After becoming attached to the bile salts, the lipids are absorbed through the intestinal walls, with the salts selectively excluded. The bile salts are recycled from the distal end of the small bowel, through the liver and bile and back to the intestine.

Up to 95 percent of dietary lipids are digested and absorbed, with the remainder removed by fecal excretion. The maximum absorption occurs during the period of six to eight hours after ingestion.[2]

Fatty acids with short chains of twelve or fewer carbons are absorbed directly into the blood and are transported to the liver attached to the blood protein albumin. Long-chained monoglycerides, diglycerides and fatty acids, having carbon chains of fourteen or more, are converted into triglycerides in the walls of the intestine. These lipids must be combined with a water-soluble substance (protein, carbohydrate or phosphate) for transport in the watery medium of the blood. These triglycerides are made soluble by incorporation into chylomicrons or very low density lipoproteins. Chylomicrons, one of the four or five types of lipoproteins, is the name for a complex of lipid surrounded with a protein coat. These complexes of protein surrounding the insoluble fats can travel easily in the watery medium of the blood. They are dumped into the lymph from the mucosal lining and finally into the bloodstream through the thoracic duct. From there, they are carried to the liver.

METABOLISM

Contrary to popular opinion, lipids are in a dynamic state of metabolism. Even stored fat is not an inert mass; it is extremely active.

Basic tissue lipid is a constant requirement of the human body, independent of diet. Even after extensive starvation, lipids are still found in tissues (primarily as phospholipid and cholesterol, instead of triglyceride).

Metabolically, lipids work with other nutrients to perform life-supporting functions in every human cell. They are integrally involved in cell membrane structure, blood and tissue structure, enzyme reactions, the manufacture and utilization of the sterol hormones and the hormone-like prostaglandins, and in memory and nervous system operations.

Lipids within the body combine with carbohydrates to form glycolipids, with proteins to form lipoproteins and with phosphate to form phospholipids. Perhaps the best-known phospholipid is lecithin. A component of lecithin is choline (which may influence the synthesis of neurotransmitters in the human brain).

The liver is the primary site of lipid metabolism. Lipoproteins are removed from the blood by the liver, which breaks down triglycerides to form new ones, and synthesizes new lipoproteins.

In the blood, the most active forms of fat are the free fatty acids bound to plasma albumin. The other fats (triglycerides, phospholipids and cholesterol) are carried by high- or low-density lipoproteins.

High-density lipoproteins (HDL) contain more protein than lipids. Low-density lipoproteins (LDL) and very low-density lipoproteins (VLDL) have more lipid than protein in their makeup. These labels make sense in light of the fact that protein is more dense than fat.[28]

HDLs are sometimes referred to as the carriers of the "good" kind of cholesterol. HDLs help prevent atherosclerosis by removing cholesterol from artery walls and transporting it to the liver for removal as bile.

Lipids also are necessary for the formation of cholesterol and 7-dehydrocholesterol, which the body requires for the synthesis of vitamin D.

The pathways for the metabolism of lipids are intertwined with the metabolic pathways for carbohydrates and protein. If carbohydrate is lacking, ketone bodies (which are potentially toxic) are formed during lipid metabolism. In response to increased levels of ketones, the kidneys draw water from the cells in an attempt to flush the ketones out. The result is dehydration, possible kidney failure, possible circulatory failure and even coma.

Three subcellular systems are responsible for the synthesis of fatty acids. Cytoplasm synthesizes palmitate; mitochondria elongate available fatty acids; and microsomes synthesize unsaturated fats. The liver and adipose tissue are the chief sites of fatty acid biosynthesis.

Prostaglandin production is one function of fatty acid metabolism that has received considerable attention in recent years. Prostaglandins play a role in the etiology of heart disease, psychosocial behavioral patterns, and the activity of almost all body tissues. Figure 9 portrays some of the metabolic pathways of essential fatty acids and prostaglandin synthesis.

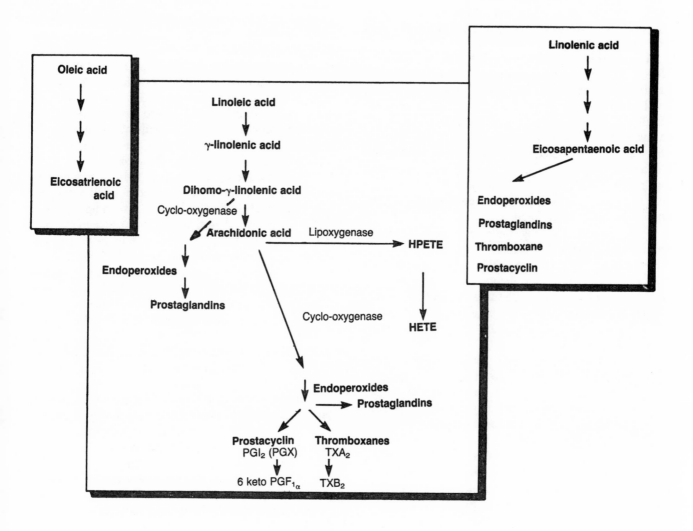

Figure 9
*Simplified pathways of essential fatty acid metabolism
and prostaglandin production*

Adapted from Anderson, L., Dibble, M., Turkki, P., et al. *Nutrition in
Health and Disease*, 17th ed. Philadelphia: J. B. Lippincott Co., 1982,
p. 44.

LIPIDS: A SUMMARY

Lipids are a group of fats and oils all of which are insoluble in water and soluble in fat solvents such as ether and benzene. They are composed of carbon, oxygen and hydrogen. The primary classes of lipids are triglycerides, phospholipids and sterols.

Triglycerides comprise 95 percent of the lipids in foods; they are the storage form of fat in the body and a primary fat in blood. They are composed of a glycerol molecule with three fatty acids of various lengths. If all the carbons on the fatty acid chains are bound to a maximum number of hydrogens, the triglyceride or fatty acid is "saturated." If two adjacent carbons are linked by a double bond and could accept additional hydrogens, the fat is "unsaturated." A triglyceride can be mono- or polyunsaturated depending on the number of points of unsaturation.

Fats that contain long fatty acid chains and are unsaturated, such as vegetable oils, are liquid at room temperature. The shorter the chains and the more saturated the fat, as with lard, the greater the likelihood of its being hard at room temperature. When hydrogen is added to vegetable oils, as in margarine and shortening, they become more saturated and solid and are called "hydrogenated" fats.

Triglycerides are the primary storage form of concentrated energy in the body, providing nine calories in the diet and about 3500 calories per pound of body fat. Fat is derived from excess intake of dietary fat, protein or carbohydrate. Deposits of fat beneath the skin help to insulate the body, and fat deposits surrounding vital organs cushion them from physical trauma. Triglycerides are a carrier of the fat-soluble vitamins A, D, E and K and are a source of the essential fatty acid linoleic acid. They are precursors for the the hormone-like prostaglandins and are essential constituents of all cell membranes. In the diet, fats increase the satiety value and palatability of a meal.

Phospholipids, such as lecithin, resemble triglycerides except that one fatty acid is replaced by a phosphate (PO-4) group and either a nitrogen-containing or a carbohydrate-like molecule. Phospholipids play an important role in membranes by transporting fats in and out of the cell's watery medium.

Cholesterol is the primary sterol present in all animal tissues. The amount synthesized by the body depends on the quantity needed and available in the diet. Cholesterol supplies no calories and is not burned for energy. It is a constituent of bile acids and salts and a precursor for the sex hormones and vitamin D. Cholesterol is needed for proper formation and function of brain and nerve cells and is found in every cell in the body. Excess cholesterol, whether endogenous or exogenous, is strongly linked to the development of atherosclerosis, heart disease and stroke.

Some digestion of fat begins in the stomach but the primary site of fat digestion is the small intestine. Here, bile acids emulsify the fats, providing a greater surface area for digestive enzymes. Pancreatic and intestinal lipase reduce the complex molecules to the absorbable forms—fatty acids, glycerol, monoglycerides and cholesterol. Once across the intestine's mucosal lining, long-chain fatty acids and glycerol are recombined to form new triglycerides. These fats and cholesterol are packaged with protein to form chylomicrons for release into the blood. Short-chain fatty acids and glycerol are dumped directly into the lymph and eventually enter the bloodstream through the thoracic duct.

Within the body, fats travel in water-soluble carriers called lipoproteins. The liver is the primary organ for lipid synthesis and degradation. Adipose tissue is the main and unlimited storage depot for fat.

No RDA exists for fat. A minimum of 10 percent of calories should come from fat to assure absorption of the fat-soluble vitamins and linoleic acid. To prevent cardiovascular disease and cancer, fat should comprise no more than 30 percent of daily calories.

Visible dietary fats include butter, lard, margarine, cream cheese, vegetable oils and the fat surrounding and marbling meat. Hidden fats include the fat in such foods as pie crust, pastries, chicken skin, whole milk, nuts and avocados.

REFERENCES

1. Select Committee on Nutrition and Human Needs. *Dietary Goals for the United States,* 2nd Edition. Washington, D.C.: 95th Congress of the United States, December 1977.

2. Goodhart, R. S. and Shils, M. E. *Modern Nutrition in Health and Disease,* 6th edition. Philadelphia: Lea & Febiger, 1980.

3. Harlan, J. R. "The Plants and Animals That Nourish Man," in *Human Nutrition: Readings from Scientific American.* San Francisco: W. H. Freeman and Company, 1978.

4. Eagles, J. A. and Randall, M. N. *Handbook of Normal and Therapeutic Nutrition.* New York: Raven Press, 1980.

5. Kolata, G. Dietary dogma disproved. *Science*, 220:487–488, 1983.

6. Vaaler, S., Hanssen, K. F. and Aagenases, O. Effect of different kinds of fibre on postpradial blood glucose in insulin-dependent diabetics. *Acta Med. Scand.*, 208:389–391, 1980.

7. Jenkins, D.J.A. and Wolever, T.M.S. Slow release carbohydrate and the treatment of diabetes. *Proc. Nutr. Soc.*, 40:227–234, 1981.

8. Johnson, I. T. and Gee, J. M. Effect of gel-forming gums on the intestinal unstirred layer and sugar transport in vitro. *Gut*, 22:398–403, 1981.

9. Holt. S., Heading, R. C., Carter, D.C., et al. Effect of gel fibre on gastric emptying and absorption of glucose and paracetamol. *Lancet*, 1: 939–639, 1979.

10. Jenkins, D.J.A., Leeds, J. R., Wolever, T. M. S., et al. Unabsorbable carbohydrates and diabetes: Decreased postprandial hyperglycemia. *Lancet*, 2: 172–174, 1976.

11. Jenkins, D.J.A., Reynolds, D., Slavin, B. et al. Dietary fiber and blood lipids: Treatment of hypercholesterolemia with guar crispbread. *Am. J. Clin. Nutr.*, 33:575–581, 1980.

12. Handler, S. Dietary fiber: Can it prevent certain colonic diseases? *Postgraduate Medicine*, 73:301-307, 1983.

13. Robinson, C. H. *Normal and Therapeutic Nutrition*. New York: Macmillan, 1972.

14. Orten, J. M. and Neuhaus, O.W. *Human Biochemistry*. 10th edition. St. Louis: The C.V. Mosby Company, 1982.

15. Food and Agriculture Organization/World Health Organization. "Energy and Protein Requirements." WHO tech. report no. 522. 1973.

16. Food and Nutrition Board. *Recommended Dietary Allowances*. Washington, D.C.: National Academy of Sciences, 1980.

17. Pfeiffer, C. C., M.D. *Mental and Elemental Nutrients: A Physician's Guide to Nutrition and Health Care*. New Canaan, Conn.: Keats Publishing, Inc., 1975.

18. Harlan, J. R. "The Plants and Animals That Nourish Man," in *Human Nutrition: Readings from Scientific American*. San Francisco: W. H. Freeman and Company, 1978.

19. Jeffers, J. D., Laufer, R.S., Cowell, M. W., et al., eds. *Blakiston's Gould Medical Dictionary*. New York: McGraw-Hill, 1979.

20. Garrison, R., Jr. *Lysine, Tryptophan and Other Amino Acids*. New Canaan, Conn.: Keats Publishing, Inc., 1982.

21. Wenck, D. A., Baren, M. and Dewan, S. P. *Nutrition*, 2nd edition. Reston, Va.: Reston Publishing Company, Inc., 1983.

22. Hamilton E. M. N. and Whitney, E. N. *Nutrition: Concepts and Controversies*. St. Paul, Minn.: West Publishing Co., 1982.

23. Munro, H. N. Metabolism and functions of amino acids in man, in *Amino Acids: Metabolism and Medical Applications*. G. L. Blackburn, J. P. Grant, V. R. Young, eds. Littleton, Mass.: PSG, Inc., 1983.

24. Eagles, J. A. and Randall, M. N. *Handbook of Nutrition and Therapeutic Nutrition*. New York: Raven Press, 1980.

25. National Research Council. *Recommended Dietary Allowances*, 9th edition. Washington, D.C.: National Academy of Sciences, 1980.

26. Anderson, L., Dibble, M. V., Turkki, P. R. et al. *Nutrition in Health and Disease*, 17th edition. Philadelphia: J. B. Lippincott, 1982.

27. Katz, D., and Goodwin, M. T. *Food: Where Nutrition, Politics, and Culture Meet*. Washington, D.C.: Center for Science in the Public Interest, 1976.

28. Goodman. L. S., and Gilman, A. *The Pharmacological Basis for Therapeutics*, 5th edition. New York: Macmillan, 1975.

3

·············· VITAMINS ···

A VITAMIN is an organic substance, needed in minute amounts, that is essential for life and cannot be synthesized in the body. Vitamins cannot be metabolized for energy, although some are necessary for energy production. They usually perform a regulatory rather than a structural function.

Vitamins are obtained from foods; however, some vitamins are ingested in their provitamin or precursor form and are converted to the active substance within the body. Although considered a single substance, several vitamins are actually a group of chemically related compounds. One of these compounds is generally the metabolically active form to which the others are converted.

Vitamins are organized into two groups: fat-soluble and water-soluble. Vitamins A, D, E and K are fat-soluble; the B vitamins and vitamin C are water-soluble. The fat-soluble vitamins require protein carriers in the blood and are not readily excreted. They are stored in the liver and fatty tissues and have the potential for toxicity. The water-soluble vitamins, on the other hand, are more easily lost during storage and cooking. They travel unattached in the blood and lymph, are excreted in the urine and are unlikely to cause toxicity symptoms except at high dosages. A daily dietary source of water-soluble vitamins is recommended because these vitamins are stored in limited amounts.

All the B vitamins have recognized coenzyme roles, but a similar role has not been identified for vitamin C or the fat-soluble vitamins.

Extensive research is accumulating on the roles and interrelationships of these essential compounds. Dietary requirements for most vitamins have been established to prevent clinical deficiency symptoms. Vitamin research, however, has only scratched the surface in understanding subclinical deficiency states, bioavailability, nutrient-nutrient interactions, and therapeutic roles beyond the prevention and treatment of recognized clinical deficiencies.

FAT-SOLUBLE VITAMINS

VITAMIN A (retinol; aldehyde form = retinal; precursors = carotenes)

Vitamin A, the first fat-soluble vitamin to be identified, is the general name for a group of substances that include retinol, retinal and the carotenoids. The active forms of vitamin A are found in animal tissue, whereas the provitamin or precursor forms, such as beta-carotene, are found in dark green and orange vegetables, and fruits.

While the carotene-precursors of vitamin A may require the presence of bile and fats in the intestines for absorption, the preformed vitamin A is not as fat-dependent and thus is a better candidate for absorption.

Vitamin A is stable to light and heat, with minimal losses from cooking or canning; however, it is destroyed by the ultraviolet rays of sunlight and by air (oxidation). This oxidation can be prevented by vitamin E, which sacrifices itself to protect vitamin A.

Once vitamin A is absorbed, it is stored in the liver and released as needed. Normal blood values of retinol are 15 to 60 mg/100ml serum.

Functions

Vitamin A plays an important role in eyesight. In this function, the retinal form of vitamin A combines with the protein opsin to form rhodopsin (visual purple). Rhodopsin occurs in the rod cells of the retina and is responsible for visual dark adaptation. When light strikes the retina this molecule is split, generating an electrical impulse that relays information to the brain. Each time rhodopsin is split, a small amount of retinal is destroyed and a constant supply of circulating retinal is needed for resynthesis of the visual purple. Other light-sensitive pigments also require vitamin A, including iodopsin, cyanopsin and porphyropsin (color pigments in cone cells of the retina).

Vitamin A is essential for the maintenance of epithelial tissue, hence it is necessary for the proper function of the cornea, all mucous membranes, the lining of the gastrointestinal tract, the lungs, the vagina, the urinary tract, the bladder and the skin. In the absence of vitamin A, these specialized tissue cells secrete a hard protein (keratin) rather than the mucus needed for protection and lubrication. Although keratin is a normal protein of hair and nails, it dries and hardens epithelial tissues, resulting in a condition called keratinization. When this occurs, cell function is impaired or halted. The tissue wastes away and becomes susceptible to bacterial infection.

Because of its role in epithelial tissue maintenance, vitamin A plays a secondary role in the prevention of infectious diseases. By maintaining healthy epithelium, vitamin A can also interrupt the process by which some cancers are initiated.

Vitamin A is important in growth, in the formation and modeling of the endochondral tissue of long bones and in the normal spacing of teeth. It is also necessary for the synthesis of certain proteins and compounds that can inhibit the formation of tumors.

Deficiency

Clinical vitamin A deficiency is second only to protein-calorie malnutrition among nutrition disorders in developing countries. In industrial countries, subclinical deficiency symptoms have been reported. Diabetics have a diminished capability to convert carotene to retinol, and, if placed on a restricted diet without insulin, the diabetic can develop a low-grade deficiency. An early symptom of vitamin A deficiency is follicular keratinosis. In this condition, keratin deposits accumulate around the hair follicles and surfaces of the upper and lower extremities, creating hardened, pigmented goose bumps. The shoulders, neck, back, buttocks and lower abdomen are common sites for this condition. Vitamin A deficiencies also occur in diseases where absorption is impaired, such as celiac disease and tropical sprue, and in diets devoid of fat.

In addition to keratinosis, a chronic lack of vitamin A in the diet results in:

- Nyactalopia (night blindness—a condition commonly seen with cirrhosis of the liver).
- Xeropthalmia (inflammation of the eyes).
- Bitot's spots (dry patches on the conjunctiva).
- Blindness.
- Hyperkeratosis.
- Reduced resistance to infection.
- Impaired growth.
- Weight loss.
- Diminished saliva and histological changes in taste buds.
- Anorexia.
- Reduced steroid synthesis.
- Improper tooth and bone formation and crooked teeth.

Requirements

Vitamin A requirements depend on body weight. Because this vitamin is fat-soluble and readily stored, daily sources are not critical. The RDA for vitamin A is expressed in retinol equivalents (RE). One RE = 1 mcg retinol or 6 mcg beta-carotene. One RE = 3.33 International Units (IU) of vitamin A activity from retinol or 10 IU of vitamin A activity from beta-carotene. An average of 1 RE = 5 IU is used for convenience.

To maintain blood concentration and prevent overt clinical deficiencies, an average daily intake of 500 to 600 mcg of retinol (1000 to 1200 mcg beta-carotene) is required. Intakes above this amount build liver stores of the vitamin.

The typical American diet derives half its vitamin A from the preformed active retinol. The other half comes from the carotene precursors.

Requirements for infants are based on the normal vitamin A content of breast milk. The RDA for women is based on 80 percent of the RDA for men because women generally weigh less and therefore need a smaller intake of the vitamin.

The RDAs are:

Infants

0–0.5 year	420 RE	2100 IU
0.5–1.0 year	400 RE	2000 IU

Children

1–3 years	400 RE	2000 IU
4–6 years	500 RE	2500 IU
7–10 years	700 RE	3300 IU
Males 11+ years	1000 RE	5000 IU
Females 11+ years	800 RE	4000 IU
Pregnant	+200 RE	+1000 IU
Lactating	+400 RE	+2000 IU

Sources

Good sources of vitamin A include whole milk, vitamin A-fortified skim milk, yellow and dark green vegetables (such as carrots, pumpkins, squash, sweet potatoes, broccoli, peas, collard greens, endive, kale, lettuce, peppers, spinach, turnip greens), orange fruits (such as apricots, cantaloupe, papayas, peaches), watermelon and cherries. Vitamin A content varies depending on the color intensity of the fruit or vegetable; a pale carrot contains less vitamin A than a dark orange carrot. Liver is also a good source of vitamin A, containing 45,000 IU in a three-ounce serving.

Butter, fish oils, egg yolk and fortified margarine all contain some vitamin A. Small amounts are contributed to the diet by corn, green beans, beets, cabbage, cauliflower, onions, parsnips, apples, cranberry sauce, dates, grapefruit, pears, strawberries and pineapple. Grains, meat, raisins, potatoes, radishes, unfortified dairy products and mushrooms are poor sources of vitamin A.

Toxicity

Vitamin A is not excreted, so overdoses can produce toxic affects. In adults, prolonged intakes of 15,000 RE-30,000 RE (50,000-100,000 IU) per day can cause transient hydrocephalus; vomiting; weight loss; joint pain; stunted growth; vague abdominal pain; irritability; bone abnormalities; amenhorrea; nausea and gastrointestinal disturbances; itching; anorexia; cracking, drying, scaling and bleeding lips; fissures at the corners of the mouth; enlargement of the spleen, liver or lymph nodes; hair loss; and liver enlargement. In animals, overdoses during pregnancy result in congenital malformations. In humans, the risk of birth defects may occur with maternal doses of 31,818 IU to 36,364 IU for a 100-pound woman. Toxicity symptoms are more pronounced in children than adults.

Excessive intake of beta-carotene does not appear to be toxic, but carotenemia (a yellowish discoloration of the skin) may occur. The condition has no adverse effects and disappears when carotene intake is reduced.

Overdoses of vitamin A from food consumption are uncommon except when large amounts of polar bear liver are consumed. Supplementing the diet with 50,000 IU or more of vitamin A daily may result in toxicity.

VITAMIN D (cholecalciferol = D3; ergocalciferol = D2)

Vitamin D is a crystalline white substance that is soluble in fat. Because of its use as a treatment for rickets, it is called the antirachitic vitamin. Ten different compounds have antirachtic characteristics; they are labeled D1, D2, D3, etc. The most important of these are D2 (ergocalciferol derived from plant sources) and D3 (cholecalciferol found in animal sources). Vitamin D3 is the form found in fish oils and eggs, and is produced in human skin.

Vitamin D is a sterol derivative. When irradiated by the sun's ultraviolet rays, an inactive sterol formed from cholesterol (7-dehydrocholesterol) converts to cholecalciferol. This enters the blood and is converted to the form (25 hydroxycholicalciferol [25,D3]) in the liver. The compound is then converted to the predominant, active form 1, 25 dihydroxycholicalciferol (1, 25–D3) in the kidney.

Vitamin D plays a dual role as both a vitamin and a hormone. Its active metabolites are produced in one tissue (the liver and kidney) and affect another (the intestinal mucosa and bone tissue). As with other hormones, a feedback mechanism controls the rate of synthesis and secretion of vitamin D's active form. Vitamin D is resistant to heat and oxidation, and stable in mild acids and alkalis.

Vitamin D conversion in the skin is restricted by skin pigments and keratin (which screens ultraviolet light). Smog, fog, smoke, clothing, screens and most glass interfere with vitamin D formation.

Functions

Vitamin D promotes calcium absorption from the intestines, calcium resorption from the bone and calcium deposition into osseous tissue. Vitamin D monitors renal excretion of calcium and maintains normal blood levels of this mineral. Vitamin D has two primary functions:

• To increase absorption of calcium, and subsequently phosphorus, in intestinal mucosal cells.

• To increase mobilization of calcium and phosphorus from bones.

Because of vitamin D's regulatory action on calcium and phosphorus, normal calcification does not occur in its absence, even if calcium and phosphorus intake are adequate. Conversely, when vitamin D is adequate, even if calcium and phosphorus are low, calcification does occur. Vitamin D facilitates the rate of calcium absorption and the rate of facilitated transfer in the intestine by its stimulation of a protein component of the calcium transport system in intestinal mucosa cells.

Vitamin D also enhances bone mineralization, perhaps by its ability to transport calcium through osteoclastic and osteoblastic cell membranes. In calcium transport and bone calcium mobilization, 1,25-D3 has greater action than 25,D3, and is ten times more potent in the prevention and treatment of rickets.

The synthesis of 1,25-D3 is sensitive to a feedback regulation. When blood calcium levels decline, parathyroid hormone stimulates the synthesis of 1,25-D3 in the kidneys. The two hormones work together to increase absorption of calcium from the intestines and increase resorption from bone. When blood calcium levels are elevated, parathyroid hormone ceases to stimulate this synthesis and 1,25-D3 production declines. In the absence of vitamin D, bone resorption and plasma calcium decline. The form 1,25-D3 encourages resorption of calcium from kidneys, and deposits of calcium and phosphorus in the teeth. Bone mineralization is affected by cadmium because of the influence of cadmium in vitamin D synthesis.

Deficiency

A vitamin D deficiency is responsible for rickets in children and osteomalacia in adults. Both conditions are a result of defective ossification leading to reduced rigidity in bones, and ultimately causing bones to become soft and pliable and to bend readily.

Rickets is characterized by bowed legs, knock knees, enlarged epiphysis, rachitic rosary (columns of beadlike swellings at rib junctures), contracted pelvis, temporal bone malformations and abnormal enlargement of the head due to retarded fontanel closure in infants. The first tooth seldom erupts before six to nine months because of delayed dentition. Ten types of vitamin D-resistant rickets have been identified, some having hereditary origins. All types are caused by metabolic abnormalities in absorption or metabolism of vitamin D, or end-organ responsiveness.

Osteomalacia is softening of the bones in adults. This condition is found in women with closely-spaced, multiple pregnancies and in confined individuals not exposed to sunlight. In osteomalacia, the calcium-to-phosphorus ratio changes, and calcium losses outweigh those of phosphorus. Serum calcium levels drop, sometimes resulting in tetany.

Celiac disease (gluten-sensitive enteropathy) is indirectly related to vitamin D deficiency. The impaired mineralization that results in structural deformities is due to steatorrhea. Because vitamin D absorption depends on normal bile secretion and fat absorption, a deficiency results from unabsorbed fats, calcium soaps and vitamin D that are flushed out in the steatorrheic stool.

All vitamin D deficiency diseases respond to vitamin D therapy. Some damage cannot be rectified, but further deformities can be prevented.

Requirements

The RDAs for vitamin D are:

	mcg	IU
Infants		
0–0.5 year	10 mcg	400 IU
0.5–1 year	10 mcg	400 IU
Children		
1–10 years	10 mcg	400 IU
Males		
11–18 years	10 mcg	400 IU
19–22 years	7.5 mcg	300 IU
23+ years	5 mcg	200 IU
Females		
11–18 years	10 mcg	400 IU
19–22 years	7.5 mcg	300 IU
23+ years	5 mcg	200 IU
Pregnant	+5 mcg	200 IU
Lactating	+5 mcg	200 IU

Sources

Vitamin D is found in cod liver oil, fish oils and the edible portion of oily fish (such as salmon, herring and sardines). Egg yolk, butter and liver have varying amounts depending on the vitamin D content of the foods the animals consumed. If fortified, milk is a good source. Other dairy products, however, are not fortified and do not contain adequate amounts of the vitamin. Plants are a poor source, with mushrooms and dark green leafy vegetables containing minute amounts. Strict vegetarians have few dietary choices in meeting vitamin D requirements. Vitamin D can be obtained by irradiating some of the above-mentioned foods containing the precursors, and by the body's exposure to ultraviolet light.

Toxicity

Vitamin D is not readily eliminated by the body because it is fat-soluble. After a large dose, the vitamin is found circulating in the body for months, and can be stored in adipose tissue, skeletal muscle and liver and kidney tissue. Toxicity is most likely to occur in infants and young children, but has been reported in all ages. Symptoms include nausea, anorexia, weakness, headache, polyuria, mental retardation, digestive disturbances, narrowing of the aorta due to calcium deposition, dermatitis, irreversible kidney damage, oxidation of tissue lipids, calcification of soft tissue and hypercalcemia due to an increased withdrawal of calcium from the bones. The threshold for toxicity is 500 to 600 mcg/kg body weight per day. Excretion is gradual through the bile.

VITAMIN E (alpha, beta and gamma tocopherol)

Vitamin E refers to a family of compounds known as tocopherols. Alpha-tocopherol, commonly referred to as vitamin E, is the form widely distributed in nature and the most biologically active. Other naturally occurring tocopherols are named according to the number and position of the methyl groups, and are labeled beta, gamma, delta, etc. Vitamin E is a light yellow oil that is predisposed to oxidation. It is stable to heat and acids, and somewhat unstable to alkalis. Rancid fats and oils destroy this vitamin.

Functions

Vitamin E is an antioxidant and is enhanced by other antioxidants, such as ascorbic acid and selenium. Along with the enzymes glutathione peroxidase, catalase and superoxide dismutase, it protects polyunsaturated fats in the body from oxidative destruction by peroxides, superoxides and other free radicals. Free radical damage to critical enzyme sites and structural membranes results in cell destruction in the absence of vitamin E. Tissues such as the testes accumulate polyunsaturated fats, and are the first to deteriorate when vitamin E is deficient. Ceroid pigmentation (a yellow-brown discoloration of tissue) accumulates over time in the presence of increased polyunsaturated fats and decreased vitamin E.

As an antioxidant, vitamin E functions:

- to stabilize membranes and to protect them against free radical damage;
- to protect the lungs against oxidative damage from air pollutants;
- to prevent tumor growth. Both free radicals and lipid peroxidation have been associated with the development of cancer;
- to protect tissues of the skin, eye, liver, breast and calf muscle;
- to maintain the biological integrity of vitamin A and increase the body's stores of this vitamin.

Deficiency

Vitamin E deficiency can be classified in two categories: (1) conditions that respond to an antioxidant as well as to the vitamin, and (2) conditions that respond to the vitamin but are not influenced by other antioxidants. The antioxidant-sensitive symptoms include encephalomalacia, in vitro erythrocyte hemolysis, formation of ceroid pigments, and reproductive failure in some species. The symptoms that respond to vitamin E, but not to antioxidants, include muscular dystrophy in most species, testicular degeneration in rats and anemia in monkeys.

Vitamin E deficiency is difficult to diagnose because the deficiency manifests itself in diverse ways. Although the major influence of the deficiency is on the reproductive system, nervous system, muscle tissue and blood erythrocytes, not all species manifest a deficiency in one or all of these areas. Some symptoms are amplified by dietary polyunsaturated fatty acids. Other symptoms may be prevented by nonspecific antioxidants (such as selenium or the sulfur-containing amino acids).

The role of vitamin E in the prevention of premature aging is a topic of current interest. The theory is that aging is due to a progressive accumulation of cellular deteriorations caused by free radical damage, and that vitamin E retards this process. This association has not been proven.

Because vitamin E is necessary for the structural and functional maintenance of all skeletal, cardiac and smooth muscle, "nutritional muscular dystrophy" is seen in animals fed a vitamin E-deficient diet. This condition is a result of injury to the lysosomal membrane of muscle cells. The skeletal muscle can be pale, ischemic and gritty because of calcium deposition.

The inability to use creatine may cause increased creatinuria.

Irreversible reproductive system damage occurs in rats fed a vitamin E-deficient diet. If the female does become pregnant, spontaneous abortion or resorption of the embryo results. Ceroid tissue has been found in the uterus and fallopian tubes of vitamin E-deficient rats. This suggests that fat peroxidation leads to tissue damage and the irreversible loss of fertility. Damage to the human reproductive system because of a vitamin E deficiency has not been identified.

Encephalomalacia (a nervous system disorder) and its clinical signs of ataxia, spasms and paralysis are seen in vitamin E-deficient chicks. The condition appears to be a result of an imbalance in the dietary ratio of tocopherol to polyunsaturated fats. The disorder, not seen in chicks fed a fat-free, vitamin E-deficient diet, can be alleviated or prevented by a nonspecific antioxidant. Brain damage in deficiency states results from the antioxidant effect of the vitamin. The peroxides, if left unchecked, alter the membrane structure of nerve cells and perhaps interfere with normal enzymatic function.

Vitamin E is important in the synthesis and maintenance of red blood cells and their constituents. Hemorrhage is a common symptom of vitamin E deficiency because of erythrocyte membrane susceptibility to peroxidation. Hemolytic anemia results if these membranes are broken and the oxygen-carrying capacity of the blood is reduced. Newborns are susceptible to this condition if there are poor placental transport of vitamin E and low stores at birth. Breast milk is an adequate source of vitamin E to alleviate this condition, but cow's milk is not. Vitamin E conserves iron stores by protecting erythrocyte membranes from hemolysis, thus reducing the turnover rate of iron.

Vitamin E may have a direct effect on the synthesis of hemoglobin, as deficiencies in the rat lead to decreased activity of some enzymes required for heme biosynthesis.

In children with cystic fibrosis, creatinuria (a condition found in vitamin E-deficient rats) is reduced with vitamin E therapy.

Although animals demonstrate a wide variety of deficiency symptoms, there is no evidence that healthy humans eating a mixed diet are susceptible to a clinical vitamin E deficiency.

Vitamin E absorption is dependent on the presence of both pancreatic secretions and bile. Pancreatic insufficiency or biliary obstruction can result in vitamin E deficiency.

Requirements

The requirement for vitamin E is proportionate to body size and polyunsaturated fat intake. Vitamin E is needed in small amounts when dietary polyunsaturated fats are minimal. Increasing polyunsaturated fats in the diet increases their concentration in the tissues. The need to protect these fats from oxidation results in an increased need for vitamin E.

Because of the close association with the type and amount of fat in the diet, dietary amounts are difficult to recommend for all people. The RDA is an average value based on the necessary amount of vitamin E needed for a balanced and mixed diet (1 mg = 1.49 IU of d-alpha tocopherol). Intake must maintain blood tocopherol levels of 0.5 mg to 0.9 mg/100 ml, adequate stores in all tissues and a suitable ratio of vitamin E to polyunsaturated fat. Taking into account the varying potencies of the tocopherols, the RDAs for healthy individuals are:

Infants	3–4 mg
Children	5–7 mg
Adolescents	8 mg
Adult Males	10 mg
Adult Females	8 mg
Pregnant	+2 mg
Lactating	+3 mg

Sources

The tocopherols are distributed in plant and animal foods, with vegetable and seed oils being the greatest contributors. Different tocopherols are not uniformly distributed in foods: the vitamin E content of safflower oil is 90 percent alpha-tocopherol; the content of corn oil is only 10 percent. Vitamin E content is often related to the linoleic acid content of the oil. Thus, safflower oil, which has a high linoleic acid content, is also one of the best sources of vitamin E.

Animal products are medium to poor sources of vitamin E. The variations are large, however, and depend on the fat composition of the animal's diet. Cooking and processing foods can substantially reduce their vitamin E content. Tocopherols are removed during the milling of white flour, and, in making white bread, all the vitamin E can be lost if chloride dioxide is used in the bleaching process. Vitamin E is also lost in substantial amounts in the refining and purification of vegetable oils. The by-products of this processing contain so much of the vitamin that they are used in producing vitamin E supplements.

Other dietary source of vitamin E are whole grains, green leafy vegetables, margarines and shortenings made from vegetable oils, wheat germ oil, egg yolk, butter, liver and nuts.

Toxicity

In humans, there appears to be little danger of toxicity from vitamin E. Toxicity has been reported in animals and is manifested as growth retardation, poor bone calcification, reduced hematocrit levels and reduced skeletal muscle respiration. Increased prothrombin times are also reported. Because of the hypervitaminosis effects in animals, large doses of this fat-soluble vitamin are discouraged in humans.

VITAMIN K (phylloquinone = K1; menaquinones = K2)

The two naturally occuring forms of vitamin K are vitamin K1 (phylloquinone) and vitamin K2 (the menaquinones). Vitamin K1 is derived from the alfalfa leaf. Vitamin K2 is produced by microorganisms such as bacteria in the intestinal tract of many animals. A third form is the synthetically derived vitamin K3 (menadione). Vitamin K3 has the basic structure of the naturally occurring vitamins and is twice as active biologically. All three forms are fat soluble and stable to heat and reducing agents. The synthetic compound is soluble in boiling water. Alkalis, strong acids, irradiation and oxidizing agents will destroy vitamin K activity.

Functions

Vitamin K plays a role in blood clotting. The vitamin contributes to the liver's synthesis of prothrombin, which converts to thrombin in the initial steps of blood coagulation. Three other factors in blood clotting are also vitamin K-dependent: Factor IX, Factor VII and Factor X.

Vitamin K functions in carboxylation of the glutamic portion of prothrombin to form calcium-binding sites. This contribution to the carboxylation of glutamic acid may also aid in bone mineralization by forming another calcium-binding protein, esteocalcin.

Deficiency

A vitamin K deficiency is uncommon in man because of the vitamin's wide distribution in plants and animals, and the microbial synthesis in the intestinal lumen. Vitamin K, in water- or fat-soluble forms, is effective in raising prothrombin levels and controlling hemorrhage in newborns. Newborns will show reduced plasma prothrombin concentrations because of the placenta's poor transmission of fats and the sterility of the gut in the first few days. (These levels begin to rise to normal by the third or fourth day.) To prevent hemorrhage, expectant mothers are given supplemental vitamin K for several days prior to delivery. The infant is given supplements during the first days of life.

Animals deficient in vitamin K tend to bleed profusely, and small bruises can escalate into major hemorrhages. Blood clotting time is slowed due to a lack of prothrombin and other factors important in blood clotting.

Ingestion of antibiotics or other agents that interfere with microbial activity will curtail intestinal synthesis. However, unless adults are given bowel sterilizing agents and fed a vitamin K-deficient diet for several weeks, vitamin K deficiency is not likely.

Vitamin K in the intestinal lumen is absorbable from two sources: ingested food and intestinal microbial synthesis. Vitamin K absorption is dependent on normal fat absorption including the presence of bile and pancreatic juice. Non-absorbable fats (such as mineral oil) greatly reduce vitamin K absorption by binding the vitamin and carrying it out of the body. Malabsorption problems (such as sprue, pellagra, bowel shunts, ulcerative colitis or regional ileitis) can also cause secondary vitamin K deficiency.

Several antagonists can interfere with the vitamin's absorption and use in the body. Coumarin (isolated from sweet clover) competes directly with vitamin K at its biologically active site. Warfarin (the rodenticide) is a dicoumaral derivative. Phylloquinone and menaquinones can reverse the effects of thse compounds; menadione cannot. Heparin (an anticoagulant) diminishes the amount of available prothrombin, thus acting as a vitamin K antagonist. Salicylates, administered over a long time, increase the need for vitamin K.

Requirements

Half of the daily need for vitamin K is supplied by dietary plant sources, the remainder from biosynthesis in the intestine. A normal, mixed diet will contain from 300 to 500 mcg daily, and individual variation results in 10 to 70 percent absorption. No specific RDA exists for the vitamin; rather, a recommended adequate and safe range has been estimated to be 2 mcg/kg body weight per day.

Infants
0–0.5 year	12 mcg
0.5–1 year	10–20 mcg

Children
1–3 years	15–30 mcg
4–6 years	20–40 mcg
7–10 years	30–60 mcg
11+ years	50–100 mcg

Adults
	70–140 mcg

These amounts are easily supplied by a varied diet. The water-soluble substitutes, such as vitamin K3, are useful for those unable to absorb fats.

Sources

Vitamin K is found in dark green leafy vegetables.

Toxicity

Hemolytic anemia is a result of vitamin K overdose. This condition is due to an accelerated breakdown of red blood cells and has been reported in low-birth-weight infants. Vitamin K1 does not appear to produce these effects.

THE WATER-SOLUBLE VITAMINS

VITAMIN B1 (thiamin)

Thiamin, also known as vitamin B1, is a water-soluble white crystalline substance that has the odor and flavor of yeast. It is somewhat soluble in ethyl alcohol and insoluble in ether and chloroform. Thiamin is stable to dry heat up to 100°C but is easily destroyed by moist heat (especially in the presence of alkalis such as baking soda). Sulfur dioxide, a compound used in the drying of fruits, destroys thiamin.

Functions

Thiamin pyrophosphate (TPP), a combination of thiamin and two molecules of phosphoric acid, is the coenzyme form of thiamin. This coenzyme is critical in several metabolic functions, including:

- The removal of CO_2, or oxidative decarboxylation reactions. The decarboxylation of alpha-keto acids is critical in the conversion of amino acids, fats and carbohydrates to energy. TPP converts pyruvic acid to acetyl CoA for entry into the Krebs cycle, and converts alpha-keto-glutarate to succinyl CoA within the Krebs cycle. Both of these reactions require the presence of lipoic acid, niacin and pantothenic acid.
- The transfer of two carbon units, or transketolation.
- The conversion of glyoxylate to carbon dioxide. This conversion drains off excess glyolic acid, thereby removing precursors to oxalates.
- The conversion of carbohydrate to fat.

Thiamin's coenzyme form is also implicated in the synthesis of acetylcholine, a lack of which causes polyneuritis or inflammation of the nerves. The mental, cardiac and circulatory defects characteristic of beri-beri may be due to diminished acetylcholine synthesis. Some symptoms of thiamin deficiency may be caused by the build-up of partially metabolized substances (such as pyruvic acid and methyl glyoxal) that cannot be catabolized further without thiamin. Exercise, carbohydrate foods and alcohol worsen symptoms because of the increased demand on the body's need for thiamin.

If the diet overemphasizes foods high in fats and sugar, thiamin intake may be inadequate. Mild forms of neurosis have been reported on such diets. A thiamin deficiency can develop during dieting or fasting or when eating a limited variety of foods, because thiamin requirements remain the same no matter how restrictive the diet.

Deficiency

Deficiency symptoms are seen when thiamin intake drops below 0.2–0.3 mg/1000 kcalories. A diet low in thiamin, such as one composed of unenriched white flour or polished rice, will result in beriberi. Early symptoms of this disease include fatigue, anorexia, weight loss, gastrointestinal disorders and weakness. Muscles may become tender and atrophied. Bradycardia (slowing of the heart rate), an enlarged heart and nausea occur in later stages. Impairment of nerve function results in numbness or increased sensitivity, tingling in the extremities, loss of reflexes or peripheral paralysis. Blood levels of pyruvate and lactic acid increase. Personality changes (such as memory loss, reduced attention span, irritability, confusion and depression) may develop. Constipation may result from reduced gastric muscle tone. Prolonged thiamin deficiency results in permanent damage to the nervous system.

Wet beriberi, a type of thiamin deficiency, is characterized by edema, with the accumulation of fluids in the ankles, feet and legs, finally progressing up the body. These excess fluids interfere with heart function and can be fatal. Edema is not seen in another type of thiamin deficiency, dry beriberi, but is replaced by severe muscle wasting and emaciation.

Childhood beriberi stunts growth. Infants may be cyanotic, developing a bluish skin color because of the reduced oxygen availability to the tissues. These infants have a piercing, high scream or may cry silently. The heartbeat is accelerated; vomiting and convulsions may occur prior to death. Within hours of thiamin ingestion, symptoms diminish.

Some gastrointestinal disturbances can be attributed to thiamin deficiency, although caution must be exercised because of numerous other factors that may be involved, and the vagueness of the symptoms. Symptoms frequently identified as a thiamin deficiency include anorexia, low gastric hydrochloric acid, atony of the stomach and intestines, constipation and intestinal inflammation.

A thiamin deficiency caused by alcohol abuse can leave the user with permanent memory impairment, inaccuracies in reality perception and motor and eye movement deficiencies. Alcohol abuse is associated with poor dietary habits and inadequate thiamin intake. In addition, thiamin is necessary for the metabolism of alcohol, and alcohol reduces the intestinal absorption of thiamin. The accumulated effect of alcohol on thiamin status is alcoholic neuritis.

A related condition, Wernicke's encephalopathy, is found in alcoholics and also in patients with pernicious vomiting. Manifestations range from mild confusion to coma. Death is not uncommon and, if the patient survives, damage to the cerebral cortex may result in psychosis (Korsakoff's). If permanent damage has not occurred, many symptoms are reversible with thiamin therapy.

Requirements

Because thiamin and its metabolites are not stored and are lost through the urine, thiamin must be frequently supplied in the diet. A small, temporary reserve may be stored in the heart, liver, kidney and brain if more than the daily requirement is ingested.

These stores can serve as a reservoir for a few weeks if thiamin supplies dwindle.

The need for thiamin depends primarily on calorie intake—0.5 mg/1000 kcalories with a minumum of 1.0 mg/day. When calculating the RDA for a twenty-five-year-old woman with a requirement of 2000 kcalories a day, thiamin needs are 1.0 mg. This requirement acknowledges the relationship of thiamin to energy metabolism.

Other factors must be considered in determining thiamin need, such as age and, in the case of a woman, whether she is pregnant or lactating. Infants and children require more thiamin for each kilogram of body weight than adults. The developing fetus and newborn demand a greater thiamin intake by the mother. Thiamin needs will increase during times of physical and emotional stress. The RDAs for thiamin are:

Infants	
0–0.5 year	0.3 mg
0.5–1 year	0.5 mg
Children	
1–3 years	0.7 mg
4–6 years	0.9 mg
7–10 years	1.2 mg
Young Adults	
Males 11–18 years	1.4 mg
Males 19–22 years	1.5 mg
Females 11–22 years	1.1 mg
Adults	
Males 23–50 years	1.4 mg
Males 52+ years	1.2 mg
Females 23+ years	1.0 mg
Pregnant	+0.4 mg
Lactating	+0.5 mg

Thiamin is lost during food preparation when water and drippings are discarded.

Sources

Few foods other than pork supply thiamin in amounts greater than a tenth of a milligram per serving. Other good sources of thiamin are beef, organ meats, whole-wheat or enriched cereals, nuts and legumes (especially peas and beans).

Moderate thiamin sources include milk, avocados, cauliflower, spinach and dried fruits. Poor sources are unenriched white flour and pastas, polished rice, molasses, blueberries, corn and cheese.

Toxicity

Because it is water-soluble, thiamin is not stored in appreciable amounts. There are no known toxic effects from oral overconsumption. However, anaphylactic shock has been reported after repeated intravenous injections of thiamin.

VITAMIN B2 (riboflavin)

Riboflavin, or vitamin B2, is an orange-yellow, crystalline substance that gives watery mediums (including urine) a yellow-green fluorescent glow. It is slightly soluble in water or acid and very soluble in an alkaline solution. Riboflavin is stable to heat in neutral or acid mediums, but easily destroyed by strong alkaline solutions and by visible and ultraviolet light.

Functions

Riboflavin is a component of two enzymes: flavin mononucleotide (FMN) and flavin adenine dinucleotide (FAD). These coenzymes are important in energy production. They play a role as hydrogen carriers for the oxidation-reduction reactions in the electron transport system leading to the formation of ATP. The coenzymes' role is in dehydrogenations. As a result of these reactions, the coenzyme is reduced. Following this reduction, the coenzyme serves as a substrate for other electron acceptors, and the oxidized form is regenerated.

Riboflavin is essential for normal fatty acid and amino acid synthesis. FMN is a component of the L-amino acid oxidase that oxidizes L-alpha amino acids and L-alpha hydroxy acids to alpha-keto acids. FAD serves with succinic dehydrogenase, xanthine oxidase, glycine oxidase, lipoyl dehydrogenase, NAD+-cytochrome C reductase, and D-amino acid oxidase. Flavin enzymes are also important in the deamination of amino acids. Cellular growth cannot take place in the absence of riboflavin.

Deficiency

Riboflavin deficiency does not occur in isolation, but is found as a component of multiple-nutrient deficiency states. While no specific disease has been attributed to riboflavin deficiency, several symptoms have been associated with an inadequate intake. These include:

- Cheilosis (cracks at the corners of the mouth) and inflammation of the mucous membranes in the mouth accompanied by a smooth, purple-tinged glossitis.
- Reddening of the eyes (due to increased vascularization), and eyes that tire easily, burn, itch, and are sensitive to light. Vision may also be dimmed.
- An unusual dermatitis characterized by simultaneous dryness and greasy scaling.
- Nerve tissue damage that may manifest itself as depression and hysteria.
- Malformations and retarded growth in infants and children.

Deficiency symptoms are reported when daily intake falls below 0.6 mg. The symptoms are rare except in alcohol abusers.

Requirements

Because the riboflavin requirement is related to energy metabolism, it reflects kcalories consumed (0.6 mg riboflavin per 1000 kcalories). When intake drops below 1.2 mg, a tissue reserve of riboflavin cannot be maintained. Therefore, riboflavin consumption should not drop below this amount, regardless of calorie intake.

Riboflavin is not stored in appreciable amounts, with only minute reserves in the heart, liver and kidneys. Consequently, a frequent supply is needed. The RDAs for riboflavin are:

Infants	
0–0.5 year	0.4 mg
0.5–1 year	0.6 mg
Children	
1–3 years	0.8 mg
4–6 years	1.0 mg
7–10 years	1.4 mg
Young Adults	
Males 11–14 years	1.6 mg
Males 15–22 years	1.7 mg
Females 11–22 years	1.3 mg
Adults	
Males 23–50 years	1.6 mg
Males 51+ years	1.4 mg
Females 23+ years	1.2 mg
Pregnant	+0.3 mg
Lactating	+0.5 mg

Sources

The Ten State Survey on the nutritional status of Americans found riboflavin intake to be a potential problem for young persons and certain ethnic groups. If milk products and other animal protein sources are curtailed, a deficiency is possible.

Excellent sources of riboflavin are liver, milk and milk products. Moderate sources are oysters, meat, dark green leafy vegetables, eggs, mushrooms, asparagus, broccoli, avocado, brussels sprouts and fish (such as tuna and salmon). Poor sources are apples, grapefruit, unenriched pastas, cereals and grains, cabbage and cucumbers.

Because riboflavin is destroyed by light, milk and enriched pastas should be stored in opaque containers. Fresh vegetables should be stored in a dark, cool environment and cooked in a covered pot. Some riboflavin is lost when cooking water and drippings are discarded.

Toxicity

Relatively large doses of riboflavin do not create adverse effects. When riboflavin intake exceeds 1.3 mg/day, the vitamin and its metabolites are excreted in proportionately greater amounts in the urine. The limited storage and easy excretion contribute to the nontoxic properties of the vitamin.

NIACIN (nicotinic acid, niacinamide)

Niacin, or vitamin B3, is the common name for two compounds: nicotinic acid (which is easily converted to the biologically active form) and nicotinamide (niacinamide). Neither compound is related to the drug nicotine. Niacin is a needlelike white crystalline substance, soluble in water and alcohol. It is one of the most stable B vitamins, withstanding temperatures up to 120° C and unaltered by exposure to oxygen. Losses occur if cooking water is discarded.

Functions

Niacin is a component of two coenzymes: nicotinamide adenine dinucleotide (NAD+) and nicotinamide adenine dinucleotide phosphate (NADP+). Like the flavin coenzymes, NAD and NADP function in oxidation-reduction reactions (the transfer of hydrogen, or electrons, from one compound to another). In their reduced forms, the coenzymes are NADH and NADPH.

Niacin functions in over fifty metabolic reactions. It plays a key role in glycolysis, the conversion of pyruvic acid to acetyl CoA and reactions of the Krebs Cycle and the hexose monophosphate shunt. All of these reactions are important in the release of energy from carbohydrates. Niacin is also important in the deamination of amino acids, fatty-acid synthesis, and beta oxidation of fatty acids. It is essential for the formation of steroids, the metabolism of several drugs and toxicants and in the formation of red blood cells. Because of its diverse and critical role in so many metabolic pathways, niacin is vital in supplying energy to, and maintaining the integrity of, all body cells.

Deficiency

Niacin deficiency, known as pellagra, affects every cell, but is most critical in tissues with rapid cell turnover, such as the skin, the gastrointestinal tract and the nerves. The initial symptoms are weakness, lassitude, anorexia and indigestion. The classic symptoms of pellagra are "the 3Ds": dermatitis, diarrhea and dementia. The fourth "D" is death.

The dermatitis found in pellagra is a scaly, dark pigmentation that develops on areas of the skin exposed to sunlight, heat or mild trauma (such as the face, arms or elbows, back of the hands, feet or parts of the body exposed to body secretions or mild irritations). Other parts of the body are pale in color. All parts of the digestive tract are affected. The tongue is swollen, corroded and brilliant red. Diarrhea, if it develops, may be accompanied by vomiting and severe inflammation of the mouth. In addition, diarrhea results in faulty fat and fat-soluble vitamin absorption. Achlorhydria contributes to intestinal infection and lesions.

Nervous system disorders include irritability, headache, insomnia, pain in the extremities, loss of memory, and emotional instability. In advanced stages, delirium and catatonia may develop. Shortly before death, convulsions and coma may occur. Because of its effect on the nervous system, niacin therapy has been used in the treatment of some schizophrenias.

Deficiency symptoms are seen in diets containing less than 7.5 mg/day. A niacin deficiency seldom occurs alone, and treatment of pellagra with this B vitamin will not cure all symptoms. Often, deficiencies of riboflavin, thiamin and other B vitamins, protein and iron simultaneously compound the condition and must be included in the therapy.

Requirements

To cure pellagra, ample amounts of the vitamin are

needed, in addition to good-quality protein. Although labeled a vitamin, niacin can be synthesized from the amino acid tryptophan. Fifty percent of the daily requirement is obtained from the conversion of tryptophan to niacin. This conversion occurs primarily in the liver and requires the presence of pyridoxine (vitamin B6).

The total amount of niacin in the diet can be expressed as milligram equivalents, which includes the niacin in the diet plus the amount converted from tryptophan. Food tables list only the milligrams of niacin and do not consider the niacin-tryptophan conversion. To estimate total milligram equivalents, assume that tryptophan comprises one percent of dietary protein and every 60 mg of tryptophan is equivalent to 1 mg of niacin. The conversion of tryptophan plus the niacin content of food provides the total niacin available in the diet.

The RDA for adults is based on calorie intake, 6.6 mg/1000 kcalories. The diet should include no less than 13 mg, even if food intake is below 2000 kcalories. The RDAs are:

Infants
0–0.5 year	6 mg
0.5–1 year	8 mg

Children
1–3 years	9 mg
4–6 years	11 mg
7–10 years	16 mg

Adults
Males 11–18 years	18 mg
Males 19–22 years	19 mg
Males 23–50 years	18 mg
Males 50+ years	16 mg
Females 11–14 years	15 mg
Females 15–22 years	14 mg
Females 23+ years	13 mg
Pregnant	+2 mg
Lactating	+4 mg

Small stores of niacin in the liver, heart and muscles are not adequate in times of increased need; therefore, a frequent supply is necessary. To meet this increased need, women in their last trimester of pregnancy can convert tryptophan to niacin three times as readily. Normal blood values are 0.6 mg/100 ml.

Sources

The best dietary sources are protein foods such as organ meats, peanuts, muscle meats, poultry, legumes, milk and eggs. Milk and eggs are especially good sources because of their high protein and tryptophan content. Moderate sources are wholegrain cereals and breads. Milling and processing of white flour, rice and other products removes 90 percent of the niacin. If the product is labelled "enriched," the niacin has been added back to preexisting levels. Except for orange juice, fruits are a poor source of this vitamin.

Toxicity

Large doses of nicotinic acid produce cutaneous vasodilation and resultant flushing and itching of the skin. These symptoms cease when the dosage is reduced. Nicotinamide does not produce this effect. Prolonged and excessive overdoses of nicotinic acid can produce gastrointestinal irritation, possible liver damage with a subsequent decrease in glucose tolerance, glycosuria, hepatic fibrosis and multiple enzyme changes. These symptoms are uncommon and humans have reported doses of 2 g/day with no ill effects other than flushing and itching. Excesses are excreted in the urine and feces, which may account for the vitamin's low toxicity.

VITAMIN B6 (pyridoxine)

Vitamin B6 is a family of compounds that includes pyridoxine, pyridoxal and pyridoxamine. The vitamin is soluble in water, acetone and alcohol. Pyridoxine is stable to heat in acid solutions, but not as stable in alkaline solutions. Pyridoxal and pyridoxamine are less stable to heat. Vitamin B6 is destroyed by visible and ultraviolet light, especially in neutral and alkaline mediums. All three forms of vitamin B6 are found in foods.

Functions

Pyridoxal phosphate (PLP), the vitamin's coenzyme form, is important in protein metabolism, more specifically in nitrogen metabolism. Because of its ability to transport several functional groups, it provides the mechanism for numerous amino acid reactions. The metabolically active PLP assists in the transport of amino acids across the intestinal mucosa and in the blood. In conjunction with other enzymes, pyridoxal phosphate performs the following functions:

- Builds amino acids (amination).
- Removes amine groups from amino acids (deamination).

- Removes sulfur from sulfur-containing amino acids (desulfhydration).
- Transfers amine groups from one amino acid to another (transamination).
- Functions in dehydration and amine oxidation.
- Participates with folic acid in the methylation of choline, methionine and serine.
- Metabolizes cysteine to pyruvic acid and oxalate to glycine.
- Plays a role in decarboxylation reactions (such as converting precursors into serotonin and gamma amino butyric acid [neurotransmitters important in brain function]). Norepinephrine, acetylcholine and histamine are also dependent on vitamin B6.

PLP is important in the biological conversion of tryptophan to niacin. In its absence, large amounts of xanthurenic acid (a product of faulty tryptophan metabolism) are excreted in the urine. The presence of this abnormal urinary metabolite is a test for B6 deficiency.

PLP is necessary for porphyrin formation and therefore for normal synthesis of hemoglobin. Vitamin B6 is also important in normal function and growth of red blood cells. Lipid and carbohydrate metabolism depend on vitamin B6, as do fatty acid synthesis, linoleic acid conversion to arachidonic acid, and cholesterol metabolism.

The coenzyme of pyridoxine works with phosphorylase in the conversion of glycogen to glucose. Without this vitamin, the body could not use glycogen as an energy supply. Vitamin B6 is primarily stored in the muscle, where it can readily mobilize glycogen.

Deficiency

A vitamin B6 deficiency produces profound effects upon amino acid metabolism, resulting in a wide spectrum of possible effects ranging from a reduced synthesis of niacin to impaired production of neurotransmitters and hemoglobin.

The symptoms of a vitamin B6 deficiency are vague and hard to reproduce. No particular disease has been associated with a vitamin B6 deficiency although weakness, mental confusion, irritability and nervousness, insomnia, poor coordination in walking, hyperactivity, convulsions, abnormal electroencephalogram, declining blood lymphocytes and white blood cells, anemia and skin lesions—symptoms similar to those of riboflavin and niacin deficiencies (seborrheic dermatitis, glossitis, cheilosis and stomatitis)—have been reported.

Increased vitamin B6 is needed during and after pregnancy, as indicated by increased amounts of xanthurenic acid excreted in the urine. Administration of the vitamin eliminates the abnormal metabolite, Infants consuming a vitamin B6-deficient diet also show symptoms, including irritability, abdominal distention, diarrhea, vomiting and convulsions.

Some drugs can impair vitamin B6 absorption or utilization. Amphetamine, chlorpromazine, reserpine and oral contraceptives affect either the concentration of the vitamin in tissues or its enzyme form. Tryptophan metabolism is impaired in women using the birth control pill, possibly due to reduced circulating vitamin B6.

Some genetic diseases are related to abnormalities in vitamin B6 metabolism. These include:

- Infant convulsive seizures caused by a reduced glutamic decarboxylase activity and resulting in decreased synthesis of GABA.
- Vitamin B6-responsive anemia due to decreased formation of aminolevulinic acid in heme synthesis.
- Cystathionuria from reduced activity of cystathionase.
- Xanthurenic aciduria resulting from decreased conversion of kynurenine to anthranilic acid because of reduced kynureninase activity.
- Homocysteinuria caused by reduced conversion of homocysteine to crysthathionine.

Requirements

Vitamin B6 requirements are dependent on protein metabolism. The adult RDA is established for a diet containing 100 g of protein. If larger protein amounts are consumed, vitamin B6 requirements increase proportionately. Women using oral contraceptives may also need to increase B6 consumption. The RDAs for vitamin B6 are:

Infants	
0–0.5 year	0.3 mg
0.5–1 year	0.6 mg
Children	
1–3 years	0.9 mg
4–6 years	1.3 mg
7–10 years	1.8 mg
Adults	
Males 15+ years	2.2 mg
Females 15+ years	2.0 mg
Pregnant	+0.6 mg
Lactating	+0.5 mg

Sources

The following protein foods are good sources of vitamin B6: meats and organ meats, poultry, fish, egg yolk, soybeans and dried beans, peanuts and walnuts. Other good sources are bananas, avocados, cabbage, cauliflower, potatoes, wholegrain cereals and bread, and prunes. Poor sources include egg whites, fruits, refined grains, lettuce, milk and beer. Significant amounts can be lost during cooking and improper storage of foods.

Toxicity

Incidents of vitamin B6 toxicity are very rare. Doses over 1.0 g are tolerated by animals, and no adverse effects have been found in humans at this level.

FOLACIN (folic acid, pteroylglutamic acid)

The B vitamin folacin, or folic acid, is a dull yellow substance, sensitive to light. It is slightly soluble in water and stable to heat in neutral and alkaline solutions. Folic acid is destroyed at a pH below 4. Significant losses also occur in cooking, storage, improper handling, exposure to light and preparation of foods.

Structurally, this B vitamin consists of a pteridine nucleus, para-aminobenzoic acid, with glutamic acid attached (hence the chemical name for this nutrient is monopteroylglutamic acid). Other biologically active forms contain three or more glutamic acid molecules. Although no method has been discovered to measure all the active forms of folic acid in foods, the vitamin is commonly found as a polyglutamyl derivative known as folacin. Once in the body, folic acid is converted to the biologically active form, tetrahydrofolic acid (THFA), in the presence of NADPH (niacin's coenzyme form) and ascorbic acid.

Functions

As with vitamin B12, THFA functions as a carrier for single-carbon groups from one substance to another. In conjunction with vitamin B12, THFA participates in amino acid conversions and the methylation of choline, methionine, serine (also requiring pyridoxal phosphate or B6), and histidine. THFA participates in the methylation of nicotinamide to N_1-methylnicotinamide.

The form of folacin most commonly found in the liver and serum is methyl folate. Methyl folate can return to the body's pool only through a vitamin B12-dependent pathway. If a B12 deficiency exists, folic acid is trapped as methyl folate and is useless to the body. Consequently, a deficiency of either vitamin B12 or folic acid will result in identical symptoms. In both cases, the characteristic anemia results from a lack of 5,10-methylene THFA for use in the synthesis of pyrimidines and purines for DNA formation.

Deficiency

Folic acid deficiency is one of the most common vitamin deficiencies. The symptoms are similar to those of a vitamin B12 deficiency: megaloblastic anemia, irritability, weakness, weight loss, apathy, anorexia, dyspnea, sore tongue, headache, palpitations, forgetfulness, hostility, paranoid behavior, glossitis, gastrointestinal tract disturbances and diarrhea. However, inadequate folacin intake does not result in the irreversible nerve damage seen in vitamin B12 deficiency. Because of the vitamin's vulnerability to destruction, as much as 100 percent may be lost if foods are improperly stored, cooking water is discarded or foods are reheated or overcooked.

Deficiency can result from poor dietary intake, defective absorption or abnormal metabolism. These can in turn result from sprue, pellagra, intestinal dysfunction or gastric resection. Many medications, including aspirin and anticonvulsants, may also interfere with folacin absorption and metabolism.

One of the symptoms of folic acid deficiency, megaloblastic anemia, is not uncommon during pregnancy, especially during the last trimester. Elevated blood levels in the fetus at birth suggest an increased drain on maternal stores. Hormonal changes during pregnancy may also play a role in folacin status since polyglutamate absorption is reduced by as much as 50 percent in women taking the birth control pill, a medication that mimics the hormonal status of pregnancy.

Dietary restriction of folacin will result in depressed serum levels in less than a month. Erythrocyte and liver stores are depleted within three months and formiminoglutamate, urocanate, formate and aminoimidazole carboxamide urinary excretion increases.

The symptoms of a folic acid deficiency quickly respond to therapy. If necessary, doses up to 1 mg may be administered. Maintenance therapy is 100 mcg for one to four months, including the amounts obtained from folacin-rich foods in the diet. In most cases, folacin deficiency may be prevented by the ingestion of one to two folacin-rich fruits or vegetables daily.

Requirements

Fifty micrograms of folacin will reduce megaloblastic anemia symptomology; 100 to 200 mcg will maintain tissue stores. The amount stored in the liver is not adequate to cover increased demands during stress, alcoholism, pregnancy, lactation or during ingestion of some medications (including oral contraceptives). The average American diet contains 220 mcg of folacin. Of this, 20 to 50 percent is absorbed and made available to the tissues. Normal blood values for folacin are 3.4 mcg/100 ml. The RDAs for folacin are:

Infants	
0–0.5 year	30 mcg
0.5–1 year	45 mcg
Children	
1–3 years	100 mcg
4–6 years	200 mcg
7–10 years	300 mcg
11+ years	400 mcg
Adults	
Pregnant	+400 mcg
Lactating	+100 mcg

Sources

Folic acid is found in a wide variety of foods, especially dark green vegetables (folic derives its name from foliage). For this reason, a dark green leafy vegetable should be included in the diet daily. Good sources also include: organ meats, kidney beans, asparagus, broccoli, beets, cabbage, yeast, cauliflower, orange juice, cantaloupe, green peas, sweet potatoes, wheat germ, wholegrain cereals and breads and lima beans. Poor sources are root vegetables, bananas, refined grains and breads, pork and lamb.

Toxicity

Large doses of folacin can mask an underlying vitamin B12 deficiency. Although folacin is effective in DNA synthesis and normal red blood cell formation, it cannot aid in the B12-dependent regeneration of the myelin sheath necessary for nerve transmission. If a B12 deficiency remains undetected, the result can be irreversible nerve damage. For this reason, folacin dosage is restricted in over-the-counter vitamin preparations.

The vitamin has a low toxicity. A one-thousand-fold increase in the daily requirement may be consumed with no harmful effects. Daily doses of 15 mg are non-toxic. Excesses are excreted in the urine.

VITAMIN B12 (cobalamin)

Vitamin B12 is a crystalline compound that is soluble in water, alcohol and acetone. It is heat-stable in neutral solutions but destroyed by heat in acid and alkaline mediums. The vitamin is somewhat sensitive to light, and is destroyed by heavy metals and by strong oxidizing and reducing agents. Vitamin B12 contains phosphorus, nitrogen and cobalt, the latter giving it a dark red color.

Vitamin B12 is the most complex of the vitamins ($C_{63}H_{90}CoN_{14}O_{14}P$). It contains a cobalt atom that is structurally similar to the position of iron in hemoglobin. B12 is the only naturally occurring organic compound that contains cobalt. Cyanocobalamin, the commercially available form of vitamin B12, has a cyanide group attached to the central cobalt atom. This cyanide is present because of contamination during manufacturing and is not found naturally. The name cobalamin signifies the vitamin without the cyanide group. Other forms of the vitamin are hydroxycobalamin (vitamin B12a, which contains a hydroxyl group attached to the cobalt atom), aquacobalamin (vitamin B12b) and nitrocobalamin (vitamin B12c, found in certain bacteria).

The biologically active coenzymes are coenzyme B12 (5'-deoxyadenosylcobalamin) and methyl-cobalamin (methyl-B12). They are the predominant forms found in animal tissues.

Functions

Vitamin B12 plays a role in the activation of amino acids during protein formation, and in the anaerobic degradation of the amino acid lysine. The coenzyme of vitamin B12 is a carrier of methyl groups and hydrogen, and is necessary for carbohydrate, protein and fat metabolism. Because of its methyl transfer role, vitamin B12 is active in the synthesis of the amino acid methionine from its precursor, homocysteine. The coenzyme-dependent synthesis of methionine occurs by first removing a methyl group from methyl folate, a derivative of the biologically active form of folic acid. Then this methyl group is transferred to homocysteine and methionine is formed.

Because methionine is needed in choline synthesis, B12 plays a secondary role in this lipid pathway. A choline deficiency that causes fatty liver can be prevented by vitamin B12 or the other methyl donors (betaine, methionine, folic acid).

Impaired fatty acid synthesis, observed in vitamin B12 deficiency states, can result in impairment of brain and nerve tissue. The insulation around nerve cells, the myelin sheath, is misformed in a vitamin B12 deficiency, and this contributes to faulty nerve transmission. Ultimately, neurological disturbances result from prolonged vitamin B12 deficiency.

Proper DNA replication is dependent on the function of coenzyme vitamin B12 as a methyl group carrier. Megaloblastic anemia (characterized by large, immature red blood cells) and changes in bone marrow associated with a vitamin B12 deficiency are due to the vitamin's role in DNA synthesis. Improper cell replication and inadequate DNA translation cause the large cells observed in this disorder. The result is anemia, leukopenia, thrombopenia and fewer, but larger and less mature, blood cells. Poor cell division in the gastrointestinal tract and other epithelial tissues produces glossitis and megaloblastosis. General growth and repair are curtailed as well.

Deficiency

Pernicious, or megaloblastic, anemia is the characteristic symptom of a vitamin B12 deficiency. This condition is caused by either inadequate intake or reduced gastric secretion of a mucoprotein called intrinsic factor that is necessary for proper vitamin B12 absorption. Intrinsic factor is produced by the parietal cells of the stomach, binds onto the vitamin and transports it into the small intestine. In the presence of calcium, this transport complex attaches to the intestinal wall, facilitating absorption of the vitamin.

Pernicious anemia may also develop from several other conditions, including:

- Gastrectomy (surgical removal of the stomach).
- Surgical removal of the portion of the lower ileum responsible for vitamin B12 absorption.
- The development of antibodies to intrinsic factor.
- Hereditary malabsorption.
- A diet devoid of animal products (strict vegetarianism).

In addition to anemia, deficiency symptoms include glossitis, degeneration of the spinal cord, loss of appetite, gastrointestinal disturbances, fatigue, pallor, dizziness, disorientation, numbness, tingling, ataxia, moodiness, confusion, agitation, dimmed vision, delusions, hallucinations and, eventually, "megaloblastic madness" (psychosis).

Vitamin B12 deficiency symptoms are generally found in mid- to late life, and are often a result of the reduced secretion of intrinsic factor. This condition can be corrected by vitamin B12 injections.

The vitamin is stored in appreciable amounts (1.0 to 10.0 mg), primarily in the liver. One-third of the body's stores are in the muscle, skin, bone, lung, kidney and spleen. Because daily needs are small, and little vitamin B12 is excreted except through the bile, a deficiency takes years to manifest.

Vitamin B12 absorption can be inhibited by many gastrointestinal disorders, such as gluten-induced enteropathy, tropical sprue, regional ileitis, malignancies and granulomatous lesions in the small intestine, tapeworm, bacteria associated with blind loop syndrome, and other disorders that impair normal intestinal function. The need for vitamin B12 is increased by hyperthyroidism, parasitism and pregnancy.

Requirements

The body's need for vitamin B12 is small. The RDAs for the vitamin are:

Infants	
0–0.5 year	0.5 mcg
0.5–1 year	1.5 mcg
Children	
1–3 years	2.0 mcg
4–6 years	2.5 mcg
7–10 years	3.0 mcg
Young adults and adults	
11+ years	3.0 mcg
Pregnant	+1.0 mcg
Lactating	+1.0 mcg

Sources

The only source of vitamin B12 in nature is microbial synthesis. The vitamin is not found in plants, but is produced by bacteria in the digestive tract of animals, or by microbial fermentation of foods.

Sources containing more than 10 mcg/100 g serving are organ meats (liver, kidney, heart), clams and oysters. Good sources (3 to 10 mcg/100 g serving) are nonfat dry milk, crab, salmon, sardines and egg yolk. Moderate amounts (1 to 3 mcg/100 g serving) are found in meat, lobster, scallops, flounder, swordfish, tuna and fermented cheese. Other sources include fermented soybean products, poultry and fluid milk products.

Deficiency is more often caused by improper absorption than by dietary lack. Because vitamin B12 is affected at temperatures above 100° C, some of the vitamin is lost when meat is cooked on a hot grill.

Toxicity

The minimum daily requirement for vitamin B12 can be exceeded by ten thousand-fold with no signs of toxicity. Excesses are excreted in the urine.

BIOTIN

Biotin is a simple monocarboxylic acid. It is soluble in ethanol, acetone and ether; salts of the acid are soluble in water. Biotin is more stable to acids and alkalies than the other B vitamins, and is stable in heated solutions.

Functions

Biotin enzymes function in carboxylation reactions where carbon dioxide is added to various substrates. (This is a two-step process: CO_2 binds to the biotin portion of the enzyme with simultaneous hydrolysis of ATP; transfer of the CO_2 to a receptor follows.) Biotin enzyme systems include: acetyl CoA carboxylase, beta-methyl crotonyl CoA carboxylase, propionyl CoA carboxylase, pyruvate carboxylase, and methylmalonyl-oxalacetic transcarboxylase.

Biotin affects the metabolism of protein, fats, and carbohydrates. It plays a role in several functions, including:

- Incorporating amino acids into protein.
- The synthesis of fatty acids.
- Deriving energy from glucose.
- The synthesis of pyrimidines (nucleic acids).
- The conversion of folic acid to its biologically active form.
- Reducing the symptoms of a zinc deficiency.

Deficiency

Deficiency symptoms are uncommon, even if a biotin-deficient diet is consumed. However, the ingestion of large quantities of raw egg whites will produce deficiency symptoms by inhibiting absorption in the intestinal tract. (Avidin, a protein-carbohydrate compound in raw egg white, binds with biotin to inhibit absorption.)

As a result, a non-pruritic dermatitis, hypercholesterolemia, electrocardiograph changes, anemia, anorexia, nausea, lassitude and muscle pain can develop. Avidin is deactivated by cooking the egg white, thus eliminating its biotin-binding capabilities.

Infants may develop a deficiency from poor absorption of biotin or from improper binding to mucosal cell receptors. In these cases, infants develop hepatomagaly, lactic acidosis and skin rash. Biotin supplementation produces prompt cessation of symptoms.

Requirements

The average American diet contains 150 to 300 mcg of biotin per day. This amount, plus what is absorbed from microbial synthesis in the intestines, alleviates clinical deficiency symptoms. The RDAs for biotin are:

Infants	
0–0.5 year	35 mcg
0.5–1 year	50 mcg
Children	
1–3 years	65 mcg
4–6 years	85 mcg
7–10 years	120 mcg
11 + years	100–200 mcg
Adults	100–200 mcg

Sources

Intestinal synthesis is a significant source of biotin unless antibiotics or other agents that interfere with microbial action are present. Both plant and animal foods contain biotin. Good dietary sources include liver and other organ meats, molasses and milk.

Toxicity

As with other B vitamins, biotin excretion reflects intake; when the dosage exceeds biological needs, the urinary excretion of biotin and its metabolites increases proportionately. Easy elimination allows ingestion of large doses of biotin with no reported toxic effects.

PANTOTHENIC ACID

Pantothenic acid is a pale yellow, water-soluble, viscous oil that is commercially available as a white crystalline calcium or sodium salt. This B vitamin is stable to moist heat as well as to oxidizing and reducing agents; however, it is destroyed by dry heat and by heating in an alkaline or acid solution.

Functions

Pantothenic acid is converted to coenzyme A, its only known biological form. Coenzyme A is an important catalyst of acetylation reactions. Coenzyme A is important in:

- Acetylation of choline and specific aromatic amines.
- Oxidation of fatty acids, pyruvate, alpha-ketoglutarate, and acetaldahyde.
- Synthesis of fatty acids, sphingosine, citrate, acetoacetate, phospholipids, and cholesterol (and all substances made from it, such as bile, vitamin D and steroid hormones).

Pantothenic acid participates in a variety of pathways involved in the metabolism of carbohydrates, fats and protein. In addition, coenzyme A functions in the synthesis of porphyrin, a heme-component of red blood cells, and the neurotransmitter acetylcholine.

Deficiency

Pantothenic acid deficiency has not been reported in humans. A laboratory-induced deficiency can be created if subjects are fed a synthetic diet complete in all nutrients except pantothenic acid and are simultaneously given a pantothenic acid antagonist that further depletes the body. The resultant deficiency produces fatigue, cardiovascular and gastrointestinal problems, upper respiratory infections, depression, and numbness and tingling in the extremities. The gastrointestinal disturbances are further complicated by a reduction in bile synthesis.

In animals, deficiency symptoms include dermatitis, greying or rusting of hair, hemorrhaging, neurological lesions, inflammation of the nasal mucosa, adrenal cortex atrophy, corneal vascularization and sexual dysfunction.

Requirements

The American diet provides between 6 mg and 16 mg of pantothenic acid a day. Because no known deficiency symptoms have been reported, this amount is sufficient to prevent a clinical deficiency. Stressful situations, including pregnancy and lactation, increase requirements. The RDAs for pantothenic acid are:

Infants	
0–0.5 year	2 mg
0.5–3 year	3 mg
Children	
4–6 years	3–4 mg
7–10 years	4–5 mg
Young adults and adults	4–7 mg

Sources

The word "pantos" means "everywhere" and reflects the vitamin's ubiquitous role in the body as well as its presence in the diet. This B vitamin is found in a wide variety of foods representing all four food groups. Good sources include liver and organ meats, fish, chicken, eggs, cheese, wholegrain cereals and breads, avocados, cauliflower, green peas, dried beans, nuts, dates and sweet potatoes. Other foods contain pantothenic acid in smaller but contributory amounts. Fruits are not a good source. Because refined grains are not enriched with pantothenic acid, the significant losses in milling make processed grains a poor source.

Toxicity

Pantothenic acid is relatively nontoxic because excesses are excreted in the urine.

VITAMIN C (L-ascorbic acid)

An Overview

Ascorbic acid is a water-soluble vitamin found in the watery medium of fruits and vegetables. It leaches into the cooking water of boiled foods. Because of its sensitivity to oxidation, ascorbic acid is destroyed whenever foods are cut or torn, exposing the cells to air. Copper accelerates this oxidation, and alkalis (baking soda or antacids) destroy ascorbic acid. Vitamin C is stable at temperatures below 0°F or in weak acids.

Functions

Ascorbic acid plays a major role in collagen formation. Collagen (an intracellular cementing substance) is a protein that forms the basis for connective tissue, the most abundant tissue in the body. Collagen binds muscle cells together, gives support and maintains shape in intervertebral discs and eustachian tubes, and provides movement in joints. Collagen is found in adipose tissue, bones, teeth, tendons, skin and scar tissue. In the capillaries, it is the supporting material that prevents bruising. The symptoms of scurvy are primarily due to a lack of ascorbic acid in the formation of collagen.

TABLE 7
Summary of Fat-Soluble Vitamins

Vitamin	Best food source	RDA (1980)*	ODA**	Principal functions	Major deficiency symptoms
A (retinol; retinal = aldehyde form; precursors = carotenes)	Green and yellow vegetables, yellow fruits, butter, whole milk	1000 mcg RE	10,000–35,000 IU	Maintenance of epithelial tissues; constituent of visual pigments	Nyctalopia, xerophthalmia, hyperkeratosis; faulty tooth formation
D (cholecalciferol = D3; ergocalciferol = D2)	Fish liver oils; fortified or irradiated milk	7.5 mcg	200–400 IU	Transport of Ca; intestinal and renal absorption of phosphate	Rickets (children); osteomalacia (adults)
E (d-alpha tocopherol)	Vegetable oils; dark green leafy vegetables	10 mg (alpha-TE)	50–400 IU	Protects cell membranes against lipid peroxidation and destruction	Hemolytic anemia; degenerative changes in muscle.
K (phylloquinone = K1; menaquinones = K2)	Green leafy vegetables, liver, egg yolk, meat, dairy products	70–140 mcg (estimated range)		Required for proper blood clotting	Hemorrhagic disease in newborn and in biliary disease; anemia

*For American men, 19 to 22 years of age, of average activity.
**Optimal Daily Allowance is a theoretical range based upon the authors' literature research. If no range is listed, the authors felt that there was insufficient evidence to make a recommendation at this time.

Adapted from Orten, J. and Neuhaus, O. *Human Biochemistry*. St. Louis: C. V. Mosby Co., 1982.

TABLE 8
Summary of Water-Soluble Vitamins

Vitamin	Best food source	RDA (1980)*	ODA**	Principal functions	Major deficiency symptoms
C (l-ascorbic acid)	Citrus fruits, tomatoes	60 mg	250–2000 mg	Collagen formation; capillary walls; metabolism of Tyr, Phe, folic acid; iron absorption	Scurvy, petechial hemorrhages, anemia, delayed wound healing, bone fragility
B1 (thiamin)	Pork, liver, yeast, whole or enriched grains, legumes	1.5 mg	5–10 mg	Decarboxylation and transketolation	Beriberi (polyneuritis), cardiovascular problems; anorexia, nausea; fatigue, paralysis

Vitamin	Best food source	RDA (1980)*	ODA**	Principal functions	Major deficiency symptoms
B2 (riboflavin)	Milk, organ meats, animal protein, enriched grains, brewer's yeast	1.7 mg	6–15 mg	Coenzyme of electron transfer system; cell respiration; metabolism of carbohydrates, fat, protein	Cracks and sores at corner of mouth (cheilosis), dermatitis, conjunctivitis, photophobia, glossitis
B3 (niacin, nicotinic acid, niacinamide)	Meat, enriched or whole grains, poultry, fish, peanuts, milk products	19 mg equiv (1 mg equiv per 60 mg Trp)	25–100 mg	Coenzyme of electron transfer system; dehydrogenase reactions; oxidation to produce ATP (NAD+); biosynthesis of fatty acids, steroids, etc. (NADP+)	Pellagra, diarrhea, scaly dermatitis, dementia, stomatitis
B6 (pyridoxine)	Meat, whole grains, poultry, fish	2.2 mg	10–20 mg	Coenzyme in amino acid metabolism; transamination, decarboxylation, transsulfuration, tryptophan synthetase, amino acid transport	Cheilosis, glossitis, stomatitis, seborrheic dermatitis, convulsions, anemia
Folacin (folic acid, peteroyl-glutamic acid)	Liver, greens, mushrooms, whole grains, legumes	400 mcg	2000–4000 mcg	Transfer of 1-carbon fragments (formyl); biosynthesis of purines, choline, methionine, etc.	Macrocytic and megaloblastic anemias, sprue, malabsorption, leukopenia, thrombocytopenia
B12 (cobalamin)	Animal protein, meats, milk, egg	3 mcg	10–100 mcg	Transfer of 1-carbon fragments (methyl); biosyntheis of purines, choline, methionine, etc.; mutase reactions	Pernicious anemia, neurological lesions, sprue
Biotin	Egg yolk, organ meats, yeast, whole grains, nuts; widely distributed	100–200 mcg		Carboxylation and transcarboxylation	Dermatitis, alopecia, anemia; experimentally only in humans
Pantothenic acid	Liver, meat, cereal, milk, legumes; widely distributed	4–7 mg	10–50 mg	Acylation reactions (acetyl group transfers)	Anemia, achromotrichia; human deficiency most unlikely

*For American men, 19 to 22 years of age, of average activity
**Optimal Daily Allowance is a theoretical range based upon the authors' literature research. If no range is listed, the authors felt that there was insufficient evidence to make a recommendation at this time.

Adapted from Orten, J. and Neuhaus, O., *Human Biochemistry*. St. Louis,: C.V. Mosby Co., 1982.

Ascorbic acid is a coenzyme for proline hydroxylase and lysyl oxidase (enzymes that convert the amino acids proline and lysine into hydroxyproline and hydroxylysine, respectively). These amino acids are important in maintaining collagen's tertiary structure.

Ascorbic acid plays a role in amino acid metabolism and hormone synthesis. It contributes to the formation of the amino acid tyrosine (the precursor for the neurotransmitters/hormones epinephrine and norepinephrine) and is associated with the release of these hormones from the adrenal glands. During periods of stress when these hormones are mobilized, the small stores of ascorbic acid in the adrenals are depleted. In the presence of ascorbic acid, tryptophan is converted to 5-hydroxytryptophan, which is decarboxylated to form the neurotransmitter serotonin.

Ascorbic acid is associated with cholesterol metabolism by its role in the hydroxylation of cholesterol to cholic acid. This is the principal metabolic pathway for the excretion of excess cholesterol.

Vitamin C plays a role in the metabolism and utilization of other nutrients, such as folic acid and iron. Folic acid is converted to its biologically active form (tetrahydrofolic acid) in the presence of ascorbic acid. Because ascorbic acid plays a part in the absorption and utilization of iron, a lack of the vitamin can result in anemia.

Ascorbic acid has strong reducing properties, and is capable of being oxidized by glutathione. Therefore, it may function in respiratory enzyme systems.

Deficiency

The classic symptom of an ascorbic acid deficiency is scurvy, a condition characterized by petechial hemorrhages, anemia, joint tenderness and swelling, poor wound healing, weakness, and defects in skeletal calcification. Scurvy also manifests in the mouth with hemorrhaging of the gums, lost teeth, gingivitis, ulceration, reddening and, occasionally, gangrene. Scurvy is rarely seen in the United States. However, chronically low intakes of ascorbic acid have been reported, resulting in delayed wound healing, reduced resistance to infection, and curtailed synthesis of some amino acids.

A lack of ascorbic acid during bone development produces many adverse conditions. Among these are lesions of the epiphyseal junctions and thinning of the alveolar bone resulting in loose teeth, spongy gums and resorption of dentine.

Requirements

Of the total dietary ascorbic acid ingested, 80 to 90 percent is absorbed. Requirements increase with acute environmental or emotional stress, and are affected to a lesser degree by age, smoking, drugs and oral contraceptives. The RDAs for vitamin C are:

Infants	35 mg
Children	
1–10 years	45 mg
Adolescents	
11–14 years	50 mg
Adults	
15+ years	60 mg
Pregnant	+20 mg
Lactating	+40 mg

Scurvy can be prevented by 10 mg of ascorbic acid daily. Requirements increase in the following conditions: diarrhea, rheumatic fever, rheumatoid arthritis, infections, trauma and surgery. Ascorbic acid levels have been found to be low in burn victims and the conditions of congestive heart failure, kidney and liver disease, gastrointestinal disturbances, purpura, endocrine cases, and malignancies. An increased need for ascorbic acid is implied during these illnesses.

Sources

Ascorbic acid is found primarily in fruits and vegetables such as citrus fruits, tomatoes, green peppers, parsley, fresh dark green leafy vegetables, broccoli, cantaloupe, strawberries, cabbage, potatoes, fresh peas, lettuce and asparagus.

Toxicity

As of this writing, research suggests that ascorbic acid is not appreciably stored in the body. When tissues are saturated, additional intake is excreted in the urine. Up to this saturation threshold, however, the vitamin is not eliminated. Even with large doses, the blood levels of ascorbic acid do not rise above 1.5 to 2 mg/100 ml because of reduced absorption from the intestines and increased excretion through the kidneys.

Large doses of ascorbic acid can cause nausea, diarrhea, increased susceptibility of red blood cells to hemolysis and reduced leukocyte bactericidal activity.

Tables 7 and 8 summarize the fat- and water-soluble vitamins.

Additional Reading

Goodhart, R. S. and Shils, M. E. *Modern Nutrition in Health and Disease*, 6th edition. Philadelphia: Lea & Febiger, 1980.

Orten, J. M. and Neuhaus, O. W. *Human Biochemistry*, 10th edition. St. Louis: The C. V. Mosby Co., 1982.

4

·············· MINERALS···

MINERALS ARE THE INORGANIC substances that remain when living tissue (plant or animal) is burned. Minerals are components of body tissues and fluids that work in combination with enzymes, hormones, vitamins and transport substances. Some are cofactors for enzymes, others activate molecules in metabolic pathways. Minerals participate in nerve transmission, muscle contraction, cell permeability, tissue rigidity and structure, blood formation, acid-base balance, fluid regulation and osmolarity, protein metabolism and energy production. Minerals work either in combination with each other or as antagonists to each other. Some minerals compete with each other for absorption, while certain minerals actually enhance the absorption of other minerals.

A mineral is considered essential when:

- A dietary lack creates specific deficiency symptoms that respond when the mineral is reinstated.
- The addition of a mineral to a purified diet improves health.
- It plays a role as a necessary component of tissue, fluids or a regulatory process (such as an enzymatic reaction).
- It is a necessary constituent of some other essential nutrient.

Minerals compose 4 percent of the body's weight. The bulk of the body's minerals reside in the skeletal structure, with calcium and phosphorus composing three-quarters of the average adult's bodily mineral content. To classify as a major mineral or macronutrient, a mineral must make up no less than 0.01 percent of body weight. Calcium, phosphorus, magnesium, potassium, sodium and chloride meet this criterion. Trace minerals that fall below the "major mineral" percentage include arsenic, chromium cobalt, copper, fluoride, iodine, iron, manganese, molybdenum, nickel, selenium, silicon, tin, vanadium and zinc. Research continues to add to, and update, information on these and other trace minerals. The biological significance of many of the trace minerals has not yet been determined.

Classifying a mineral as either major or trace does not reflect its importance. A deficiency of either a trace or a major mineral can be equally devastating.

The body's concentration of many minerals is maintained within narrow limits through absorption from the gut; excretion through the kidneys and through bile and other intestinal secretions; storage; utilization; and mineral-mineral competition. Even though daily intakes vary enormously from one individual to another, the average adult male excretes 20 to 30 g of inorganic substances each day. Chronic low-grade and acute deficiencies can occur, as well as overdoses from air, water and food. Some trace minerals (such as iron, selenium and zinc) are essential in small amounts but toxic in larger doses.

Minerals can be found in their free ionic state, or bound to a variety of substances ranging from proteins (such as the iron in porphyrin or hemoglobin) to vitamins (such as cobalt in vitamin B12). This flexibility allows for a greater versatility of biological roles.

Absorption of the divalent ions is slower than absorption of the monovalent ions. For example, sodium (a monovalent ion) is absorbed twice as fast as calcium (a divalent ion). Absorption also depends on the body's need for the mineral, as well as on other substances in the gut that may enhance or impede intestinal uptake.

CALCIUM

Calcium is the most abundant mineral, and the fifth most abundant substance, in the body. Bone tissue comprises about 99 percent of the 1200 g of calcium in the average body. The mineral is found along with magnesium, sodium, phosphorus, strontium, carbonate and citrate, and plays a key role in the strengthening and in the structural integrity of skeletal tissue. The remaining 1 percent of the body's calcium is used in nerve transmission, muscle contraction, blood clotting and numerous other functions.

Functions

Bone and tooth development and maintenance are dependent on normal, adequate calcium absorption and metabolism. There is a lifelong need for dietary calcium. Strenuous physical exercise as well as adequate dietary intake of calcium, vitamin D, protein and other nutrients are necessary for proper development of bone density.

Bones act as a calcium reservoir, supplying calcium when blood values decline and absorbing excesses when blood values are elevated above the normal value of 10 to 11 mg/100 ml. Bones are a metabolically active tissue and their status reflects the dynamic equilibrium of the entire body as well as the equilibrium between bone and blood calcium. This status quo can be maintained by slight shifts from one compartment to another. When blood calcium levels drop below 10 mg/100 ml, calcium in the bone intercrystalline material is mobilized and dissolves into the surrounding fluid, finally moving into the blood. This process insures blood levels of around 7 mg/100 ml. The remaining 3 mg/100 ml are supplied by the feedback mechanism, involving parathyroid hormone. Calcium blood levels are independent of dietary intake; abnormalities resulting in blood excesses or inadequacies are rare because of hormone control.

Over half of the calcium found in serum is ionized and the rest is bound to protein (mainly albumin or globulins) or incorporated with organic acids (such as citrate) or inorganic acids (such as sulfate or phosphate) in a non-ionized form. The protein-bound calcium acts as a weak electrolyte. Metabolically available, ionized calcium (the body's miscible calcium pool) is found in soft tissues, extracellular fluid and blood. It is the ionized form that is controlled by parathyroid secretion and is active in all aspects of calcium metabolism.

When blood calcium falls, parathyroid hormone (PTH) stimulates vitamin D to increase circulating calcium. Intestinal absorption and bone resorption of calcium increase. When proper blood values are reached, PTH synthesis stops and calcitonin (a thyroid hormone) is released to diminish bone resorption.

Besides providing structure and strength to skeletal tissue, calcium is integral in nerve transmission. If blood calcium concentrations fall, the nerves become hypersensitive, resulting in tetany. In contrast, high calcium concentrations depress nerve irritability because of the role of calcium in neurotransmitter release from synaptic vesicles. The amount of neurotransmitter released is proportionate to the calcium ion concentration in the terminal membrane, and inversely proportionate to the magnesium concentration. The neurotransmitters affected by calcium include serotonin, acetylcholine and norepinephrine. Calcium also facilitates acetylcholine synthesis by activating the enzyme choline acetylase in synaptic vesicles.

Calcium, along with magnesium, is directly responsible for activating the mechanisms in striated and smooth muscle contraction. Calcium activates the enzyme glycogen phosphorylase kinase, which in turn triggers glycogenolysis (the breakdown of glycogen to glucose-6-P for use in energy production). In the presence of calcium, adenosine triphosphatase (ATPase) is activated to hydrolyse ATP, and provides an available energy source for muscle contraction.

Calcium plays an essential role in the cells. Small amounts of calcium are a vital part of intracellular fluids as well as fluids bathing the cells. Calcium is essential to the integrity of intracellular cement. An intracellular protein, calmodulin, regulates the intracellular calcium level for various reactions by pumping accumulated calcium excesses out of the cells. As a component of membranes, calcium also regulates ion transport.

Calcium is an important contributor to blood clotting because of its roles in prothrombin activation (as a cofactor with Factor XIII-a) and in the conversion of fibrinogen to fibrin. Calcium is also a constituent of platelets. In addition, it activates saliva and pancreatic alpha-amylases, plasma lipoprotein lipase, phosporylase-A and succinate dehydrogenase. It also plays a role in maintaining proper blood pressure.

Deficiency

Bone is the primary tissue that suffers in a calcium-deficient state because of its role in maintaining plasma levels and providing calcium reserves. Bone fractures and osteoporosis are common in the elderly, especially in postmenopausal women. These conditions are promoted by consuming inadequate dietary calcium and/or excessive dietary phosphorus over many years, coupled with limited strenuous physical activity. After a 40 percent loss of calcium, decreased bone density becomes apparent in X rays. Long before this, however, symptoms of poor calcium status can be detected. Increasing calcium intake through diet and mineral supplementation, limiting phosphorus intake, estrogen therapy and exercise can reduce the incidence of fractures and retard or prevent osteoporosis in postmenopausal women. Vitamin D and small amounts of fluoride are also useful in treating this condition.

Unlike the calcium in osseous tissue, that in teeth is stable. Once formed, it is relatively insensitive to calcium deficiency. Deficiencies during the period of tooth formation, however, can have irreversible effects on tooth structure and resistance to decay.

Calcium metabolism and bone formation are influenced by other nutrients. Because calcium absorption is vitamin D-dependent (via an active and passive mechanism), calcium deposition is impaired in rickets because of inadequate vitamin D intake or synthesis. Bone growth is retarded by excessive vitamin A (especially endochondral bone formation), and aided by ascorbic acid through its participation in the formation of tropocollagen.

Calcium absorption requires the presence of bile salts, bile and dietary fat. Excessive dietary fat, however, curtails calcium absorption. An interference in calcium absorption may result from either steatorrhea or the following conditions:

- Poor fat absorption that reduces vitamin D uptake by mucosal cells.
- Impermeability of intestinal mucosa.
- Fatty acids forming insoluble soaps with calcium and carrying them out of the body.

Calcium absorption may also be reduced by physical and emotional stress, and may result in unexplained dumping of calcium into the intestinal tract. A net loss of as much as 900 mg may occur each day during times of worry and tension. Fecal excretion can be twice the dietary intake.

Calcium must be soluble to be absorbed. Acids (such as hydrochloric, ascorbic and citric acid) and some of the amino acids (such as glycine and lysine) can increase solubility, thus increasing absorption. The sugars lactose, sorbose, cellobiose, xylose, raffinose and mannitol facilitate calcium absorption, whereas excess dietary fat, protein, phosphorus, phytates in unleavened grains, and oxalates in spinach, swiss chard, beet greens, rhubarb and cocoa interfere with calcium uptake. Phytates, oxalates and phosphorus increase fecal excretion either by forming insoluble salts with calcium or disrupting the intestinal pH. The levels of phytates and oxalates in the typical diet do not substantially interfere with calcium status. In fact, there is evidence that animals adapt to the presence of low oxalate levels in the diet, regaining positive calcium balance within days of oxalate supplementation.

Calcium status is affected by need. If need is low, absorption from the intestines may be as low as 10 percent. During growth, pregnancy and lactation, absorption may increase to 50 percent or more.

Calcium is excreted primarily through the intestines, but also through the urine. Excretion by the intestines occurs whether calcium is provided in the diet or not, so a negative calcium balance is possible. Fecal excretion partially reflects unabsorbed dietary intake although calcium may also enter the intestinal tract through digestive juices. Calcium precipitates out as calcium phosphate, carbonate, oxalate, phytate or sulfate salts, or as calcium soaps.

Daily urinary excretion values of calcium for an average male adult range from 85 to 420 mg, with an average of 175 mg. Because 4.5 g of calcium are pumped through the kidneys each day, conservation of this mineral is still commendable. Intestinal absorption is reduced in patients with chronic renal insufficiency, which may explain the osteodystrophy characteristic of renal disease.

Calcium may also be lost in sweat, but this loss is insignificant unless an individual engages in heavy physical labor in dry, hot environments, and sweats profusely. In these cases, as much as 1000 mg may be lost in a day.

An excessive protein intake results in urinary overexcretion of calcium, perhaps because of two conditions: the increased acidity of amino acid metabolites in the urine, and the increased glomerular filtration rate and calcium clearance along with a decreased ability of the kidneys to resorb calcium.

High dietary protein also may increase bone resorption, predisposing an individual to osteoporosis. This may be a problem especially in the United States, where the typical American consumes two to three times the necessary daily requirement of protein.

Calcium interacts with other minerals, one being phosphorus. The dietary phosphorus:calcium ratio should be 1:1 or 1:1.5. The average American diet contains two parts phosphorus for every one part calcium. At this ratio, excess calcium is removed from bone tissue and blood levels are depressed, resulting in increased calcium excretion and bone demineralization. These conditions are promoted by high-phosphorus foods such as soda pop, diet pop, processed foods (cheese spreads, meats and convenience foods), peanuts, eggs, meat, organ meats, as well as by a low intake of calcium-rich foods. In such a diet, the phosphorus:calcium ratio may be as high as 4:1. Diets high in phosphorus and low in calcium have been linked to soft tissue calcification and bone loss in some animals.

Hypocalcemia has been associated with a magnesium deficiency. The condition does not respond to therapeutic administration of calcium alone, but requires concomitant magnesium therapy.

Requirements

The ability of the human body to adapt to low intakes of calcium makes establishing an RDA difficult. Populations in other parts of the world thrive, grow and maintain normal skeletons on intakes of less than 200 mg/day, whereas in the United States, osteoporosis can develop on a diet of 600 mg. Apparently, adaptation to low intakes is best initiated early in life. Negative calcium balance occurs when calcium intake is restricted after adaptation to a high dietary intake. The adaptive process, whenever initiated, must be gradual.

The adult allowance of 800 mg is viewed with uncertainty because calcium intake and absorption may not be adequate to prevent the development of osteoporosis, and because smaller amounts of calcium are needed in the diet if protein consumption is adequate but not excessive. An intake of 800 to 1000 mg of calcium over the years may prove beneficial in the prevention of osteoporosis.

The RDAs are based on average daily losses of the mineral, and are adjusted for the percent of dietary calcium that is absorbed. Because average losses total approximately 320 mg/day and the estimated absorption rate is 20 to 40 percent, 800 mg are required to replace daily losses. As previously mentioned, the absorption rate for some people may be 15 percent or less, resulting in a negative calcium balance even when intakes exceed 800 mg. Calcium needs increase during periods of growth, pregnancy and lactation. The RDAs for calcium are:

Infants	
0–0.5 year	360 mg
0.5–1 year	540 mg
Children	
1–10 years	800 mg
11–18 years	1000 mg
Adults	800 mg
Pregnant	+400 mg
Lactating	+400 mg

Sources

Excellent sources of calcium (providing approximately 300 mg per serving) are: milk and yogurt (1 cup), hard cheeses (1½ ounces), cottage cheese (1¼ cup), dark green leafy vegetables (1 to 2 cups cooked) and broccoli (2 cups cooked). Butter, sour cream, cream cheese and other high-fat dairy products contain minimal calcium. Citrus fruits, canned fish with edible bones, and dried peas and beans are good calcium sources. Meats and nuts that are excellent sources of many other nutrients are poor sources of this mineral. Whole grains are not a good source unless they comprise a large portion of the diet, in which case they can be a major contributor. Hard water provides some calcium; commercial mineral waters are a poor source.

Toxicity

Normally, large doses of calcium show no toxic effects; the body rids itself of excesses by reducing absorption through the intestines and increasing urinary excretion. In magnesium deficiency, overdoses of parathyroid hormone, vitamin D or calcium can result in soft tissue calcification.

Several clinical conditions are associated with unusually high serum, urinary and soft tissue calcium levels. These include idiopathic hypercalcemia of infancy, hypercalciuria and renal stones. Dietary calcium does not appear to be causally related to these conditions.

CHLORIDE

Chloride is an essential anion that accounts for just 0.15 percent of total body weight. There are 450 to

600 mg of chloride for every 100 ml of blood; there is minimal variation in this concentration. Chloride is found primarily in extracellular fluids and is especially abundant in gastrointestinal secretions and cerebrospinal fluid. Less than 15 percent of the body's total chloride content is found in intracellular fluids; erythrocytes have the highest concentration, with lesser amounts in the skin, gonads and gastric mucosa. Small amounts of chloride are found in bone and connective tissue, and lesser amounts in muscle and nerve tissue. Chloride is closely associated with sodium and water in foods, body secretions, fluids, tissues and excretions. It is also found loosely bound to protein and other substances.

Functions

Chloride is a constituent of gastric hydrochloric acid, and an active participant in the chloride shift. The chloride shift permits plasma transport of tissue CO_2, as bicarbonate, to the lungs for excretion. It is important in regulating the body's acid-base balance.

Chloride is readily absorbed from the intestines. Intake is usually in excess of sodium, and amounts that are not needed are excreted. Excretion of the anion is through the kidneys, primarily as sodium chloride. Some losses occur through sweat and feces.

Deficiency

A deficiency of chloride can result from diarrhea or vomiting, adrenal insufficiency, and acidosis. Chloride losses usually reflect sodium losses, except in the case of chronic vomiting. In this case, chloride and, to a lesser extent, other electrolytes that are derived from intestinal secretions (such as pancreatic juice, hydrochloric acid and bile) are secreted into the gastrointestinal tract and lost. Disturbances in acid-base balance result.

In rats, chloride deficiency results in growth retardation. When chloride is unintentionally neglected in infant formula preparations, infants develop metabolic alkalosis, hypovolemia and significant urinary potassium loss. Psychomotor defects, memory loss and growth retardation also occur. All symptoms are alleviated with the administration of chloride.

Requirements

Nutritional concern for chloride has been minimal because the mineral is found in abundance in the food supply. The sodium and potassium to chloride ratio should be maintained at a range of 1.5:2 for adequate acid-base regulation in infants. Estimated safe and adequate intakes for chloride are:

Infants	
0–0.5 year	0.275–0.7 g
0.5–1 year	0.4–1.2 g
Children	
1–3 years	0.5–1.5 g
4–6 years	0.7–2.1 g
7–10 years	0.925–2.775 g
11 + years	1.4–4.2 g
Adults	1.7–5.1 g

Sources

Chloride is obtained from table salt (sodium chloride) or from salt substitutes (such as potassium chloride). It is found in abundance in vegetable and animal foods.

CHROMIUM

The body contains about 6 mg of chromium, and the blood contains 20 ppb. Despite its small concentration, this mineral is gaining recognized importance in carbohydrate metabolism.

Functions

Chromium is a critical component of the glucose tolerance factor (GTF). GTF contains niacin, glycine, glutamic acid, cysteine and chromium in the trivalent form. The insulin-enhancing properties of this compound imply that adequate chromium is necessary in the diet for normal carbohydrate metabolism. The mineral may also facilitate the binding of insulin to the cell membrane. Chromium and insulin administration to rats increases glucose uptake in the eye and utilization of glucose for fatty acid production and energy.

Chromium in drinking water in amounts as low as 0.2 ppm has been shown to lower cholesterol levels in sugar-fed rats. Body concentrations of chromium are known to decline with age. Excretion of the mineral occurs primarily through the kidneys.

Deficiency

A chromium deficiency can result in reduced peripheral tissue sensitivity to glucose, a condition similar to diabetes. Glucose ingestion raises serum chromium levels and increases its urinary excretion. Research has demonstrated an improved glucose tolerance in some adult-onset diabetics who were given chromium. Poor glucose tolerance in some children with protein-calorie malnutrition has also responded to chromium therapy. Those children who respond may be deficient in the mineral, whereas those resistant to chromium therapy may have other underlying problems.

Most chromium is removed from grains when they are refined. Low chromium levels in a highly refined diet, combined with an increased intake of sugars and other processed carbohydrates that require chromium for metabolism, may predispose some individuals to a chromium deficiency and may aggravate adult-onset diabetes.

Requirements

Little information is available for determining chromium requirements, so normal intakes are used. The RDAs for chromium are:

Infants	
0–0.5 year	0.01–0.04 mg
0.5–1 year	0.02–0.06 mg
Children	
1–3 years	0.02–0.08 mg
4–6 years	0.03–0.12 mg
Young adults and adults	
7+ years	0.05–0.20 mg

Sources

Good sources of chromium are whole grains, brewer's yeast, pork kidney, meats and cheeses. Little information exists on the chromium content of vegetables. Hard water can supply from 1 to 70 percent of the daily intake. Chromium is poorly absorbed in any form other than the trivalent form found in the glucose tolerance factor.

Toxicity

The range of concentration at which chromium is effective is narrow. If exceeded, the function of chromium reverses to inhibit, rather than enhance, insulin activity.

COBALT

Cobalt is a constituent of vitamin B12 (cobalamin). Normal cobalt concentrations in the blood are 80 to 300 mcg/ml.

Functions

Cobalt is essential to erythropoiesis in the human body because it is a constituent of cobalamin. Cobalt has several functions, including:

- Acting as a substitute for manganese in the activation of several enzymes (such as glycylglycine dipeptidase).
- Replacing zinc in some enzymes (such as carboxypeptidase A and B; and bovine, human and monkey carbonic anhydrase).
- Activating phosphotransferases and other enzymes (even though these enzymes are activated in the presence of other metals or in the absence of any metal).
- Participating in the biotin-dependent oxalacetate transcarboxylase.

Because of its relationship with vitamin B12, cobalt must be absorbed as a component of B12. The amount absorbed is stored in the liver and kidney, with a reserve of 0.2 ppm of dry weight. The majority of ingested cobalt is excreted in the feces, with an average of 0.26 mg being excreted daily.

Deficiency

Low cobalt levels create different reactions in animals. Cattle and sheep grazed on cobalt-deficient lands become emaciated and anemic, whereas horses raised on the same land show no deficiency symptoms. Any deficiency is ultimately a vitamin B12 deficiency, and administration of the vitamin alleviates the condition. An excess intake of molybdenum may interfere with vitamin B12 synthesis in the rumen of cattle.

Requirements

The average intake of cobalt is 5 to 8 mcg/day. No RDA or safe and adequate amount has been established for cobalt at this time.

Sources

Foods containing about 0.2 ppm cobalt are figs, cabbage, spinach, beet greens, buckwheat, lettuce and watercress.

Toxicity

When fed a pharmacological dose of cobalt, many animals, as well as humans, develop polycythemia because of increases in the hormone erythropoietin in the blood. Elevated erythrocyte and hemoglobin levels, reticulocytosis, increased red blood cell mass and normoblastic hyperplasia in the bone marrow have also been reported.

Congestive heart failure due to cardiomyopathy has been reported when beer containing 1.2 ppm of cobalt was consumed. Pericardial effusion, thyroid hyperplasia and neurological disorders have also been noted.

Large doses of cobalt may interfere with decarboxylation reactions (by binding to lipoic acid), impair pyruvate and fatty acid metabolism, and enhance iron absorption and globin synthesis.

COPPER

The human body contains 75 to 100 mg of this trace mineral. Although copper is found in all tissues, its greatest concentrations are in the brain and liver. Because copper competes with zinc for entry from the intestines, an increase in dietary zinc may precipitate a copper deficiency.

Serum copper is bound to the protein ceruplasmin, with 5 percent attached to alpha-albumin. Copper in red blood cells is bound to erythrocuprein, a protein known to have superoxide dismutase activity. During growth, the largest concentrations of copper occur in developing tissues. Estrogens tend to markedly increase serum copper and ceruplasmin concentrations, which explains copper increases observed during pregnancy.

Functions

Copper performs many functions in the body. This mineral:

- Acts as a cofactor for several enzyme systems, eleven of which are oxidases (including cytochrome oxidase, superoxide dismutase, ferroxidase, uricase, lysyl oxidase, dopamine beta-hydroxylase, tyrosinase, spermine oxidase, tryptophan pyrolase and diamine oxidase).
- Is a catalyst in the synthesis of hemoglobin.
- Influences iron absorption and mobilization from the liver and other tissue stores; facilitates the electron shift of iron from the $+2$ to the $+3$ state, thus playing a crucial role in respiration. (In a copper deficiency, the red blood cells that are formed have a shortened life span.)
- Produces energy by oxidizing cytochrome c in the respiratory chain.

- Aids in collagen formation for bone and connective tissue.
- Is involved in the synthesis of phospholipids needed to maintain the myelin sheath around nerve fibers.

Copper is found in the enzymes participating in the oxidation of mono- and diamines, uric acid and galactose, as well as in ribonucleic acid.

Copper absorption takes place in the stomach and duodenum, and averages 30 percent of intake. Absorption of the mineral is increased by acids and inhibited by calcium. Copper availability is inhibited by molybdenum in combination with sulfate by either blocking usage, encouraging excretion, or both.

Copper is incorporated into bile and eliminated through the intestines.

Deficiency

A clinical copper deficiency is rare, but has been reported in children with kwashiorkor, chronic diarrhea or iron-deficiency anemia. Subadequate copper intakes are common, as are subclinical deficiencies (especially in hospital and parenteral feedings). Because copper is important to the normal development of nerve, bone, blood and connective tissue, deficiency can result in a decline in red blood cell formation and subsequent anemia.

A copper deficiency may result in:

- a low white blood cell count associated with reduced resistance to infection.
- faulty collagen formation.
- fragile connective tissue that is easily damaged, resulting in damage to blood vessels, epithelial linings and numerous other tissues.
- bone demineralization.
- central nervous system impairment because of reduced energy metabolism, disintegration of nerve tissue or alterations in neurotransmitter concentrations.
- diminished skin pigmentation because of the role of copper in synthesizing melanin from tyrosine.
- copper deficiency anemia (seen in infants fed a cow's milk diet exclusively after the first three months).
- Menke's syndrome, a malabsorption problem leading to steely or kinky hair, aneurisms, impaired growth, cerebral degeneration, and death.

Requirements

The RDAs for copper are:

Infants
0–0.5 year	0.5–0.7 mg
0.5–1 year	0.7–1.0 mg

Children
1–3 years	1.0–1.5 mg
4–6 years	1.5–2.0 mg
7–10 years	2.0–2.5 mg

Young adults and adults
11+ years	2.0–3.0 mg

Sources

Good dietary sources of copper are wholegrain cereals and breads, shellfish, nuts, organ meats, eggs, poultry, dried beans and peas, and dark green leafy vegetables. Fresh and dried fruits and vegetables are moderate to poor sources. Milk and milk products are poor sources.

Toxicity

Wilson's disease, a genetic disorder, results in excessive accumulation of copper in soft tissues with low serum levels. In this disease, irreversible liver, kidney and brain damage occurs if chelating agents are not administered to bind copper in the gut. In addition, this disorder leads to central nervous system damage, cirrhosis of the liver and corneal degradation.

Hemolytic anemia, hemoglobinuria and jaundice result from a sudden release of copper into the bloodstream. In humans, toxicity results in nausea, vomiting, epigastric pain, headache, dizziness, weakness, diarrhea and a characteristic metallic taste. In severe (but rare) cases, tachycardia, hypertension, jaundice, uremia, coma and death can result. Copper levels also increase in hemochromatosis, a disease characterized by an accumulation of iron in soft tissues.

FLUORIDE

The body's fluoride content depends on the diet and water intake. Normal blood levels for the mineral are 0.28 mg/100 ml. Up to 3 mg of fluoride are excreted by the body each day through the urine and sweat.

Functions

Fluoride is essential to the teeth and bones. It is necessary for replacing the hydroxy portion of their crystalline structure, creating a less water-soluble fluoride salt called fluorapatite. As a result, bone and tooth structure is harder, larger, more uniform and more resistant to decay by acids and demineralization.

A reduced incidence of osteoporosis is found in areas with naturally occurring or added fluoride in the drinking water. With adequate fluoride intake, some elderly patients show a reduced excretion of calcium, improved bone density and alleviation of osteoporosis symptoms. Fluoride may also prevent the most common cause of hearing loss in the elderly by recalcifying the inner bone structure of the ear.

Tooth decay is less prevalent when the concentration of fluoride in the water is above 1 ppm (or 1 mg per liter). The benefits are most pronounced in those consuming fluoridated water from infancy and during tooth development. All ages, however, benefit from the mineral. The reduction in dental caries may be as high as 58 percent when adequate fluoride is available.

Deficiency

A low fluoride intake results in a significant increase in dental caries. No other deficiency symptoms have been reported, even at minimal intakes.

Requirements

The range for fluoride consumption is 0.2–3.4 mg. Although no established RDA value has been set, ranges of estimated safe and adequate daily intakes are:

Infants
0–0.5 year	0.1–0.5 mg
0.5–1 year	0.2–1.0 mg

Children
1–3 years	0.5–1.5 mg
4–6 years	1.0–2.5 mg
7+ years	1.5–2.5 mg

Adults
	1.5–4.0 mg

Sources

Fluoridated water is the most convenient and effective source of the mineral. For those living in areas without access to fluoridated water, bottled fluoridated water or fluoride tablets can be used. Topical application to the teeth is less effective than fluoride circulating in the body, but does provide some benefit. Fluoridated toothpaste is also helpful.

Foods vary in fluoride content depending on the fluoride in the soil and water on which they were grown. Fish, tea, milk and eggs are usually fair sources of fluoride.

Toxicity

Drinking water that contains 2 to 8 ppm fluoride can cause mottling, dulling and pitting of teeth. Although esthetically unpleasing, this preliminary toxicity sign is harmless, and the teeth are strong and caries-free. At 8 ppm, bone fluorosis occurs, with arthritis-like symptoms. More extensive damage requires an intake of 20 to 80 mg over several years. The amount of the mineral consumed from fluoridated water (either naturally occurring or supplemented) is 1 mg/day.

IODINE

Of the 20 to 50 mg of iodine present in the body, 50 percent is found in the muscles, 20 percent in the thyroid gland, 10 percent in the skin and 7 percent in the skeletal structure. The remaining 13 percent is found in other endocrine glands (such as the ovaries and central nervous system). Normal values for protein-bound iodine (PBI) in plasma and serum are 0.004 to 0.008 mg/100 ml.

Functions

The primary role of iodine is as a component of thyroid hormone, and ultimately the regulation of cellular oxidation. Thyroid hormone accelerates cellular reactions, increases oxygen consumption and basal metabolic rate and influences growth and development, energy metabolism, differentiation and protein synthesis. The concentration of iodine in the thyroid gland is 1000 times that in the muscle, and 10,000 times that in blood. One-quarter of the iodine in the thyroid gland is found in thyroxine (T_4) and triiodothyronine (T_3). The remaining three-quarters is in the precursors of thyroxine, and in small amounts as the inorganic form.

Iodine can be absorbed from the skin surface or from the intestinal mucosa. In the intestinal tract, dietary iodine is converted to iodide and absorption is quick and complete. Iodine is excreted primarily through the kidneys, with minor amounts lost in sweat, tears, saliva, and bile. There is no feedback mechanism for conserving iodine in the presence of a deficiency.

Deficiency

In adults, inadequate dietary iodine over several months results in simple endemic goiter or hypothyroidism. Endemic goiter is caused by enlargement of the thyroid gland with follicular epithelial cell hypertrophy, hyperplasia or both.

If iodine intake diminishes, hormone secretion remains constant until available stores of the mineral are depleted. The pituitary gland releases quantities of Thyroid Stimulating Hormone (TSH) and thyroid activity increases accordingly. The end result is enlargement of the thyroid gland, or goiter. Goiter is common in areas with low water concentrations of iodine (such as the Great Lakes region or areas removed from the ocean or ocean winds). Water supplies vary in iodine content from 0.01 to 73.3 ppb. Ocean water, which is high in iodine, enriches soil and water supplies exposed to its spray.

Goitrogens are substances that can induce goiter. If consumed in quantity from areas where the soil and water are iodine-deficient, endemic goiter can be precipitated. Natural goitrogens are found in cabbage, rutabagas, cauliflower, turnips, peanuts, mustard seeds and soybeans. Synthetically, goitrogens are drugs such as thiourea, thiouracil, sulfonamide and perhaps antabuse. Goitrogens can induce goiter by interfering with thyroglobulin synthesis. Endemic goiter is usually reversible by administration of thyroid hormone or iodine.

In infants deprived of iodine during gestation, iodine deficiency results in cretinism. Cretinism is much more serious than iodine deficiency in adults. Inadequate maternal iodine stores result in impaired physical and mental development of the fetus. The basal metabolic rate is lower, the muscles are flabby and bones are poorly formed. Severe and irreversible mental retardation is common.

Requirements

To prevent goiter, about 150 mcg of iodine are needed daily. The RDAs for iodine are:

Infants	
0–0.5 year	40 mcg
0.5–1 year	50 mcg
Children	
1–3 years	70 mcg
4–6 years	90 mcg
7–10 years	120 mcg

Young adults and adults

11 + years	150 mcg
Pregnant	+ 25 mcg
Lactating	+ 50 mcg

Sources

Iodized salt and water containing adequate amounts of iodine are good sources of the mineral. Enrichment is 76 mcg per gram of salt. If salt consumption averages 3.4 g/day, 260 mcg of iodine will be ingested, more than meeting the RDA. The iodine content of foods will vary depending on the soil and water supply, fertilizers, animal feed and processing methods. If a low sodium diet is consumed, iodine intake must be considered. If a bakery adds iodine to dough as a stabilizer, a slice of bread may provide as much as 150 mcg of iodine.

Toxicity

Doses greater than ten times the normal requirement result in little or no toxic effects in individuals with a normal thyroid gland. The gland initially absorbs more iodine, but within weeks the iodine concentration resembles normal intake and hormone synthesis remains constant regardless of excess intake. When plasma levels exceed 20 to 35 mcg/100 ml, thyroxine synthesis ceases, but adaptation results in normal hormone synthesis within weeks.

In cases of hyperthyroidism, doses as small as 1 mg result in cessation of hormone release and significant amelioration of thyrotoxicosis symptomatology.

IRON

Iron is found in two forms in the body: in functional forms (such as hemoglobin and enzymes), and in transport and storage forms (transferrin, ferritin and hemosiderin). The amount of iron in the storage forms (ferritin and hemosiderin) reflects dietary absorption and body demands.

The iron pool varies from 1000 mg in a healthy male to 200 to 400 mg in women prior to menopause, but may be even lower in iron-deficient individuals. In the male, 70 to 80 percent of iron is found in hemoglobin, with myoglobin containing 5 percent. One percent is associated with the enzyme systems, and the remainder is in storage. Iron is seldom found free, but prefers to be protein-bound.

The iron available for biological needs is from en-dogenous recycling or exogenous dietary sources. Iron is stored in the liver, spleen and bone marrow. Pregnancy or blood loss (such as menstruation or injury) can remove iron from these stores at a rate of 10 to 40 mg a day.

Functions

The three to five grams of iron in the body are found primarily as a component of hemoglobin and myoglobin, which are oxygen carrying and releasing substances. Because iron can convert from the ferrous ($+2$) to the ferric ($+3$) form, oxygen may be held or released as needed. Therefore, iron is the main determinant of the oxygen supply to cells. Hemoglobin is the oxygen-carrier in the blood. Myoglobin, which has a greater capacity for holding oxygen, serves as an oxygen reservoir within the cells (especially heart and skeletal muscle). The presence of myoglobin within a cell tends to draw oxygen into the cell from surrounding fluids.

Iron participates in energy production as a transporter of hydrogen to oxygen in cellular electron transport systems. Catalases and other enzymes in the Krebs cycle, as well as the cytochromes of the respiratory chain, benefit from the ability of iron to convert to and from the reduced state.

Iron is also required for collagen synthesis by enzymes important in the hydroxylation of proline and lysine.

Deficiency

Of the many types of anemia, iron-deficiency anemia is best known. In this condition, red blood cells contain less hemoglobin, have a reduced capacity to carry oxygen, and are small and pale in color, hence the name microcytic hypochromic anemia. The reduced iron supply to tissues results in diminished energy production and the characteristic symptoms of lethargy, tiredness, apathy, reduced brain function, pallor, headache, heart enlargement, spoon-shaped nails, depleted iron stores and a plasma iron of less than 40 mcg/100 ml.

Iron-deficiency anemia is a major nutritional concern worldwide, and its prevalence may range as high as 50 percent in some segments of the population. In the United States, vulnerable populations include women of childbearing years, older infants, children, the elderly, low-income groups, and minorities, although every sector of the population (including males) is a candidate for a potential deficiency. One in every four college women has depleted iron stores.

Iron deficiency can be caused by low-grade, constant blood loss (from bleeding ulcers or hemorrhoids, parasites or cancer), poor dietary intake or absorption, or an increased demand. Growth periods and repeated pregnancies are associated with increases in blood volume, thereby raising the iron need.

Reduced iron in the blood is one of the final stages in iron deficiency. Iron deficiency and its effect on body processes have been progressing long before this stage. For instance, iron is found in the brain as a cofactor in neurotransmitter synthesis. The brain stores are diminished long before blood levels decline. This reduction of body stores produces no overt symptomatology.

Women are close to the deficiency borderline. Monthly blood loss from menstruation means a 28 mg loss of iron. This loss, combined with reduced food intake, results in a double-fold need for iron. Blood donations (a pint of blood contains 200 to 300 mg of iron), lactation (1 to 2.5 mg lost daily) and pregnancy (from 500 to 1000 mg of iron donated to fetal growth and storage) can all warrant close attention to iron status.

Unusual cravings are common in iron deficiency. An appetite for ice, clay, starch and other nonfood items in iron-deficient populations has been termed "pica." This condition responds to iron therapy more rapidly than do red blood cells.

Children with iron deficiency show signs of hyperactivity, decreased attention span and reduced IQ. These behavioral changes manifest prior to a diagnosed iron deficiency and disappear with iron administration.

Only 10 percent of dietary iron is absorbed. Approximately 10 to 30 percent of heme iron (the iron found in meat) is absorbed, but only 2 to 10 percent of the iron found in beans, vegetables and fruits is absorbed. Heme iron increases the absorption of non-heme iron if the two are consumed simultaneously.

Iron absorption increases as a reflection of individual iron status. For example, when plasma transferrin levels are low, absorption increases, and when they are high, less iron is absorbed from the intestines. Absorption also reflects the type of dietary iron ingested and the presence or absence of enhancing substances. The iron absorption rate increases during infancy, pregnancy, childhood and adolescence because of increased protein needs. Because the adaptive mechanism does not effectively counteract increased needs, anemia is frequent in these populations.

Substances that reduce iron from the $+3$ state (found mostly in foods) to the $+2$ state (the form most readily absorbed from the gut) increase iron absorption up to four-fold. Stomach acid and ascorbic acid serve this purpose. Because iron supplements are poorly absorbed, vitamin C is frequently added to oral iron preparations. (Antacids reduce the stomach's acidity, counteract the effects of ascorbic acid and predispose the user to iron-deficiency anemia.) Chelating substances, including the sulfur-containing amino acids, may increase absorption.

Absorption is reduced with rapid intestinal transit time, achylia and malabsorption syndromes. Antibiotics, phosphates, carbonates (such as calcium carbonate found in prenatal vitamins) and phytates inhibit iron absorption. Aspirin plays a secondary role in iron loss because of blood lost through low-grade gastrointestinal bleeding.

Once iron is absorbed, it is well conserved. Red blood cells are manufactured at a rate of 1 percent a day, requiring 25 mg of iron. The body recycles 90 percent of the iron from ruptured and dead red blood cells for hematopoeisis. Only minute amounts are lost in nail clippings, hair, urine and sweat, through the digestive tract, or by the sloughing of dead skin cells. Daily losses average 1 mg; however, large amounts may be involved in hemorrhage or blood loss.

Requirements

Assuming a 10 percent absorption, the RDAs for iron are designed to replace daily losses and maintain stores of 500 mg or more in healthy adults. Normal hemoglobin levels for males should be maintained at or above 14 to 15 g/100 ml of blood; normal values for females are 13 to 14 g/100 ml. The average American diet contains about 6 mg of iron/1000 kcalories. A woman with an RDA of 18 mg who consumes 2000 kcalories a day may consume only two-thirds of her daily needs. The iron-to-kcalorie ratio must be doubled in this case to meet iron needs.

Women show an increased need for iron because of monthly losses during menstruation. During pregnancy, and for three months postpartum, a 30 to 60 mg supplement is recommended. Larger doses may be required if the iron supplement also contains calcium carbonate. Teenage males require the same amount of iron as women because of significant growth spurts during these years.

The RDAs for iron are:

Infants

0–0.5 year	10 mg
0.5–1 year	15 mg

Children

1–3 years	15 mg
4–6 years	10 mg
7–10 years	10 mg

Young adults and adults

Males 11–18 years	18 mg
Males 19+ years	10 mg
Females 11–50 years	18 mg
Females 51+ years	10 mg
Pregnant	+30–60 mg
Lactating (2–3 months postpartum)	+30–60 mg

Sources

Excellent sources of iron are liver and other organ meats, beef, dried fruits, lima beans, ham, legumes, dark green leafy vegetables, sardines, prune juice and oysters. Good sources are wholegrain cereals and breads, tuna, green peas, chicken, strawberries, egg, tomato juice, enriched grains, brussels sprouts, winter squash, blackberries, pumpkin, nuts, canned salmon and broccoli.

Other dietary contributions come from potatoes, applesauce, corn muffins, peanut butter, watermelon, corn, pears and peaches. The iron in iron-fortified foods is poorly absorbed, but does contribute to daily needs.

Cooking acidic foods in cast iron pots can increase the iron content thirty-fold. Iron intake can also be increased by combining heme and non-heme food sources, consuming vitamin C-containing foods with each meal and selecting iron-rich foods.

Toxicity

The body has no effective means of excreting excesses of iron, so accumulation is possible. Hemosiderosis results from ingestion, absorption or intravenous administration of excess iron. With excess iron, transferrin becomes saturated and the iron is then deposited in soft tissue. Genetically susceptible individuals are more likely to develop this disorder from over-ingestion of iron-fortified foods.

The pathological condition called hemochromatosis is a more severe deposition of iron in soft tissues. Tissues such as the liver and spleen accumulate pronounced pigment, the tissue is damaged, and its func-

tion is depressed. Alcoholism predisposes an individual to this disorder by altering iron absorption. People with chronic liver disease or pancreatitis absorb excess amounts of iron from the intestines. However, this may or may not result in hemochromatosis.

MAGNESIUM

Although considered a major mineral, magnesium accounts for only 1.75 ounces of a 130-pound individual. The muscles contain approximately 27 percent of the body's magnesium, and the serum concentration is 1 to 3 mg/100 ml. The bones contain 60 percent of the body's magnesium, providing a reservoir to guarantee adequate supplies in times of need. One-third of magnesium in the bones is bound to phosphate; the rest is loosely absorbed on the surface of the mineral structure. Over a third of the magnesium in the body is not available for transfer into the bone because it is bound to protein or other molecules.

Functions

Magnesium is the most bountiful cation in soft tissues other than potassium, and its loss is associated with tissue breakdown and cell destruction. Magnesium also functions:

- In energy production. Magnesium is a cofactor in the decarboxylation of pyruvic acid and is required for oxidative phosphorylation in the production of ATP. Magnesium is found in all phosphate transferring systems and is frequently complexed with ATP, ADP and AMP. Calcium ions interfere with some magnesium-dependent enzymes, including pyruvate phosphokinase, ATPase and pyrophosphatase. All reactions requiring the thiamin coenzyme (TPP) depend on magnesium.
- In some lipid and protein synthesis pathways, including the transfer of CoA to acetate and to cholic acid, creating acetyl CoA and cholyll CoA. Protein synthesis requires magnesium for ribosomal aggregation, for binding RNA to 70S ribosomes, and in the synthesis and degradation of DNA.
- In the formation of urea, in conjunction with glutamine synthetase. As such, it is important in removing excess ammonia from the body.
- In muscle relaxation and neuromuscular transmission and activity.
- In the prevention of tooth decay by binding calcium to tooth enamel.

Approximately 30 to 40 percent of dietary magnesium is absorbed, the remainder being excreted in the feces. Absorption is dependent on intestinal transit time, rate of water absorption and luminal magnesium concentrations. Magnesium absorption is proportionate to intake but competes with dietary calcium for the same absorption site in the intestine. Absorption is also inhibited by dietary fat, phosphate, lactose, phytate and oxalate, which form insoluble compounds with magnesium.

Magnesium is conserved by the kidneys. Declining blood levels encourage renal absorption and blood excesses result in increased magnesium in the urine. The effective renal and intestinal mechanisms for conservation and excretion allow magnesium status to remain constant through a wide range of dietary intake.

Deficiency

Inadequate magnesium most severely affects cardiovascular, neuromuscular and renal tissues.

The incidence of heart attack is reduced in regions of the country having high magnesium levels in the water supply. Heart failure from defibrillation has been linked to a lack of sufficient magnesium. (See p. 108.)

A low-magnesium diet consumed for three months will lower serum magnesium, calcium and potassium. These normalize with magnesium therapy. Magnesium may also be lost by vomiting, diarrhea, long-term use of diuretics or ammonium chloride, alcoholism and protein malnutrition. Significant magnesium may be lost during diabetic acidosis.

The symptoms of a magnesium deficiency include:

- Weakness.
- Confusion.
- Personality changes.
- Muscle tremor.
- Anorexia.
- Nausea.
- Lack of coordination.
- Gastrointestinal disorders.

A severe or long-term deficiency may result in:

- Tetany similar to that seen in calcium deficiency.
- Bizarre muscle movements, especially in the face and eye muscles.
- Alopecia.
- Swollen gums.
- Skin lesions.

- Lesions of the small arteries.
- Myocardial necrosis.

Alcoholic hallucinations may be caused or aggrevated by a magnesium deficiency, and high intakes of calcium can increase the severity of deficiency symptoms.

Rats fed a magnesium-deficient diet develop vasodilatation in three to five days. The vasodilatation subsides after a week, but is followed by hyperkinetic behavior and fatal convulsions. Other deficiency symptoms in the rat include skin lesions, edema, hypertropic gums, alopecia, growth retardation, and calcification and degeneration of the kidneys and other organs.

Requirements

Establishing conclusive criteria for determining magnesium requirements is difficult because of the mineral's complex interrelationship with other dietary components (such as calcium, protein, phosphate, lactose, potassium and kcalories). A typical diet containing 120 mg/1000 kcalories will prevent a clinical deficiency, but recommended amounts will be inadequate for those suffering from renal and intestinal absorption disorders. The RDAs for magnesium are:

Infants	
0–0.5 year	50 mg
0.5–1 year	70 mg
Children	
1–3 years	150 mg
4–6 years	200 mg
7–10 years	250 mg
Young adults	
Males 11–14 years	350 mg
Males 15–18 years	400 mg
Adults	
Males 18+ years	350 mg
Females 11+ years	300 mg
Pregnant	+150 mg
Lactating	+150 mg

Sources

Good sources of magnesium are nuts, legumes, wholegrain cereals and breads, soybeans and seafoods. Magnesium is important in photosynthesis, so vegetables high in chlorophyll (such as dark green vegetables) are good sources. Milk, although not a good source of magnesium, provides approximately 22 percent of daily needs for the average American. Small amounts are supplied by pork, meat, poultry and eggs.

Toxicity

Toxicity is reduced by the kidneys' ability to excrete excesses of magnesium (up to 60 g of magnesium sulfate each day), thus providing an escape route for escalating blood levels.

In clinical renal insufficiency, hypermagnesemia can result from administration of magnesium-containing drugs (such as some antacids). Central nervous system suppression and anesthesia that result from hypermagnesemia are due to the role of magnesium in neuromuscular excitability.

Toxicity symptoms have been reported in elderly populations consuming magnesium-containing laxatives and antacids. This population is more vulnerable because of its general reduced renal function. Symptoms of the toxicity include drowsiness, weakness and lethargy.

If plasma concentrations of magnesium rise above 15 mEq/l, skeletal paralysis, respiratory depression, coma and death may result. Intravenous injections of calcium can counteract magnesium toxicity.

MANGANESE

Manganese may be found in small amounts in the bones, pituitary, pancreas, intestinal mucosa, liver and other tissues. However, storage is minimal, with a mere 12 to 20 mg present in the body at any one time. Normal blood levels of manganese are 0.005 to 0.02 mg/100 ml.

Functions

The functions of manganese are not specific, since other minerals (such as magnesium) can perform in its place. Manganese is known to play a role in:

- Mucopolysaccharide synthesis.
- Collagen formation.
- Urea formation.
- Synthesis of fatty acids and cholesterol.
- Digestion of proteins.
- Normal bone formation and development.
- The formation of prothrombin (along with vitamin K).
- Protein synthesis (by stimulating RNA polymerase activity).

Manganese is a cofactor for phosphotases, succinic dehydrogenase, peptidases, pyruvate carboxylase, arginase, glycosyltransferases, adenosine triphosphatase, phosphoglucomutase, pyruvate carboxylase (biotin-dependent), mitochondrial superoxide dismutase and cholinesterase.

Approximately 40 percent of dietary manganese is absorbed by the body. Large amounts of calcium and phosphorus in the intestine are known to interfere with absorption.

Manganese is excreted in the feces and bile, with little being removed through the kidneys.

Deficiency

A manganese deficiency or its symptoms have not been observed in humans. However, in rats, a manganese-deficient diet produces sterility and testicular degeneration. Manganese-deprived pregnant rats produce weak offspring with poor survival rates. The surviving offspring show growth retardation and abnormal otoliths of the inner ear, resulting in poor balance, convulsions and epileptic-like seizures. Lactation is also impaired. Guinea pigs deprived of manganese in utero develop a dwarfed pancreas and reduced glucose tolerance. In chicks, shortened legs and vertebral columns are the result of a manganese deficiency.

Requirements

Although specific manganese requirements are unknown, the average adult intake ranges from 2 to 9 mg daily with no clinical deficiency symptoms. This average intake may or may not eliminate a subclinical deficiency. Estimated safe and adequate daily dietary intakes for manganese are:

Infants	
0–0.5 year	0.5–0.7 mg
0.5–1 year	0.7–1.0 mg
Children	
1–3 years	1.0–1.5 mg
4–6 years	1.5–2.0 mg
7–10 years	2.0–3.0 mg
Young adults and adults	
11+ years	2.5–5.0 mg

Sources

The richest sources of manganese are liver, kidney, lettuce, spinach, muscle meats, tea, wholegrain cereals and breads, dried peas and beans, and nuts. Moderate amounts are found in leafy green vegetables, dried fruits, and the stalk, root and tuber parts of vegetables.

Small amounts are provided in meats, fish and other animal products.

Toxicity

An excessive intake of manganese interferes with iron absorption and can precipitate iron-deficiency anemia. This condition is reversible by administration of iron.

Toxicity symptoms have been observed in miners who inhale large amounts of the mineral, with increased amounts of manganese found in the lungs. Initial symptoms of this toxicity include pulmonary changes, asthenia, anorexia, apathy, impotence, leg cramps, headaches and speech impairments. In more advanced stages, the condition resembles Parkinson's disease or viral encephalitis. The facial expression is blank and the voice tone is monotonous; muscle rigidity and spasms may occur.

MOLYBDENUM

The body contains small amounts of the trace mineral molybdenum, with 3.2 ppm found in the liver and 1.6 ppm in the kidney. Other tissues, including muscle, brain, lung and spleen, contain amounts ranging from 0.14 to 0.2 ppm.

Functions

Molybdenum is essential in the function of two enzyme systems: the catalytic role of xanthine oxidase in uric acid formation, and the aldehyde oxidase role in the oxidation of various aldehydes. Both enzymes contain FAD (a riboflavin enzyme), and are important in electron transport. Xanthine oxidase is also important in converting iron from the ferrous to the ferric form. Therefore, molybdenum, like copper, is necessary in iron metabolism.

Molybdenum is sensitive to sulfur metabolism; inorganic sulfate or endogenous sulfur from amino acids can affect the mineral's tissue concentration. An increased sulfur intake causes a decline in molybdenum status.

Molybdenum can interfere with copper absorption, as the two minerals compete for similar absorption sites in the intestines. It is excreted in the urine and bile.

Deficiency

No deficiency is known in humans. In animals, intakes of less than 0.005 mcg/g cause weight loss, anorexia, reduced life expectancy and disturbed microbiological processes in the rumen.

Requirements

Molybdenum intakes considered safe and adequate are:

Infants	
0–0.5 year	0.03–0.06 mg
0.5–1 year	0.04–0.08 mg
Children	
1–3 years	0.05–0.10 mg
4–6 years	0.06–0.15 mg
7–10 years	0.10–0.30 mg
Young adults and adults	
11+ years	0.15–0.50 mg

Sources

Dietary intake of molybdenum depends on the status of the soil on which grains and vegetables are raised. Plants grown on molybdenum-rich soil may contain 500 times as much of the mineral as plants grown on depleted soil. Hard water can provide up to 41 percent of daily intake. Meats, whole grains, legumes, leafy vegetables and organ meats are other good sources of molybdenum.

Toxicity

Toxicity symptoms vary with species, age and the amount and form of the mineral when ingested. Symptoms are also affected by dietary intake of sulfate, copper and other minerals. Growth retardation and weight loss have been consistently reported in animals. In cattle, toxicity results in "teart," a disease characterized by diarrhea and general wasting.

PHOSPHORUS

Phosphorus is the second most abundant mineral in the body; 12 grams of phosphorus are in each kilogram of fat-free tissue. About 85 percent of all phosphorus is found as inorganic calcium phosphate in a two-to-one ratio in the bones and teeth. Calcium phosphate gives bones and teeth their strength and rigidity. In plasma, the phosphorus concentration is 3.5 mg/100 ml, about half that of calcium. The total phosphorus content of blood, if red cell phosphorus is included, is between 30 and 45 mg/100 ml. This level is kept constant by renal resorption, and is responsive to plasma concentrations of calcium and phosphorus, PTH and active vitamin D3.

Functions

Unlike calcium, phosphorus is a structural component of all cells, including soft tissues (such as striated muscle). It is a part of the nucleic acids comprising the genetic code in all cells. Therefore, phosphorus (primarily as phosphoric acid) is fundamental to the growth, maintenance and repair of all body tissues, besides being necessary for protein synthesis. Phosphorus is critical for energy transfer and production in the body. The mineral plays a role in the phosphorylation of monosaccharides for energy.

Many enzymes and the B vitamins are activated only in the presence of phosphorus. Thus, the oxidation of carbohydrates, protein and fats leading to the formation of ATP requires phosphorus.

The phospholipids (such as lecithin) contain phosphorus in their structure. These lipids carry fats in watery mediums and form the part of cell membranes responsible for transporting nutrients in and out of the cell. The sphingolipids contain a fatty acid, phosphorus, choline and an amino acid.

Plasma phosphorus functions as a buffer to maintain the delicate acid-base balance in the body.

Calcium and phosphorus are closely related; fluctuations in one mineral will be reflected by subsequent fluctuations in the other. The goal of the kidneys is to maintain a stable calcium:phosphorus ratio and provide adequate phosphorus for biological needs. The hormone calcitonin causes a rapid lowering of plasma calcium and phosphorus. Plasma concentrations of phosphorus are regulated primarily by urinary excretion.

As much as seventy percent of dietary phosphorus is absorbed by the body. Absorption may be inhibited by excessive iron intake, which forms insoluble phosphates in the intestines.

Deficiency

A dietary deficiency of phosphorus in humans is uncommon; phosphorus intake is invariably higher than that of calcium. Although the significance of the calcium:phosphorus ratio is still unclear in osteoporosis, the initial symptoms (such as resorption of the alveolar bone) are associated with a low calcium intake, a high proportion of phosphorus, or both.

In rickets, serum calcium or serum phosphorus or both may be low. Rickets has developed in rats when large variations in the calcium:phosphorus ratio occur. This has not been replicated in human studies.

A phosphorus deficiency has been reported in cattle that consume grains and grasses high in calcium and low in phosphorus. In these cases, symptoms include anorexia, weakness, stiff joints and fragile bones. Similar symptoms have been produced in humans by a long-term excessive use of antacids that render phosphate unabsorbable.

A vitamin D deficiency can result in reduced serum phosphate levels.

Requirements

Recommended dietary needs for phosphorus have been set somewhat arbitrarily. Because of the relationship of phosphorus to calcium, the RDA is similar for both minerals. The RDAs for phosphorus are:

Infants	
0–0.5 year	240 mg
0.5–1 year	360 mg
Children	
1–10 years	800 mg
11–18 years	1200 mg
Adults	
18+ years	800 mg
Pregnant	+400 mg
Lactating	+400 mg

Sources

Phosphorus is a component of all cells and therefore is found in abundance in animal tissues. The major food sources are meats, fish, poultry, eggs, milk and milk products. Soft drinks contain as much as 500 mg/serving and contribute to excessive phosphorus levels. Phosphoric acid is frequently used in convenience foods as phosphate preservatives to enhance antioxidant effectiveness.

Toxicity

Overconsumption of phosphorus is possible for those choosing the typical American diet high in meats, convenience foods and soft drinks. The effects of this diet may influence calcium absorption, metabolism and utilization.

POTASSIUM

Potassium is the primary cation in intracellular fluids. Ninety-eight percent of the total body potassium is intracellular, a concentration thirty times greater than in extracellular spaces. The blood contains 16 to 22 mg/100 ml of potassium and erythrocytes contain 420 mg/100 ml.

Functions

Potassium can cross cell membranes with greater ease than sodium. This shift is probably mediated by changes in the body's acid-base balance. Potassium also performs other functions in the body:

- It plays a role in maintaining cellular integrity and water balance.
- It is important in muscle contraction.
- Glycogen formation and glucose catabolism, protein metabolism and carbohydrate metabolism are all potassium-dependent.
- It is important in nerve transmission. Stimulation of the nerves causes a migration of potassium out of the cell, altering the membrane potential and conducting a nerve impulse down the axon.

Nearly all potassium (90 percent) is absorbed by the body. Because the kidneys are the major efficient regulator of potassium, plasma levels remain relatively constant regardless of intake. Potassium regulation is also dependent on factors that maintain sodium homeostasis. Concentrations of potassium in sweat are less than half that of sodium (less than 10 mEq/liter vs. 25 to 30 mEq/liter).

Deficiency

The concentration of potassium in the body declines with age. It is also lost from burned or injured tissue or during starvation. A potassium deficiency may be precipitated by diarrhea, vomiting, diabetic acidosis, chronic renal disease, fasting and chronic use of diuretics and laxatives.

Prolonged dehydration causes potassium to be removed from intracellular compartments and subsequently the electrolyte is lost in the urine. This release of potassium is a sign of protein catabolism and tissue wasting. Potassium will also be lost from cellular spaces when an excessive loss of sodium occurs. In some disease states or surgical procedures, potassium is lost from the muscles and other organs. When renal function is normal, potassium salts are lost in the urine.

Untreated diabetes is characterized by polyuria, with increased losses of potassium and sodium. Excessive potassium is lost in the urine in diabetic acidosis because of the failure to adequately metabolize carbohydrates. Insulin can cause potassium influx into the cells and hypokalemia that can lead to paralysis of the respiratory muscles.

A potassium deficiency causes impaired growth, bone fragility, paralysis, sterility, muscle weakness, central nervous system changes, renal hypertrophy, diminished heart rate and death.

Requirements

In the healthy adult, daily potassium balance can be maintained on intakes as low as those required for infants. The typical intake of potassium is 0.8 to 1.5 g/1000 kcalories, and the estimated safe and adequate intakes are:

Infants	
0–0.5 year	0.350–0.925 g
0.5–1 year	0.425–1.275 g
Children	
1–3 years	0.55–1.65 g
4–6 years	0.775–2.325 g
7–10 years	1.0–3.0 g
11+ years	1.525–4.575 g
Adults	1.875–5.625 g

Sources

Potassium is found in a wide variety of foods including meat, milk, fruits and vegetables. Lean meats contain 0.3 to 0.5 g per serving. Potatoes, bananas, orange juice, apricots, other dried and fresh fruits and fruit juices are excellent sources.

Toxicity

Plasma levels higher than 6 mEq/liter are abnormal; levels in excess of 8 mEq/liter are dangerous. Hyperkalemia can develop from a sudden increase in dietary intake above 18 g for the average adult. If potassium excretion is impaired and potassium chloride (a salt substitute) or potassium tablets are ingested in appreciable amounts, hyperkalemia can result. No substantial increase in intracellular or total body potassium occurs, but disturbances in cardiac function and renal insufficiency can be fatal.

Other causes of hyperkalemia are: acute or chronic renal failure, acute hydration, adrenal insufficiency, severe metabolic or respiratory acidosis, major infection, hemorrhage into the gastrointestinal tract or a large and rapid catabolic use of protein. Although hypertension is primarily related to sodium intake, the ratio of potassium to sodium can be another determinant in some cases.

SELENIUM

Selenium closely resembles sulfur in its physical and chemical properties. It is found in highest concentration in the kidney, heart, spleen and liver. Once absorbed, however, selenium is deposited in all tissues except fat. The selenium concentration in the blood is 0.22 mcg/100 ml.

Functions

Selenium is a trace mineral that functions either alone or as a part of enzyme systems. The cofactor role of selenium parallels the antioxidant and free radical scavenging action of vitamin E. In fact, because of its ability to protect cell, mitochondria, microsome and lysosome membranes from lipid peroxidation damage, selenium can substitute for vitamin E in some antioxidant functions. Generally, however, vitamin E and selenium do not replace each other, but are involved in overlapping systems with similar end results. When vitamin E and selenium are jointly administered, the stabilizing effect on lysosomal membranes is potentiated.

Selenium also functions:

- As a cofactor with glutathione peroxidase in destroying hydrogen peroxide.
- As a component of sulfur amino acid metabolism.
- In binding to heavy metals and possibly reducing toxicity from mercury contamination.
- In cancer prevention.
- In the prevention of cardiac disorders.

About 90 percent of ingested selenium is absorbed by the body. Urinary excretion and excretion through the lungs reflect selenium status.

Deficiency

In animals raised on selenium-poor soil, deficiency symptoms similar to those of vitamin E deficiency have been reported. Laboratory-induced muscular dystrophy in lambs has been treated with selenium and vitamin E. And hepatic necrosis in rats, produced by a diet low in cystine and vitamin E, was found to be only partially responsive to the two nutrients, but very responsive to selenium.

In humans, a selenium deficiency in the soil and water has resulted in cardiomyopathy and myocardial deaths. Keshan cardiomyopathy in China is prevented with selenium supplementation. Low-selenium soil has also been associated with an increased risk of cancer.

Requirements

Normal intakes of 0.1 mg/day are adequate to alleviate clinical selenium deficiency symptoms. Estimated safe and adequate daily dietary intakes for selenium are:

Infants	
0–0.5 year	0.01–0.04 mg
0.5–1 year	0.02–0.06 mg
Children	
1–3 years	0.02–0.08 mg
4–6 years	0.03–0.12 mg
7–10 years	0.05–0.20 mg
Young adults and adults	
11+ years	0.05–0.20 mg

Sources

Excellent sources of selenium are liver, kidney, meats and seafood. Grains and vegetables will vary in their selenium content depending on the soil on which they were grown.

Toxicity

Selenium may interfere with sulfur metabolism, thus inhibiting several enzymes (including succinic dehydrogenase, choline oxidase and proline oxidase). In the presence of excess selenium embryonic development is impaired, and bone and cartilage develop abnormally.

In greater than trace amounts, selenium may be toxic to humans. Individuals in industrial settings have been reported to suffer from toxic symptoms of selenium overdoses, including liver disease and cardiomyopathy. Children raised in selenium-rich areas show a higher incidence of decayed, missing and filled teeth. Similar effects have been demonstrated in monkeys consuming selenium-rich water.

Animals grazed on selenium-rich soil develop "blind staggers," characterized by blindness, salivation, muscle paralysis, abdominal pain, and respiratory failure. Another condition, "alkali disease," produces hair loss, sore hoofs, liver damage, cardiac atrophy, cirrhosis, anemia, erosion of long bone joints and dry, dull coat. These symptoms are partially a result of selenocysteine's replacing cysteine in keratine formation. The animal may be protected somewhat by a diet high in protein or sulfate.

SODIUM

The body contains 1.8 g of sodium/kg of fat-free body weight, or 0.15 percent of total body weight. Sodium is found in every cell of the body, with greatest concentrations in extracellular fluids. Normal serum levels of sodium are maintained at 310 to 333 mg/100 ml.

Functions

As the primary extracellular cation, sodium is fundamental in regulating osmolarity and body fluid volume. It also acts as a buffer in maintaining the body's acid-base balance.

Other functions that depend on sodium are:

- CO_2 transport.
- Muscle contraction and nerve transmission. These functions depend on sodium's ability to permeate cell membranes and temporarily replace the intracellular cation potassium.
- Amino acid uptake from the gut, as well as transportation into all body cells, depends on sodium because the cation is critical in moving amino acids across cell membranes.

Some sodium is bound to the surface crystals of bone and acts as a labile sodium reservoir for the body.

All dietary sodium is absorbed from the gut. Sodium metabolism is mediated by the adrenal cortex hormone aldosterone. This hormone regulates sodium resorption from the kidneys, preventing overexcretion and sodium deficiency. The adrenal minerocorticoids (hydrocortisone and deoxycorticosterone) play a lesser role in regulating sodium excretion.

Sodium metabolism, uptake and excretion correlate to those of water. Water loss through skin and lungs totals between 500 and 800 ml/day, with 75 percent of this being electrolyte-free. Moderate water losses during physical exertion and humidity will result in a sodium loss of 46 to 92 mg a day.

Deficiency·

A dietary sodium deficiency is uncommon in humans. If a deficiency does occur, it is often caused by starvation (due to abrupt reduction in available carbohydrate), excess vomiting, diarrhea or profuse sweating, and is associated with a concurrent water loss. If sodium is lost, but water remains constant, the reduced sodium concentration causes water migration into the cells. The result is subsequent symptoms of water intoxication: mental apathy, muscle twitching and anorexia. If both water and sodium are lost, the extracellular fluids are depleted with resultant low blood volume, low blood pressure, muscle cramping and high hematocrit. The veins may collapse as well.

Perspiration contains 1 g of sodium per liter, which can be replaced through normal dietary sodium intake. Fluids should be replaced first, with the need to consider salt replacements (1 g [⅕ teaspoon]/quart of water) only after eight or more pounds of fluids have been lost. Salt tablets usually contain 1 g of salt each and can be used to replace losses. However, a slight increase in dietary salt during the day can adequately replace losses.

Other symptoms of a sodium deficiency are muscle weakness, poor memory and concentration, anorexia, acidosis, dehydration and tissue atrophy.

Requirements

Sodium intake is more a product of habit, taste and custom than need. Tissue formation requires 1.1 to 2.2 mg/kg of tissue formed; tissue maintenance requires less. A diet containing a daily intake of 0.5 g can maintain sodium balance in the body. However, intakes vary, averaging 2.3 to 6.0 g daily, and an intake of 15 g is not unusual.

No RDA has been established, but intakes of 1.1 to 3.3 g are assumed adequate for healthy adults. Estimated safe and adequate daily intakes for sodium are:

Infants	
0–0.5 year	0.115–0.35 g
0.5–1 year	0.25–0.75 g
Children	
1–3 years	0.325–0.975 g
4–6 years	0.45–1.35 g
7–10 years	0.60–1.80 g
11+ years	0.90–2.70 g
Adults	1.10–3.30 g

Sources

Sodium chloride (table salt) is the major dietary source of sodium. Because 40 percent of the weight of table salt is sodium, 6 g of salt sprinkled on a meal will yield 2.4 g of ingested sodium.

Sodium is found in abundance in the food supply; plant sources contain less than animal products. Many fast foods and commercially processed foods, (canned, frozen and instant) are high in sodium, contributing a quarter to a half of the daily intake. Naturally occurring sodium is found in milk products, soft water, shellfish, meats, eggs, poultry and fish. Fruits, vegetables, legumes and wholegrain cereals are low, unless sodium has been added during processing. Commercial soups, olives, pickles, sauerkraut, sandwich meats, catsup, beef broth and most prepared food items are high in sodium. Non-salt sodium contributors include baking soda, baking powder, soy sauce, monosodium glutamate (MSG), sodium sulfite, sodium alginate, sodium citrate, sodium nitrite and nitrate, sodium propionate and other sodium-containing additives.

To replace sodium and other minerals lost during athletic events or profuse sweating, electrolyte-replacement beverages have been developed. Some of these beverages contain 21 milliequivalents of sodium (about 1 g of sodium per liter). Beverages such as these provide no benefit over water for use during athletic events. Electrolytes lost during exercise are readily replaced from normal dietary sources.

Toxicity

Evidence correlates high sodium intake with elevated blood pressure and edema. Sodium restriction resulting in reduced blood pressure has been noted in 20 to 30 percent of those with essential hypertension. Because there are no known benefits to excessive sodium intake, consuming a low-to-moderate sodium diet throughout life will do no harm, and may prevent the development of hypertension (see Dietary Goals, p. 205).

SULFUR

Sulfur, which comprises 0.25 percent of the total body weight, is found in all tissues, especially those of high-protein content. Most of the sulfur is found in the three sulfur-containing amino acids methionine, cystine and cysteine. Sulfur also occurs in organic sulfates and sulfides in minor amounts and in the two B vitamins thiamin and biotin.

Functions

Sulfur compounds are metabolically important because of their ability to interconvert disulfide and sulfhydryl groups in oxidation-reduction reactions. As an example, cystine (a disulfide) can be reduced to cysteine (a sulfhydryl). Cystine incorporated into keratin in human hair is responsible for the sulfur smell when hair is burned. Nails, fur, feathers and skin also contain substantial amounts of sulfur-containing amino acids. Disulfide and sulfhydryl bonds provide the configuration and stabilization for protein molecules (for example, the permanent wave in hair or the biologically active shape of enzymes).

Glutathione activity in oxidation-reduction reactions is also dependent on cysteine's sulfhydryl group. The active sites of CoASH and lipoic acid are the sulfhydryl portions.

Besides its role in oxidation-reduction reactions, sulfur is important in many other compounds, reactions, and metabolites:

- Taurine, the precursor for the bile acid taurocholic acid, is synthesized from cystine by way of cysteine.
- The mucopolysaccharides (especially chondroitin sulfate and collagen) contain sulfur.
- Sulfur, in the presence of magnesium, is important in detoxifying metabolic sulfuric acid. The esters produced are excreted through the kidneys.
- Sulfolipids are found in the liver, brain and kidneys.

Most dietary sulfur is ingested in the amino acid forms, and excesses are excreted in the urine.

Deficiency

Deficiency symptoms of sulfur are unknown although it is conceivable that a diet severely lacking in protein could produce a deficiency.

Requirements

No RDAs or adequate and safe ranges have been set for sulfur.

Sources

Protein-containing foods such as meat, poultry, eggs, fish, legumes and milk are good sources of the mineral.

ZINC

Zinc is distributed in all tissues, with substantial concentrations in the eye (particularly the retina, iris and choroid), kidney, brain, liver, muscle and male reproductive organs (prostate, prostate secretions and spermatozoa). The majority of serum zinc is protein-bound; red blood cell zinc is associated with carbonic anhydrase; and zinc in leukocytes is bound with alkaline phosphatase. The blood contains about 900 mcg/100 ml.

Functions

The two to three grams of zinc found in the body function as a cofactor in over twenty enzymatic reactions and act as a binder in maintaining the structural configuration of some nonenzymatic molecules. Zinc is a cofactor for:

- Alcohol dehydrogenase (NAD+ is the organic cofactor for this metalloenzyme) which works in the liver to detoxify ethanol, methanol, ethylene glycol and other alcohols (such as vitamin A).
- Alkaline phosphatase; as such, zinc frees inorganic phosphates to be used in bone metabolism.
- Carboxypeptidase, functioning in the digestion of dietary proteins.
- Cytochrome C, important in electron transport and energy production.
- Glutamate dehydrogenase, necessary in the catabolism and synthesis of amino acids.
- Glyceraldehyde-3-P dehydrogenase in glycolysis.
- Lactate dehydrogenase, needed in the conversion of pyruvate to lactic acid during anaerobic energy production.
- Malate dehydrogenase, involved in the Krebs cycle and energy production.

Zinc acts as a binder to some amino acids, including histidine, cysteine and the albumins (glycoproteins in plasma) and it assists in binding nucleoproteins for the stabilization of RNA structure in protein synthesis. Zinc is also important:

- For insulin activity.
- For protein and DNA synthesis.
- For normal taste and wound healing.
- To maintain normal vitamin A levels and usage.
- In the structure of the bones.
- In the immune system.
- In some enzymatic reactions necessary for the

skin's normal oil gland function. For this reason, zinc has been implicated in the treatment of acne.

The average diet provides about 10 to 15 mg of zinc daily, one-third to one-half of which is absorbed. Zinc absorption is impaired when large amounts of calcium in the diet bind with phytates and zinc in the intestine and form an insoluble complex. Zinc, cadmium, silver and copper all compete for absorption sites in the intestine. Serum zinc declines with increases in dietary fiber.

Once zinc is absorbed, the prime avenue for its excretion is gastrointestinal and pancreatic secretions. Body stores of zinc are not readily mobilized, so a daily supply from the diet is required.

Deficiency

Because of its wide variety of functions, a zinc deficiency has extensive metabolic effects:

- Protein synthesis is impaired as is energy production.
- Collagen formation and alcohol tolerance are impeded.

These restricted functions alone result in diverse manifestations, including changes in hair and nails, dwarfism, sterility, skin inflammation, lethargy, anemia, poor wound healing and a loss of taste and smell.

Zinc levels are suppressed during acute and chronic infections, pernicious anemia, alcoholism, cirrhosis of the liver (zinc levels are 50 percent of normal), renal disease, cardiovascular disease, some malignancies, protein-calorie malnutrition and parenteral feeding.

A prenatal deficiency increases the risk of spontaneous abortion and restricts fetal growth. Congenital malformations include changes in skeletal, brain, heart, gastrointestinal tract, eye and lung tissue. The brain of a zinc-deficient infant contains less DNA than that of a healthy infant.

If a deficiency occurs during a period of rapid growth, the clinical manifestations (such as growth failure and sexual development) are more severe. Prostate gland, seminal vesicle and sperm degeneration from a zinc deficiency are reversible; testicular degeneration is not.

Zinc deficiencies seen in children in the United States suggest inadequate intake in other segments of the population as well. Zinc deficiencies may exist in preschool, hospital patient, low-income or elderly populations. Athletes and strict vegetarians may also have depressed zinc levels. Contributing factors to a low trace mineral diet are low meat consumption combined with refined grains, convenience foods and a high-fat, high-sugar intake.

A diet high in cereal and low in animal protein has produced zinc deficiency symptoms in Middle Eastern populations. The cause may be the high phytate diet, in which phytates bind with available zinc and reduce absorption. Geophagia and intestinal parasites common in these regions may also contribute to poor zinc absorption. Elevated environmental temperatures compound the problem, causing increased zinc loss through sweat.

Zinc-deficient animals demonstrate abnormal sulfur metabolism. This may explain the hyperkeratinization of the epidermis and parakeratosis of the esophagus in these animals. Animals manifest other behavioral abnormalities in a low-zinc state, including impaired learning, hypersensitivity to stress and increased aggression.

Requirements

Healthy adults require about 12.5 mg of dietary zinc each day. Nearly 6 mg are lost daily, and 40 percent of the mineral is absorbed from a mixed diet. The RDAs for zinc are:

Infants	
0–0.5 year	3 mg
0.5–1 year	5 mg
Children	
1–10 years	10 mg
Young adults and adults	
11+ years	15 mg
Pregnant	+5 mg
Lactating	+10 mg

Sources

Animal foods are a good source of zinc; excellent sources include oysters, herring, milk, meat and egg yolks. The zinc in whole grains, even though it is not well absorbed, supplies a substantial contribution to the diet, especially for the vegetarian with a reduced protein intake. Fruits and vegetables are poor sources of the mineral.

Breast milk contains a zinc-binding protein that increases absorption in the infant's intestinal tract. The zinc in infant formula is not absorbed as well as the zinc in breast milk.

Toxicity

Zinc toxicity is rare in humans. To produce toxic effects (such as muscle incoordination, dizziness, drowsiness, vomiting, gastrointestinal disturbances, lethargy, renal failure and anemia) doses of more than 2 g must be taken. Inhalation of zinc oxide produces temporary fever, cough, salivation, headache and leukocytosis. High doses of zinc may be ingested from food stored in galvanized containers.

ADDITIONAL TRACE MINERALS

Aluminum, arsenic, cadmium, lead, nickel, silicon, tin and vanadium are trace minerals identified in animal metabolism and found in human tissue. Their biological value is poorly understood and some are toxic.

Aluminum is found in abundance in the earth, but in small amounts in plant and animal tissues. Its greatest concentrations are in the brain, liver, thyroid and lungs. Dietary intakes of aluminum vary between 5 and 125 mg/day; the body effectively excretes 74 to 96 percent of this.

Major dietary sources of aluminum are food additives (such as sodium aluminum phosphate used as an emulsifier in processed cheese), table salt (with added sodium silico aluminate or aluminum calcium silicate) and potassium alum (used to whiten flour). Acidic foods (such as rhubarb) cooked in aluminum pots leech the mineral into the water and available foods. Aluminum is also found in some anatacids (as aluminum hydroxide gel), and some antiperspirants contain aluminum salts.

Large doses of aluminum have been implicated in the formation of osteomalacia in dialysis patients. Chronic renal insufficiency increases the severity of the aluminum-induced disease. Aluminum ingestion reduces total bone and matrix formation, periosteal bone and matrix formation. Aluminum toxicity causes impaired absorption of selenium and phosphorus. Low serum phosphate causes the bones to dissolve and the muscles to weaken and ache. The body adapts to higher aluminum intakes over time; however, in young people with hypophosophatemia or in individuals with abnormal bone metabolism, adaptation may not occur as readily. Large doses of the mineral also increase serum levels and increase urinary excretion two- to five-fold.

Aluminum toxicity has been implicated in brain disorders associated with aging, such as Alzheimer's disease. Aluminum-injected rats learn at a slower rate and have aluminum concentrations in their brains parallel to those found in the brains of Alzheimer's patients. (Alzheimer's is a form of senile dementia characterized by cerebral atrophy, neurofibrillary degeneration and senile plaques.)

Average amounts of aluminum in the diet (150 mg/day) do not appear to interfere with absorption or utilization of calcium, phosphorus, zinc, copper, selenium, iron or magnesium. Impairment in fluoride metabolism may occur, but this has yet to be proven. The risk of aluminum toxicity may be decreased in individuals with adequate calcium levels.

Arsenic is found throughout the human body, although its role is unknown. It is associated with the development of fatty liver. In the rat, arsenic is essential for growth and iron metabolism. This trace mineral is found in soil, water and food. Daily intake of arsenic averages 0.4 to 0.9 mg, an amount far below toxic levels.

Cadmium can accumulate to toxic levels over a lifetime because the mineral is not well excreted by the human body. However, cadmium is poorly absorbed, so normal dietary intake does not warrant concern for toxicity. Increases in dietary intake may be caused by soft water that leaches cadmium from pipes. Cadmium can also be inhaled from cigarette smoke, urban air pollution and the air near zinc refineries.

Workers exposed to copper-cadmium alloys have a high incidence of pulmonary emphysema. Anemia, proteinuria and amino aciduria are associated with high concentrations of cadmium (10 to 100 times normal) in the liver and kidneys. In the rat, toxic levels of cadmium predispose the animal to hypertension (similar effects have not been reported in humans), and lesions have been found in the kidneys and liver.

Because excretion of cadmium is slow, high concentrations can remain in the body for years after cessation of exposure. The estimated daily intake of cadmium is 13 to 24 mcg, with urinary excretion at approximately 10 mcg/liter.

Lead is found in some foods and in drinking water. It may be ingested from a variety of sources, including lead-based paint or plants grown on lead-rich soil. Lead is stored in the bones and the liver, and reacts with cell membranes in the body by altering their permeability or destroying them. This trace mineral inhibits sulfhydryl groups in molecules such as alpha-aminolevulinic acid dehydrogenase (important in hemoglobin synthesis). Lead, together with mercury, beryllium, cadmium and silver, inhibits alkaline phosphatase, catalase, xanthine oxidase and ribonuclease in fish. Body stores of lead can reach toxic levels; one of the symptoms of toxicity is anemia.

Mercury is a highly toxic, silver-white liquid metal that is somewhat volatile at room temperature. It is easily absorbed through inhalation of the fumes. Since mercury salts are used in medicine, agriculture and industry, it is not impossible to accumulate toxic levels as a result of environmental exposure.

Mercury has an affinity for the sulfhydryl groups on proteins. It alters protein structure, thus rendering it useless. Since enzymes, hormones, antibodies, hemoglobin and numerous cellular constituents are proteins, mercury can have far-reaching effects. Within minutes of ingesting a toxic dose of mercury, humans develop symptoms that include acute gastrointestinal inflammation, a metallic taste in the mouth, thirst, nausea, vomiting, and pain in the abdomen. Bloody diarrhea follows. The common first-aid remedy when a heavy metal such as mercury has been swallowed is a drink of milk. The mercury acts on the milk protein rather than degrading the protein in the mouth, esophagus and stomach. Vomiting is then induced to expel the milk and mercury.

Mercury poisoning is most common in workers exposed over long periods of time in the mining of mercury. This long-term exposure can result in acute mercury poisoning, characterized by fever, chills, loss of memory, renal damage, loosening of teeth, chest pain and weakness. In addition, nervousness, irritability, lack of ambition and loss of sexual drive are commonly reported.

The kidneys store 50 percent of the absorbed mercury. The rest accumulates throughout numerous tissues including the blood, liver, bone marrow, spleen, brain, myocardium, skin, salivary glands and muscles. Excretion occurs primarily through the urine and feces, although minute amounts are lost in sweat, hair, breast milk and exhaled air.

Fetal tissues are most susceptible to mercury toxicity. If the mother ingests substantial amounts of mercury during pregnancy, the fetus and placenta accumulate the mineral, resulting in neurological damage.

Acceptable daily intake of mercury has been established at about 0.1 mg per day or three pounds of fish containing 1 ppm methylmercury or one pound of fish containing 3 ppm per week. Dietary cadmium and zinc may accelerate accumulation of mercury in tissue mitochondria.

TABLE 9
Summary of Essential Inorganic Elements

Element*	Best food source	RDA (1980)**	ODA***	Principal functions	Major deficiency symptoms
Sodium (Na^+)	Table salt, salty foods, baking soda, baking powder	1.1–1.3 g‡		Acid-base balance, water balance, CO_2 transport, cell membrane permeability, muscle activity	Dehydration, acidosis
Potassium (K^+)	Vegetables, fruits, whole grains, meat, milk, legumes	1.9–5.6 g‡		Acid-base balance, water balance, CO_2 transport, membrane transport, neuro-muscular activity	Acidosis, renal damage, cardiac arrest
Calcium (Ca^{++})	Milk, milk products, bone meal, dark green leafy vegetables	800 mg	800–1500 mg	Formation of bones, teeth; blood clotting; cell membrane permeability; neuromuscular activity	Rickets (child), poor growth; osteoporosis (adult); muscle cramps
Phosphorus (PO_4)	Milk, milk products, egg yolk, meat, whole grains, legumes, nuts	800 mg	800–1500 mg	Formation of bones, teeth; constituent of buffers; constituent of metabolic intermediates, nucleoproteins, phospholipids, phosphoproteins; constituent of enzymes	Osteomalacia (rare); renal rickets; cardiac arrhythmia
Chloride (CL^-)	Animal foods, table salt	1.7–5.1 g‡		Electrolyte, osmotic balance; gastric acid; acid-base balance	Hypochloremic alkalosis (penicious vomiting)
Sulfur (SO_4)	Plant and animal proteins	2–3 g‡		Constituent of proteins, muco-polysaccharides, heparin, thiamin, biotin, lipoic acid; biotransformation	Cystinuria; methioninuria

Element*	Best food source	RDA (1980)**	ODA***	Principal functions	Major deficiency symptoms
Magnesium (Mg^{++})	Chlorophyll, nuts, legumes, whole grains	350 mg male; 300 mg female	400–700 mg	Constituent of bones, teeth; decreases neuromuscular sensitivity; enzyme cofactor	Muscular tremor; confusion; vasodilatation
Iron (Fe^{++} or Fe^{+++})	Liver, meats, egg yolk, green leafy vegetables, whole grains	10 mg male; 18 mg female	10–30 mg	Constituent of hemoglobin, myoglobin, catalase, cytochromes; enzyme cofactor	Microcytic-hypochromic anemia
Iodine (I^-)	Seafoods, iodized salt	150 mcg	250–350 mcg	Constituent of thyroxin; regulator of cellular oxidation	Goiter (hypothyroidism) cretinism
Fluoride (F^-)	Seafoods, some drinking water	1.5–4 mg‡ (1ppm in drinking water)		Constituent of tooth enamel; strengthens bones and teeth	Dental caries; osteoporosis
Zinc (Zn^{++})	Liver, pancreas, shellfish, most animal tissues, wheat germ, legumes	15 mg	15–35 mg	Constituent of insulin, carbonic anhydrase, lactic dehydrogenase, alcohol dehydrogenase, and other enzymes	Anemia; stunted growth; hypogonadism in male; decreased protein synthesis and wound healing; lack of taste
Copper (Cu^{++})	Liver, kidney, egg yolk, whole grains, legumes	2–3 mg‡	2–3 mg	Formation of hemoglobin; constituent of 11 oxidase enzymes	Anemia; aneurysms: CNS lesions
Manganese (Mn^{++})	Liver, kidney, wheat germ, legumes, nuts	2.5–5 mg‡		Cofactor for number of enzymes; synthesis of mucopolysaccharides	In animals – sterility, weakness
Cobalt (Co^{++})	Vitamin B12 in animal proteins	Not estab.		Constituent of vitamin B12	Anemia
Chromium (Cr^{+++})	Liver, animal and plant tissue, brewer's yeast	0.05–0.2 mg‡	0.1–0.2 mg	Necessary for glucose utilization; possible cofactor of insulin	Unknown; deficiency in diabetes claimed; decreased glucose tolerance in rats; possible relation to cardiovascular disease

Element*	Best food source	RDA (1980)**	ODA***	Principal functions	Major deficiency symptoms
Selenium (Se)	Liver, kidney, heart, whole grains, vegetables (varies with Se in soil)	0.05–0.2 mg‡	100–200 mcg	Constituent of glutathione peroxidase; inhibits lipid peroxidation	Liver necrosis and muscular dystrophy in animals; cardiomyopathy in humans
Molybdenum (Mo)	Liver, kidney, whole grains, legumes, leafy green vegetables	0.15–0.5 mg‡	250–1000 mcg	Constituent of xanthine oxidase, aldehyde oxidase	Decreased growth, food consumption, and life expectancy

*The inorganic elements included are those for which evidence exists that they are essential for humans. Other elements not included but present in the human body in trace amounts for which there is fragmentary evidence for some biochemical function, include cadmium, lithium, nickel, vanadium. Other elements present in human tissues in trace amounts as incidental constituents of no known significance include Ag, Au, Al, As, Br, Pb, Rb, Si, Ti, B.

**Recommended Dietary Allowance per day, established by the Food and Nutrition Board, National Research Council, 1980. The values given are for a normal adult male, 19 to 22 years of age.

***Optimal Daily Allowance is a theoretical range based on the authors' literature research. If no range is listed, the authors felt that there was insufficient evidence to make a recommendation at this time.

‡An estimated range recommended by the Food and Nutrition Board (1980) as a safe and adequate daily intake for healthy adults.

Adapted from Orten, J. and Neuhaus, O. *Human Biochemistry*. St. Louis: C. V. Mosby Co., 1982.

Nickel has no known specific metabolic role, although it is typically found with RNA, and may play a role in the activation of liver arginase and in maintaining cell membrane integrity. A nickel deficiency induced in animals results in retarded growth, dermatitis, pigmentation alterations, poor reproductive performance and impaired liver function. The average daily intake of nickel is 0.17 to 0.7 mg.

Silicon is the earth's most prevalent mineral and is consumed in gram quantities by humans each day. The highest concentrations of the mineral are found in the tissues of the skin, bones, tendons, trachea, aorta, lymph nodes and lungs. Lungs contain larger amounts than other tissues because of inhalation of environmental silica. Silicon content in some tissues (such as the heart, muscle, kidneys and tendons) remains constant as the tissues age. However, other tissues (including the skin, aorta and thymus) show marked reduction in the mineral with aging.

The function of silicon is poorly understood. Concentrations of the mineral are found in the area of active bone mineralization, implying an association between silicon and calcium binding with bone matrices. In chicks, silicon is essential in collagen formation, growth and bone calcification. It is necessary in the formation of mucopolysaccharides found in cartilage, bone, connective tissue and vascular walls.

Silicon intake in humans is variable and has been poorly researched; therefore, the mineral has not been proven necessary. Silicates are readily absorbed, with blood levels averaging 1 mg/100 ml. Excretion is primarily through the kidneys.

Silicosis is the best known toxicity symptom. This respiratory disease developed by miners results from silicon fibers stimulating fibrosis of the lungs and other tissues. Normal lung tissue is replaced with nodular connective tissue patches, perhaps caused by overproduction of collagen. Malignant tumor formation is not uncommon.

Tin is essential for normal growth in the rat, although its role in human metabolism is thought to be as a contaminant. High tin levels in the body can be caused by environmental contamination, such as leakage from the metal into canned foods. (Food storage, especially acidic foods, in unlacquered tin cans can result in a significant intake of the mineral.) Tin absorption is poor; it is not clear how much of the average 1.5 to 3.5 mg intake actually crosses the intestinal mucosa.

Vanadium, 20 mg of which is found in the body,

may be involved in both lipid and catecholamine metabolism. In the rat, vanadium is found in greatest concentration in bones and teeth. A vanadium-deficient diet fed to these animals results in impaired reproductive ability and increased infant mortality. These defects are passed down to offspring, with third and fourth generation descendants exhibiting reduced fertility. Dietary intake of vanadium averages 4 mg/day, and estimated requirements for adults are 0.1 to 0.3 mg/day.

Table 9 summarizes the essential inorganic elements.

Additional Reading

Goodhart, R. S. and Shils, M. E. *Modern Nutrition in Health and Disease*, 6th edition. Philadelphia: Lea & Febiger, 1980.

Orten, J. M. and Neuhaus, O. W. *Human Biochemistry*, 10th edition. St. Louis: The C. V. Mosby Co, 1982.

Part II
VITAMIN AND MINERAL RESEARCH:
SELECTED TOPICS

5

............VITAMIN RESEARCH: ....
SELECTED TOPICS

THE SCIENCE OF NUTRITION is highly dynamic. A wealth of new research data is generated daily in an attempt to answer numerous questions and satisfy the nutrition enthusiast's voracious appetite for more information. The field of nutrition began a mere fifty years ago as the study of the effects of a specific nutrient (e.g., retinol) on a specific disease (e.g., xeropthalmia), and it evolved in the 1940s into a general guide for menu planning. The establishment of the Four Food Groups served that purpose well. As new information was added exponentially to the growing body of knowledge, it became apparent that nutritional science overlapped with the social sciences and more comprehensive medical models. With advanced medical and scientific technology, subclinical deficiencies could be detected. The movement away from the medical disease model toward prevention of disease and optimal standards of health placed nutrition on the leading edge. The major killers in the United States were identified to be the degenerative diseases—cardiovascular disease, cancer and diabetes. Poor nutrition was identified as the greatest risk for these diseases. In addition, nutritional regulation of neurotransmitters, bioamines, hormones and neuromodulators opened the door to the study of the effect of nutrition on behavior. The science of nutrition also gained in complexity as more and more nutrient-nutrient and nutrient-drug interactions were identified.

Nutritional science is in its infancy. Its rapid growth is characterized by the trials and errors of youth. In this science, nothing is absolute; what was believed to be true yesterday may be disclaimed, altered or adapted tomorrow. The information in the preceding chapters is well established and generally accepted as fundamental knowledge about the functions and characteristics of vitamins and minerals. The information in the following two chapters is a summary of current research on additional roles vitamins and minerals might play in health and disease. The research studies present possible nutrient-disease correlations based on initial findings; in all cases, more research is required before final decisions are reached.

The authors feel obliged to refrain, in most cases, from voicing recommendations or conclusions. Without the firm answers that come from repeated, well-designed research studies, simple ''yes'' and ''no'' answers would be presumptuous. If the following chapters aid the reader in making personal nutrition decisions or merely keep him informed of current research trends, then they have served their purpose.

VITAMIN A

VITAMIN A AND CANCER

Vitamin A is necessary for the proper maintenance and growth of epithelial tissue. This established role for vitamin A is the basis for investigating its relationship to cancer. Epidemiological studies have shown a tendency for some human cancer risks to be higher in populations with low blood retinol.[1,2,3] (See also p. 139.)

Cancer of epithelial tissue represents 95 percent of all fetal malignancies in humans. This type of cancer always involves alterations in the normal differentiation of tissue (the ability of the tissue to develop into specialized tissues or organs). Vitamin A deficiency prevents normal differentiation of epithelial tissues. The relationship between vitamin A and cancer has therefore been studied more actively in recent years.

In animal studies, some of the retinoids have been shown to prevent or inhibit the development of cancer of the bladder, breast and skin. Complete tumor regression, using a combination of vitamin A or beta-carotene and radiation, has been achieved at Albert Einstein College of Medicine. In this study, the animals that were treated with radiation plus beta-carotene or radiation plus vitamin A showed complete tumor regression and survival beyond twenty-four months. The control mice in this study all died within three months.[4,5]

Smokers should take particular interest in a nineteen-year study published recently in Chicago showing that high dietary intakes of carotene, but not preformed vitamin A, are directly and dramatically linked to low incidences of lung cancer. The *British Journal of Cancer* reported a study that measured serum vitamin A concentration in twenty-six newly diagnosed lung cancer patients. Vitamin A levels in these patients were found to be significantly lower than levels in patients of similar age who had either nonmalignant lung disease or nonlung diseases. The authors of this study suggested that the low serum vitamin A levels might be due to low zinc levels. Zinc is necessary for the synthesis of retinol-binding protein and this protein was also reduced in the cancer patients. Without sufficient retinol-binding protein, the mobilization of vitamin A from the liver may be impaired.[6,7]

Whelan and coworkers at St. James University, Leeds, have found that serum zinc is significantly lower in patients with prostatic cancer than in controls. It is also known that there is a significantly lower serum zinc level in patients with benign prostatic hypertrophy. Hence serum zinc on its own is not a helpful predictor of the presence of prostatic cancer, but rather may be related to prostate function in general.

In this same study, vitamin A levels were noted as lower in the prostatic cancer group than in the control group. In mouse studies, deterioration of prostate tissue can be reversed by vitamin A supplementation.

The authors' correlation of vitamin A and zinc levels with prostate cancer lends further evidence that these two nutrients are intimately involved in the physiology of the prostate. Further research is needed to discover whether these elements might play a significant role in the development of the malignant prostate.[8]

A conflicting report regarding vitamin A and prostate cancer has been published by the University of Hawaii Cancer Center. The study involved analysis of 304 cases and 411 controls.

Men sixty-nine years and older had a higher incidence of prostate cancer as their vitamin A intake went up. Conversely, the subjects with the lower incidence of prostate cancer had lower intakes of vitamin A. The same relationship for total fat intake was reported. The authors suggest that vitamin A "may be a risk factor for certain human cancers and that caution against the premature promotion of vitamin A as a cancer preventive agent for the general population is needed."[9]

Investigators from the Institute of Cancer Research at the University of Bologna in Italy have studied the ability of vitamin A to inhibit UV-induced mutagenesis.

Cultures of a human epithelial-like cell line (EUE) were exposed to 3.5 J/m^2 of ultraviolet light to induce mutagenesis. The irradiated cells were grown with and without vitamin A 10^{-6} M, and the mutation frequencies were determined by selection against diphtheria toxin.

The frequency of diphtheria toxin-resistant mutants was lower in cultures treated with vitamin A, showing a clear inhibitory effect on mutagenesis induced by UV irradiation.[10]

VITAMIN A, ACNE AND PSORIASIS

Most of the research today involving vitamin A and acne is focused on either the retinol form of vitamin A or on analogs of vitamin A called retinoids. A 1982 study reported in the *Journal of the American Academy of Dermatology* proposed a mechanism of action for the clinical effectiveness of retinol and retinoids in the treatment of cystic acne and psoriasis.

Cystic acne and psoriasis are diseases in which the major components of the inflammatory cell infiltrate are neutrophils. Two to four weeks after the initiation of retinoid therapy, the neutrophils disappear. This particular study demonstrated that most retinoids, especially tretinoin and isotretinoin, inhibit superoxide anion production and lysosomal enzyme release. This is probably the mechanism whereby these agents, when applied topically or systematically, exert their anti-inflammatory effect and prevent the accumulation of neutrophils in acne lesions.[11]

An exciting side effect has been observed by researchers at the UCLA School of Medicine who have been treating psoriasis with the vitamin A derivative etretinate. The arthritis which frequently accompanies psoriasis was "greatly improved" in four of the seven patients receiving the retinoid therapy.[12]

Dr. T. G. Olsen of the Yale University School of Medicine suggests the use of oral vitamin A in "the small group of patients with grades III and IV inflammatory-cystic acne that has been unresponsive to conventional therapy." The author made an interesting statement in this 1982 review. Having commented on how well acne can be controlled today, he said that "successful acne management depends to a large extent on physician interest."[13]

VITAMIN A AND ALCOHOL

Drs. Grummer and Erdman of the Department of Food Science, University of Illinois, published a study in 1983 that investigated the effect of chronic alcohol consumption on vitamin A metabolism. The test animals showed a significant reduction in liver vitamin A levels. This reduction in hepatic vitamin A storage was not due to malabsorption of either retinyl acetate or beta-carotene, or to altered enzyme activity associated with alcohol and vitamin A metabolism.[14]

A 1982 German study has suggested a relationship between low blood levels of vitamin A in alcoholics and poor hearing. Fifty-nine patients with chronic alcoholic liver disease who had no history of ear infection, head injury, noise exposure or streptomycin usage and no hereditary deafness were tested for hearing ability. All age groups were found to have a hearing impairment.

The alcoholics in this study all had low levels of vitamin A, retinol-binding protein, beta-carotene and zinc. Recent animal studies were cited that demonstrated inner ear abnormalities following a vitamin A deficit. The authors suggested that poor hearing in alcoholics is due to a vitamin A deficit.[15]

VITAMIN A AND ATHEROSCLEROSIS

The major factors related to atherosclerosis include: (a) circulatory disturbances; (b) vasal endothelium distress; (c) alterations in plasma lipids; (d) dietary intake of saturated and polyunsaturated fatty acids; (e) alteration of mitochondrial and microsomal membranes; (f) injury of vascular membranes by immune complexes; and (g) excessive lipid peroxidations.

Vitamins A and E play a role in protecting endothelium. They also have antioxidant properties and can protect against excessive lipid peroxidation. These two vitamins can decrease platelet aggregation, affect oxygen transport and utilization, increase HDL-cholesterol and enhance the ability of nicotinic acid to low lipid levels. Thus, vitamin A and vitamin E have a positive affect on a number of factors related to atherosclerosis.[16]

Looking at associations between dietary changes and mortality rates can offer significant insight into some of the major diseases, such as heart disease. One study, reported in the *American Journal of Clinical Nutrition,* compared dietary changes and mortality in Israel between 1949 and 1977.

All of the investigated mortality rates in this study were positively associated with increasing total fat consumption. Moreover, vitamin A was consistently in negative association with mortality rates. The authors of this study suggested that "increased consumption of vitamin A may prove to reduce mortality rates due to heart disease and peptic ulcer."[17]

Scientists from the University of Parma, Italy, recently reviewed the literature regarding the use of vitamins in the prevention of hyperlipoproteinemia and atherosclerosis. Their summary stated that "the use of vitamins in metabolic disorders is justified both for the primary prevention, in order to correct the causes of hyperlipoproteinemias, and in the secondary prevention, to diminish the blood fat levels, which increase the risk of atherogenesis."[18]

VITAMIN A AND CYSTIC FIBROSIS

A number of studies have shown that many patients with cystic fibrosis (CF) have low plasma concentrations of vitamin A. The Department of Pediatrics at St. James's University Hospital in England recently assessed the levels of a number of nutrients in CF patients. Vitamin A was low in over 40 percent of the patients even though the patients were supplementing with 4,000 IU of vitamin A. When the patients were switched to a water-miscible form of vitamin A, 4,000 IU for a two-week period restored the serum vitamin A to normal.[19]

VITAMIN A AND DIABETES

Studies have shown that when non-diabetic animals are wounded, the early inflammatory response can be enhanced by vitamin A supplements. In animals treated with streptozotocin, diabetes is induced. In these animals, wound healing is impaired much as it is in human diabetics. The impaired wound healing in diabetic animals can be prevented with supplemental vitamin A.[20]

VITAMIN A, CAROTENE AND THYROID DISEASE

Austrian researchers have studied vitamin A and carotene levels in 190 patients with thyroid disease (31 hypothyroid, 53 hyperthyroid, 106 euthyroid). Serum levels of carotene were decreased only in hypothyroidism, but serum levels of vitamin A were significantly decreased in both the hypothyroid patients and the hyperthyroid patients.[21]

The effects of vitamin A in maintaining proper epithelial growth and function have been the basis for additional studies of diseases characterized by excessive accumulation of extracellular matrix material. Rheumatoid arthritis, idiopathic pulmonary fibrosis, scleroderma and cervical dysplasia might be associated with altered vitamin A activity.

VITAMIN A TRANSPORT

Zinc is necessary for the mobilization of vitamin A. In zinc-deficient children, 40 mg of zinc as a daily supplement can raise retinol and retinol-binding protein levels significantly.[22]

There are additional factors that can affect the transport of vitamin A. Dietary supply of vitamin A or beta-carotene, good quality protein and lipids all play a role in vitamin A transport. Controversy exists regarding the body's ability to absorb vitamin A and other fat-soluble vitamins without adequate dietary fat. Mead Johnson's Nutritional Division, Evansville, Indiana, has shown that vitamin A as retinyl palmitate is absorbed independently of dietary fat intake.

In another recent animal study from this group, the effects of dietary fat on the bioavailability of beta-carotene were studied. It was found that 10 percent dietary fat significantly improved the absorption and bioavailability of this nutrient. Hormonal control of vitamin A transport is effectuated by the glucocorticoids, sex hormones, and the hypothalamo-pituitary axis. Pathological conditions such as liver, kidney, intestinal and endocrine gland diseases can all affect the transport of vitamin A. [23,24]

B VITAMINS

B VITAMINS AND ALCOHOLISM

Alcoholics are frequently vitamin-deficient, although clinical evidence of this deficiency could be masked by the side effects of prolonged and excessive use of alcohol. Three major causes of this deficiency have been defined: poor dietary intake, malabsorption and increased vitamin need by the alcoholic. Vitamin B1 deficiency, in particular, is known to result in a neurologic impairment called Wernicke's syndrome.

Recently, ninety-seven patients admitted to three London hospitals for alcohol detoxification were studied to determine the influence of vitamin supplementation on the success of the alcoholic rehabilitation program. In this study, all patients had been drinking in excess of 1.5 liters of alcohol per day and were chemically dependent.

The treatment trial was placebo controlled, with individuals receiving oral vitamin supplements, intravenous vitamin therapy or a placebo during a five-day detoxification regime. Thiamin, riboflavin and pyridoxine status were assessed by measurements of specific erythrocyte enzyme activities. The results of the study were interesting in that even with vitamin B1 supplementation, the vitamin B1-dependent enzyme (transketolase) did not show normal activity in the alcoholics. The authors concluded that vitamin supplementation in chronic alcoholics undergoing detoxification might not be completely efficacious because of poor conversion of the vitamin to its coenzyme or the relative inability of specific enzymes to utilize cofactors because of acetaldehyde inhibition.

This may indicate that higher levels of vitamin therapy are needed or that specific preformed coenzymic forms of vitamins need to be administered intravenously.[25]

B VITAMINS AND PREMENSTRUAL TENSION

A review of the relationship of nutrition to premenstrual syndrome indicates that a number of patients have benefited from extra magnesium and B-complex vitamins. Women with symptoms of anxiety associated with PMS improved with increased doses of vitamin B6 daily. Those women with symptoms of headache, dizziness and craving for sweets responded to magnesium, zinc, niacin and vitamin C supplementation, whereas those who had breast tenderness responded to vitamin E supplementation.

The differential approach to the management of PMS through nutrition modification indicates the important role that nutritional status may play in the modulation of certain endocrine dysfunctions.[26]

B VITAMINS AND RADIATION THERAPY

Levels of vitamins B1, B2 and B6 have been evaluated in cancer patients treated with radiation. The method of evaluation was by prospective erythrocyte enzyme tests: transketolase for vitamin B1, glutathione reductase for B2 and AST for B6. This work indicated that radiation-treated cancer patients demonstrated normal vitamin B1 activity, but they showed depressed activities of enzymes activated by vitamins B2 and B6.

The authors of the study concluded that X-radiation of mammary, cervical or ovarian cancers results in a defect in the metabolism of vitamin B2, and a tumor-induced error in the metabolism of vitamin B6; both of these conditions can be therapeutically avoided by treatment of the patient with a vitamin B-complex supplement.[27]

THIAMIN (B1) AND RIBOFLAVIN (B2) IN NERVOUS SYSTEM DISORDERS

Two papers have been published indicating the potential of vitamin B1 and vitamin B2 therapy in specific types of nervous system disorders.

The first of these two papers presents a case report on a forty-three-year-old patient who had been treated with the oral hypoglycemic tolazamide (Tolinase). He developed symptoms which included poor coordination and balance, mental confusion and memory loss. His drug-induced condition was "tentatively" diagnosed as Wernicke's encephalopathy.

When Vitamin B1 was given at levels of 200 mg per day the patient's condition "improved dramatically within two hours." One month later his earlier nervous system problems had resolved, except for some mild difficulties in walking.

The second report is that of a girl, aged thirteen, who developed progressive exercise intolerance and a weakening of her arms and legs, but no pain or cramps. Studies indicated that she was suffering from an enzyme deficiency due to the lack of availability of a vitamin B2 derivative. Administration of vitamin B2 at high levels (100 mg per day) "resulted in a striking and sustained improvement." After several weeks, the patient could perform sustained heavy exercise, such as bicycling, with none of the adverse symptoms that she had sustained prior to supplementation.

The investigators concluded that a large dose of vitamin B2 was important in promoting optimal enzyme function in this patient, so that her muscles could continue to operate efficiently, and that the reason she required the high level was her own genetic uniqueness.[28,29]

THIAMIN (B1) AND TEA CONSUMPTION

Thiamin (B1) deficiencies, both in man and experimental animals, result in a dysfunction of the nervous system. The most common symptom is polyneuritis, which results in muscular weakness. The tannin in tea has been reported to act as an anti-B1 agent.

The Department of Biochemistry at Mahidol University, Bangkok, has reported that in animal studies that they conducted, prolonged consumption of tea led to vitamin B1 deficiency. It was also mentioned that supplementing with high doses of vitamin B1 or discontinuing the tea resulted in restoration of normal B1 levels.[30]

RIBOFLAVIN (B2) AND ANEMIA

Treatment of microcytic anemia in men with iron or iron with riboflavin has been evaluated in a group of individuals from four to sixty years of age. Eighty men and eighty children with initially poor iron status were identified and assigned to three treatment groups. The treatments consisted of a placebo, ferrous sulfate and ferrous sulfate with riboflavin.

The inclusion of riboflavin with the iron supplement greatly enhanced recovery from microcytic anemia. This was particularly true for those individuals whose initial hemoglobin levels were strikingly low. Therefore, combination therapy in the hypochromic microcytic anemia patient utilizing iron and riboflavin together seems to be far superior to administering an iron supplement by itself.[33]

RIBOFLAVIN (B2) AND PSYCHOTIC SYMPTOMS

Symptoms of riboflavin deficiency have been identified in two patients at Napa State Hospital, California. Both patients with severe psychotic symptoms received high doses of phenothiazine derivatives and lithium. Neither patient responded to the drug therapy.

Upon administration of riboflavin and a multivitamin supplement, the physical findings of riboflavin deficiency cleared. The authors noted that, "Unexpectedly, the patients' psychotic symptoms also improved or remitted."[34]

RIBOFLAVIN (B2) AND FEMALE ATHLETES

The 1980 Recommended Dietary Allowance for riboflavin (1.3 mg or 0.6 mg/1000 calories) does not appear to be adequate for healthy, physically active women. In a recent study, Cornell University researchers demonstrated that biochemical normality with respect to riboflavin status could not be achieved with current RDA levels in women who were moderately or very active.

Even when these active women were not allowed to engage in their usual physical activity programs, riboflavin deficiency developed in spite of a dietary intake at RDA levels. Boosting intake of the vitamin ameliorated the situation. However, when physical activity was again resumed, riboflavin status declined. Physical signs of riboflavin deficiency did not develop, but biochemical parameters deteriorated. (Erythrocyte glutathione reductase activity is used to measure riboflavin status.) It appears that marginal riboflavin deficiency might impair the stability of the red cell.

This study suggests that actual riboflavin requirements may be higher in physically active women than the current RDA. The authors propose an intake of 0.96 mg/1000 calories and 1.1 mg/1000 calories for those who exercise regularly.[35]

RIBOFLAVIN (B2) AND SICKLE CELL DISEASE

Sickle cell disease (SCD) is characterized by deficiencies of essential nutrients (such as zinc, folate, iron and vitamin E) and impaired growth. Treatment of SCD routinely involves folate supplementation. Zinc in therapeutic doses has also been used to accelerate body growth and sexual maturity in SCD patients.

Researchers at the Department of Pediatrics, South Alabama College of Medicine, Mobile, measured red blood cell glutathione reductase levels in SCD patients and discovered very low status of the riboflavin vitamin (B2)-derived enzyme FAD, which is necessary for glutathione reductase activity. Dietary records indicated adequate riboflavin intake. Because deficiency symptoms occurred during adequate vitamin B2 intake, there might be decreased absorption, altered metabolism, increased excretion or an increased need for vitamin B2 in SCD.

In the patients studied, damage to blood cells could have been a result of increased oxidative attack of cellular membrane lipids, resulting in the sickle cell crisis. Riboflavin stimulates FAD production; FAD is then used as part of the glutathione reductase enzyme to prevent cellular damage from superoxide. Further studies are needed to define whether the riboflavin problem in SCD is related to underconversion to FAD, to increased excretion or to impaired absorption.[36]

NIACIN (B3) AND ADRIAMYCIN TOXICITY

The chemotherapeutic agent adriamycin can have cardiac toxicity. This side effect could be a result of increased lipid peroxidation of the cardiac muscle. This relationship has led to the suggestion that alpha-tocopherol (vitamin E) might be useful in prevention of the cardiac toxicity induced by adriamycin. Studies in dogs seem to indicate that vitamin E supplementation prevents cardiac death without interfering with the chemotherapeutic potential of the drug.

A team of researchers at the University Medical School, Dusseldorf, has found that niacin, given to animals in large doses, also prevents the cardiotoxicity of adriamycin without destroying the chemotherapeutic benefit of the drug.

These findings suggest that the cardiotoxicity of adriamycin is due to a depletion of NADPH which is utilized to metabolize adriamycin. Lack of NADPH results in a reduction of sulfhydryls in the heart. Since niacin is a necessary precursor of NADPH, increasing niacin levels apparently provides the necessary level of NADPH to protect the heart adequately.[31]

NIACIN (B3) AND CHOLESTEROL

Supplementation with high levels of niacin (as nicotinic acid) is known to produce a lowering of blood cholesterol levels. Dr. William Conner at the University of Oregon School of Medicine has shown that niacin can be part of an effective cholesterol-lowering program for type 3 hyperlipoproteinemics.

In a study conducted jointly by researchers from Cairo University (Giza, Egypt) and the University of Maryland, niacin and inositol hexanicotinate (IHN) were compared for cholesterol-lowering properties. IHN combines the properties of both inositol and nicotinic acid as a lipotropic agent.

IHN was found to be much more effective in reducing blood cholesterol levels than nicotinic acid and could achieve significant clinical reduction of cholesterol at much lower doses than required when utilizing niacin alone.

This study indicates that IHN may be a more effective cholesterol-lowering substance than niacin or inositol alone, and warrants further clinical trial.[32]

PYRIDOXINE (B6) AND CARPAL TUNNEL SYNDROME

The work of Drs. Watanobi and Folkers has indicated that many individuals suffering from carpal tunnel syndrome (CTS) are responsive to vitamin B6 supplementation. Recently, researchers at the Department of Rehabilitation Medicine at the University of Washington examined the potential role of insufficient vitamin B6 as an etiological factor in the development of CTS.

In this study, subjects presenting the symptoms of CTS were categorized by electrodiagnostic criteria. A significant difference in pyridoxine metabolic activity was found in various groups of patients with and without carpal tunnel syndrome.

Study results indicated that an abnormality of vitamin B6 metabolism was a factor highly correlated with the presence of peripheral neuropathy, but not with CTS alone. Moreover, the previously suggested link between vitamin B6 and the amelioration of carpal tunnel syndrome might actually be related to unrecognized peripheral neuropathy, which is responsive to vitamin B6.[37]

PYRIDOXINE (B6) AND RUNNERS

More and more people are engaging in strenuous activity such as running. The impact these activities could have upon vitamin/mineral nutriture and turnover is thus of interest to increasing numbers of people.

Researchers at Oregon State and Loma Linda Universities found that in trained adolescent athletes who had just completed a 4500-meter run, there was a significant alteration in the blood level of the coenzyme form of vitamin B6 (pyridoxal 5-phosphate). Investigators could not conclude that there was an increased need for vitamin B6 in people who exercise, but they did show for the first time that exercise in the form of a long-distance run can dramatically alter levels of the active coenzymic form of vitamin B6.

The implications of this for glucose metabolism and other functional roles of vitamin B6 phosphate remain to be determined.[38]

PYRIDOXINE (B6) AND DEPRESSION

Current research indicates that depressed patients have disturbed serotonin production. The neurotransmitter serotonin is derived from dietary tryptophan with the aid of vitamin B6. Researchers at the National Institute of Mental Health, Bethesda, and the Department of Human Nutrition and Foods at Virginia Polytechnic Institute and State University have been studying the vitamin B6 status of depressed patients and obsessive-compulsive patients.

They found that the depressed subjects had significantly lower plasma B6 levels than the control subjects. But no significant difference was found between the controls and the obsessive-compulsive patients, although one-fourth of the obsessive-compulsive patients had inadequate vitamin B6 status.[39]

PYRIDOXINE (B6) AND PREGNANCY

Considerable controversy surrounds the use of supplemental vitamin B6 in pregnancy. Clinicians are concerned about potential toxic side effects that might result from large doses.

A study was conducted on twenty-four pregnant women who, prior to labor, had taken daily supplements of vitamin B6 at the level of 100 mg per day. Investigators studied oxygen affinity of maternal blood and of cord blood as compared to those of unsupplemented controls. The difference between supplemented and unsupplemented groups was found to be statistically significant. The supplemented group had offspring with increased oxygen affinity when measured five days after birth.

Injected vitamin B6 had a somewhat greater effect than the same amount given orally. Prolactin levels in maternal and cord blood were not affected. Vitamin B6 given to the mother at the start of labor was suggested to improve the oxygen transport function of a newborn's blood, and could help protect against thromboembolism following labor.[40]

PYRIDOXINE (B6) AND RENAL STONES

Oxalic acid concentration in the urine is a significant factor in the formation of calcium oxalate calculi. Vitamin B6 has been reported to lower oxalic acid excretion in patients with type 1 primary hyperoxaluria. Researchers at the University of Vienna, Austria, have studied the effect of pyridoxine in twelve patients suffering from calcium oxalate stones.

The patients received 300 mg of pyridoxine daily for six weeks. Mean urinary oxalic acid excretion dropped from 480.9 to 336.8 mmoles (normal range is 320 plus or minus 92 mmoles). The authors concluded that "by reducing calcium oxalate saturation, the pyridoxine-induced reduction of urinary oxalic acid excretion is beneficial in preventing the formation of idiopathic calcium oxalate calculi."[41]

CYANOCOBALAMIN (B12) AND SULFITE SENSITIVITY

Sulfite-sensitive reactions such as severe asthma attacks have been under study at the Research Institute of Scripps Clinic, La Jolla. Among asthmatics with no history of restaurant-provoked asthma, approximately 5 percent demonstrated a positive reaction to sulfite.

Cromolyn sodium, atropine and doxepin can prevent or suppress the sulfite reaction. Studies have shown that vitamin B12, an oxidation catalyzer, readily forms a sulfite-cobalamin complex with sulfite. When given orally in doses from 1 to 4 mcg, vitamin B12 can prevent or diminish the sulfite reaction.

Researchers "found that vitamin B12 (cyanocobalamin) affords the best protection against sulfite-induced hyperreactivity when given preceding the challenge. Moreover, cobalamin seems to be effective over a greater time period than the pharmacological blockers."[42]

CYANOCOBALAMIN (B12) AND THE SCHILLING TEST

One of the most common methods for determining vitamin B12 status is the Schilling test. This test measures the ability to absorb vitamin B12 from an aqueous solution. However, recent findings suggest that there is no relationship between the actual B12 status of the patient and the results of the Schilling test.

Dawson and researchers at the North Manchester General Hospital, Manchester, England, evaluated the reliability of the Schilling test in forty-nine subjects. They found that defective absorption was present in six patients who had adequate intake of vitamin B12 and normal Schilling test results but had low serum vitamin concentrations. They concluded that the malabsorption of the vitamin from protein-bound sources not detected by the Schilling test may produce this vitamin B12 deficiency syndrome. The conditions did not respond to treatment with vitamin B12.

Two forms of vitamin B12 are available for therapy, cyanocobalamin and hydroxocobalamin. Researchers from Albany Medical College and the Veterans Administration Medical Center, Albany, New York, have evaluated the relative availability of these two forms of vitamin B12. Hydroxocobalamin was found to be a more efficient form in the treatment of common vitamin B12 deficiencies, principally because of better retention and greater availability to the cells.[43,44]

CYANOCOBALAMIN (B12) AND DIABETES

The symptoms of vitamin B12 deficiency and the secondary neuropathic signs of diabetes are very similar,

if not identical. This would suggest that the neurologic symptoms of degeneration seen in diabetics may be the result of vitamin B12 deficiency.

This hypothesis has recently been studied in animals that were made diabetic and whose metabolism of vitamin B12 was examined. Diabetic animals were found to have a dramatically reduced management of vitamin B12. This suggests that tissue metabolism of cobalamines was disturbed and resulted in the buildup of substances such as methylmalonic acid, which is associated with the production of neurological disorders. The researchers concluded that a possible disturbance in vitamin B12 metabolism could be an important factor in the development of acute diabetic neuropathy.[45]

FOLIC ACID AND CERVICAL DYSPLASIA

A study was done of eighty-nine women, all of whom had mild to moderate cervical intraepithelial neoplasia (CIN) on Pap smear and a cervical lesion visible by colooscopy. All the women had been taking oral contraceptives for at least six months. After random assignment to a group that received either 10 mg of folic acid or a placebo for three months, all women were examined monthly during the three months by colposcopy and Pap smear. A punch biopsy was taken at the end of the three-month trial. Data on forty-seven women indicate that the folate had a significant beneficial effect on cervical epithelium. Pap smears revealed a decreased amount of cervical dysplasia in women in the folate group while there was no change in the control group. Punch biopsies noted significantly less cervical dysplasia in folate-treated women. CIN completely disappeared in seven women, all of whom were in the folate-supplemented group. Folic acid administration also seemed to reduce the progression of the dysplasia.

This study indicates that pharmacologic doses of folic acid can reverse cervical tissue changes. If it is determined that cervical intraepithelial neoplasia is definitely a precancerous lesion, folic acid holds great promise for cancer prevention.[46]

FOLIC ACID AND DEPRESSION

For several years, reports have suggested that one of the brain biochemical pathways contributing to affective behavior disorders is activation of the methylation process. This activation results in over-methylation of amine neuromodulators in the brain and ultimately in alteration of normal brain biochemistry. The nutrients that are important in this methylation pathway include folic acid, methionine, vitamin B12 and pyridoxine.

Folic acid deficiency has been found to cause a variety of neuropsychiatric disturbances, most commonly depression. This may be the result of interruptions to the proper methyl transfer reactions in the brain.

One additional substance involved in the control of methyl groups is the intermediate compound S-adenosyl methionine (SAM). Trials over the last five years have suggested that SAM has antidepressant properties. Recent clinical trials have shown that SAM is as effective in the treatment of depression as the standard antidepressant medications.

Current research from the Department of Neurology, Institute of Psychiatry, London, has demonstrated that folic acid and SAM, administered together, may have important functions in the management of certain affective personality disorders. The researchers concluded, "The observations that we have reviewed have important research and therapeutic implications in psychiatry."[47]

VITAMIN C

VITAMIN C AND COLLAGEN

Vitamin C (ascorbate) is essential for the biosynthesis of collagen. In the genetic disorder known as Ehlers-Danlos syndrome, collagen is not synthesized properly. This results in skin fragility, easy bruising, hyperelasticity, atrophic scars and soft pseudotumors, bleeding tendency and other symptoms.

Researchers at Emory University, Atlanta investigated the potential of pharmacologic doses of ascorbate (5 g/day) in a five-year-old boy suffering from dermal fibroblasts associated with Ehlers-Danlos syndrome. Collagen lysyl hydroxylase levels were significantly depressed in this patient. Because this enzyme and ascorbate are necessary for the production of mature collagen, vitamin C trials were undertaken. The authors concluded that "ascorbate in pharmacologic doses increases both lysyl hydroxylase activity and total collagen biosynthesis."[48]

VITAMIN C, ASPIRIN AND ARTHRITIS

A number of studies have been undertaken recently to investigate the interactions between aspirin and ascorbic acid. When animals were given vitamin C alone, peak plasma levels were reached within ninety minutes.

But when the vitamin C was given along with aspirin, the peak vitamin C plasma levels were lower and the time to reach this peak was delayed considerably. The absorption of vitamin C during the first 400 minutes of the study was reduced by half when it was given along with aspirin.

Human studies have shown similar findings. Investigators at the University of Surrey, Guilford, England, report that the normal increases in plasma, leukocytes and urine from a single oral dose of 500 mg of vitamin C is blocked by 900 mg of aspirin. It has been suggested that aspirin blocks the absorption of ascorbic acid by interfering with its active transport.

Currently, there are studies being conducted to measure the beneficial effects of vitamin C in treating arthritis. Vitamin C supplementation might be particularly beneficial for the arthritic using aspirin on a regular basis.[49,50]

VITAMIN C AND DIABETES

Vitamin C is one of many nutritional factors that influence lipid metabolism. It is necessary for the conversion of cholesterol to bile acids. A marginal deficiency of vitamin C can adversely affect serum cholesterol levels.

Diabetics have an increased incidence of atherogenic complications. Because vitamin C appears to reduce the severity of atherosclerosis, researchers have explored the relationship between vitamin C, glucose and insulin on the cellular level. Vitamin C transport is greatly enhanced by the presence of insulin. In vitro studies of cell cultures show that elevated glucose levels impair the uptake of vitamin C by the cell. This indicates that the diabetic state (low insulin, high glucose) reduces vitamin C transport into the cell, which may contribute to injury of the vessel wall and increase the risk for atherosclerosis.[51,52]

Vitamin C is also known to play an important role in leukocyte immune function. Diabetics often have problems with immune function, wound healing and peripheral vascular stability. A recent study has shown that diabetics have vitamin C-depleted leukocytes. Administration of an intravenous glucose load in diabetics or normal subjects resulted in a prompt decrease of vitamin C levels in the white blood cells in both groups. The rate of decline of vitamin C in the white cells closely correlated with the rate of change of blood glucose, suggesting that the diabetics were more prone to vitamin C depletion of the white cells than normal subjects.

The researchers in Seattle, Washington, concluded that this hyperglycemic-induced depletion of vitamin C from the white cells could be clinically important in terms of reducing immune protection. Depletion of the white cell vitamin C content could have a significant impact upon the ability of the cell to be involved in immune protection and could be related to poor blood sugar control.[53]

VITAMIN C AND BURNS

Ascorbic acid (AA) has been demonstrated to be an essential factor in certain facets of the immune system, including phagocytosis and cell-mediated immune responses. Burn patients have an increased risk of infection as a result of depressed immune system activity, and the effects of various doses of AA on anesthetized mice given murine burns have been studied at the New Jersey Medical School.

Vitamin C significantly retarded the transformation from second- to third-degree burns. The authors concluded that "this beneficial effect may, in part, be due to the improvement of immune capabilities of these animals."[54]

VITAMIN C AND COLDS

Animal studies have shown that vitamin C enhances the production of interferon, a protein that is excreted by cells which have been exposed to a virus. The role of interferon is not completely understood, but it appears that it works in the early stages of viral exposure by preventing the multiplication of the virus until other facets of the immune system take over. Though it possesses broad antiviral activity, interferon works only on a short-term basis.

During the past decade, controversy has raged over the effectiveness of vitamin C in curing the common cold.

In vitro, lymphocytes treated with ascorbic acid have been demonstrated to offer an enhanced response to lymphocyte challenge. This suggests that symptoms associated with the inflammatory process (such as those resulting from the common cold) could conceivably be reduced or obviated by supplemental ascorbic acid. Consequently, ascorbic acid might not prevent infection by the common cold virus (as suggested some years ago by Pauling), but rather might minimize the symptoms associated with the infection based upon this model.[55]

VITAMIN C AND DENTAL EROSION

Several reports have appeared in the literature from dental research studies indicating that habitual users of unbuffered vitamin C lozenges could suffer severe dental erosion.

A thirty-year-old woman showed severe dental erosion of the enamel caused by her chewable vitamin C tablets (600 mg tablets taken three times daily for three years). The upper and lower premolars were affected, with the occlusal surfaces and cusps missing.

The pH of vitamin C in the ascorbic form is less than 2, making it a very strong acid in the oral cavity. A normal extracted premolar kept in a solution of vitamin C became rough and lost 5 percent of its width in two weeks. Other acidic material, such as citrus fruits, tomatoes, bananas, fruit juices, carbonated beverages, vinegar, candy, aspirin and hydrochloric acid replacements can also contribute to dental erosion.

The authors suggest that a vitamin C supplement should be swallowed rather than chewed, or taken in a buffered, more natural ascorbate form.[56]

VITAMIN C AND STRESS

The role of vitamin C in stress conditions has been studied for over ten years. Under physical stress and in acute myocardial infarction, leukocyte and serum vitamin C levels are decreased. In addition, an increase in the serum level of cortisol has been observed under these conditions.

The benefits of high doses of ascorbate in heart disease (a severe stress condition) have been demonstrated. Because there appears to be a relationship between stress, cortical stimuli and ascorbate, scientists from the Department of Clinical Chemistry, Karolinska Hospital, Stockholm, have studied the excretion of catecholamines and cortisol in the urine of subjects with different vitamin C intakes. The research was undertaken to determine if there is any difference in response to a standardized stressor.

A low-ascorbate group of volunteers was compared to a group taking 3 g of ascorbate daily. Both groups were stressed using the color-word conflict task, and then tested for urinary excretion of catecholamines and cortisol. The group taking the high dose of ascorbate excreted significantly greater amounts of adrenaline under stress than did the low-dose group.

These results are significant for two reasons. First, the study demonstrated a different effect in humans than previously reported in rats. Rats on high intakes of ascorbate do not have altered metabolism and excretion of catecholamines. Therefore, negative animal studies on the role of vitamin C in stress cannot be applied to humans. Second, this study suggests another role of vitamin C in the biosynthesis of catecholamines in addition to its role as a cofactor for specific enzymes.

If an increased excretion of adrenaline is beneficial for humans under stress, then the results of this study imply that a high intake of vitamin C under stressful conditions may ". . . lead to a better-prepared individual."[57]

VITAMIN C AND PSYCHIATRIC PATIENTS

Plasma vitamin C levels have been studied in 885 patients in a psychiatric hospital, and compared to those of 110 healthy controls. The psychiatric patients showed significantly lower vitamin C levels (0.51 mg/100 ml) than the healthy controls (0.87 mg/100 ml). The length of stay in the hospital had little effect on vitamin C levels.

Clinical symptoms of vitamin C deficiency generally do not appear until plasma concentrations fall below 0.35 mg/100 ml. However, a significant difference in vitamin C levels clearly exists in the particular psychiatric population studied when compared to a healthy population. Further studies are necessary to determine the relationship between low vitamin C levels and psychiatric disorders.[58]

VITAMIN C AND FERTILITY

The consumption of 1000 mg of vitamin C a day may be able to restore fertility in infertile men in just four days, according to a study. Dr. Earl Dawson, with his colleagues at the University of Texas Medical Branch, Galveston, studied thirty-five male patients who could not impregnate their wives because of sperm defect.

These men were found to have low serum ascorbic acid levels and, upon supplementation with a 500 mg capsule of vitamin C every twelve hours, their sperm motility improved as their serum vitamin C level increased. As the study continued with the daily supplementation of vitamin C, it was confirmed that there were statistically significant continuous improvements in sperm function in these men.

Dawson reports that pregnancy occurred in the wives of all of the twelve men whom his group had placed on the sixty-day vitamin C regime, whereas the wives

of the eight subjects who had received the placebo did not become pregnant. This would suggest that vitamin C may play an important role in normalizing sperm motility and alleviating certain forms of male infertility.[59]

VITAMIN C: NATURAL VS. SYNTHETIC

Natural vitamin C that contains bioflavonoids may have advantages over the synthetic form of vitamin C. In animal studies, bioflavonoids have been shown to improve the utilization and storage of vitamin C. But similar studies on humans have provided conflicting reports. Drs. Vinson and Bose at the University of Scranton, Pennsylvania, have reported that in their animal studies, "The bioavailability of the natural vitamin C was significantly greater than that of the synthetic ascorbic acid." The natural vitamin C remained in the serum for a longer period of time.[60]

VITAMIN C AND CANCER

The work of Drs. Pauling and Cameron has suggested that vitamin C in high doses may be useful for the prevention of cancer and possibly in the treatment of certain forms of the disease.

However, in seeming contradiction are research findings from the University of Perugia, Italy, which suggest that vitamin C actually may accelerate solid-tumor growth in certain strains of mice. The work of Dr. Liotti and his colleagues has revealed that low doses of vitamin C seem to stimulate tumor cell multiplication in vitro, while at high doses the opposite occurs and the vitamin C is antineoplastic.

Although this work cannot be directly extrapolated to human studies, it does suggest that there may be a nonlinear relationship between vitamin C and its effect upon tumors.

Certain tumors are known to be stimulated by reducing factors other than vitamin C (such as cysteine or reduced glutathione). Therefore, low doses of vitamin C in this system may be tumor-promoting because of the vitamin's reducing characteristics, whereas high doses of vitamin C may be antineoplastic because of immune potentiation or an unknown direct tumor cytotoxic action.

Human bowel cancer appears to be caused by both dietary imbalances (high-fat, low-fiber) and environmental carcinogens. In order for the experimental carcinogen DMH to induce cancer, it must first be oxidized. Scientists at the Vince Lombardi Cancer Clinic of the Medical College of Wisconsin studied the effects of vitamin C and BHA, a preservative added to many convenience foods, in preventing experimental large bowel neoplasia.

BHA produced the most beneficial effects by decreasing the incidence and density of large bowel tumors. Vitamin C increased the ratio of adenomas to adenocarcinomas but had no affect on the incidence or density of large bowel tumors.

The maximum effects on tumor incidence were observed when BHA was administered along with vitamin C. The authors concluded that vitamin C has only a modest effect whereas BHA has a significant effect in preventing DMH-induced large bowel cancer.[61] (See also p. 140.)

VITAMIN D

DO ADULTS NEED TO SUPPLEMENT THEIR DIET?

There is considerable controversy surrounding the question of whether older individuals do or do not need vitamin D supplementation. Dr. Kummerow, Department of Food Science, University of Illinois, believes that excess vitamin D is a risk factor in atherosclerotic conditions. His work indicates that the average American is receiving excessive vitamin D in the absence of any additional supplementation, because of the level of vitamin D in our milk, cereal products and other foods. He believes that high levels of vitamin D create an excess of calcium, which plays a role in the development of atherosclerosis and in the aging process.

Dr. Kummerow concluded in a recent article that "attempting to prevent bone disease in the elderly by additional vitamin D supplementation may not only be ineffective, but may increase the risk of accelerating other diseases, resulting from excessive tissue calcium accumulation."

On the other side of the question are those investigators who feel that vitamin D nutriture is lacking in the elderly American, and that this nutrient needs to be supplemented. Omdahl and Garry, University of New Mexico, studied individuals supplementing with 400 IU of vitamin D daily. The test group showed no biochemical signs of excess vitamin D; when alkaline phosphatase was measured, a lowered rate of bone loss during vitamin D supplementation was noted. The researchers concluded: "It seems reasonable that the prudent use of vitamin D supplements could represent one of the successful modalities for the prevention and treatment of bone diseases in the elderly."

It is the authors' opinion that adults who supplement their diet with vitamin D should be monitored.[62, 63]

VITAMIN D AND DEAFNESS

Findings of vitamin D deficiency associated with bilateral cochlear deafness suggest that too little vitamin D can have debilitating affects other than rickets.

Following the 1981 preliminary findings of two cases of deafness associated with vitamin D deficiency, "Eight additional patients who presented to the London Hospital with progressive bilateral deafness have been found to have low vitamin D levels."[64]

VITAMIN E

VITAMIN E, CANCER AND CHEMOTHERAPY

Vitamin E maintains the integrity of the body's polyunsaturated fats and protects them from oxidative attack by peroxides, superoxides and other free radicals. Several tissues (including the heart) contain low levels of antioxidant defense enzymes and are particularly susceptible to these poisonous byproducts. It is interesting to note that tumors are also low in antioxidant-containing enzymes.[65,66]

Some of the anticancer drugs currently in use generate superoxides. These superoxides are believed to have some anti-tumor activity. Unfortunately, they also have undesirable side effects on the heart. Given that the nature of these useful cancer-fighting drugs is a "two-edged sword," supplementation with an antioxidant (such as vitamin E) might protect the non-tumorous tissue by scavenging the toxic byproducts produced by these drugs.

The therapeutic usefulness of Adriamycin (dioxorubicin) has been limited because of several undesirable side effects, the most serious of which is cardiotoxicity. Existing data suggest that this toxicity is caused by direct or indirect cell membrane damage through the formation of free oxygen radicals.

Studies of the effects of this antibiotic on polymorphonuclear leukocyte (PMNL) function demonstrated a marked reduction in ability to stimulate oxidative metabolism of cells exposed to Adriamycin. This study proved that human leukocytes that were pre-incubated with vitamin E before exposure to Adriamycin displayed significantly greater oxygen consumption.

Researchers at the University of Texas concluded that because vitamin E is a potent antioxidant, it may combine with natural cellular protective mechanisms to guard against Adriamycin damage to cellular membranes.[67]

Vitamin E may be helpful in decreasing lipoperoxide formation during chemotherapy. Lipoperoxides are thought to be carcinogens that enhance the activation of other carcinogens.

Free radicals, such as singlet oxygen, superoxide, hydroxyl and hydrogen peroxide, can form lipoperoxides during normal metabolism. Certain drugs can also increase the formation of these lipoperoxides.

There are enzyme systems and nutrients which act as antioxidants to detoxify these lipoperoxides; these include superoxide dismutase (SOD), glutathione peroxidase, catalase, vitamins A, C, and E and the mineral selenium.

A number of studies have demonstrated that cancerous tissue is deficient in all components of this antioxidant defense system. And many of the anticancer drugs create more lipoperoxides, which further increases the need for antioxidant defense.

Recent research from England has demonstrated that when rats are given vitamin E supplements along with the popular anticancer drug 5-fluorouracil, the levels of liver and plasma lipoperoxides are significantly lower than when the anticancer drug is given alone.[66]

In addition to being a protective partner of anticancer drugs, vitamin E appears to have an inhibitory effect on tumor growth. Scientists from the Department of Radiology at the University of Colorado Health Sciences center studied the effects of vitamin E on cultures of cancerous (melanoma) and non-cancerous mouse cells.

Natural d-alpha tocopherol succinate induced morphologic alterations and growth inhibitions in these cancer cells. When the vitamin E was removed four days after treatment, the changes remained irreversible for a period of twenty-four hours, after which the resistant and partially affected cells renewed cell division.

Other forms of vitamin E such as synthetic dl-alpha tocopherol or dl-alpha tocopherol acetate were ineffective in producing the same effects as the d-alpha tocopherol acid succinate. The authors concluded that vitamin E succinate might be a potentially useful therapeutic agent for tumors.[68]

It has been demonstrated that the nitrates and nitrites commonly used in processed foods and beer can cause cancer. But recent testing in animals showed that vitamin E can prevent the formation of nitrosamines, the cancer causing agent formed by the interaction of nitrates and nitrites with an amino group. In addition vitamin E also prevents the liver toxicity that is caused by the nitrosamines.[69]

VITAMIN E: ANTIOXIDANT PROPERTIES

Published reports note that vitamin E supplementation can result in protection against sickle cell and thalassemic crisis. These conditions are characterized by the oxidative breakdown of red blood cells. Investigations at the Louisiana State University School of Medicine have found that vitamin E protects against the peroxidative damage to phospholipids in red blood cell membranes by way of its antioxidant capabilities. Because vitamin E is fat soluble, it is localized in the fat-rich membranes of cells awaiting the arrival of oxidants. Before these oxidants can chemically induce damage to critical membrane phospholipids, the vitamin E diffuses them, thereby preventing free radical pathology.[70]

VITAMIN E, PREMENSTRUAL SYNDROME AND BENIGN BREAST DISEASE

Researchers have studied the effect of vitamin E in a double-blind, randomized protocol on premenstrual syndrome in seventy-five women with benign breast disease (fibrocystic disease). The women were given vitamin E at levels of 150, 300 or 600 IU per day, or a placebo control.

Controlling for age and pretreatment scores, vitamin E had a significantly greater affect on controlling symptoms of premenstrual syndrome than the placebo. The effective dosage ranged from 150 IU to 600 IU daily, depending on the particular symptoms and other characteristics of the group studied.

The authors concluded that vitamin E supplementation may be of value in women with severe premenstrual syndrome.[71]

VITAMIN E, SELENIUM AND BREAST CANCER

Epidemiological studies have demonstrated a potential role for the trace element selenium in protecting humans from certain types of cancer. In animal studies, selenium's anticarcinogenic activity has been shown to inhibit the growth of mammary tumors.

The Department of Breast Surgery and Breast Cancer Research Unit, Roswell Park Memorial Institute, Buffalo, New York, recently reported that vitamin E, although apparently ineffective by itself, is able to "potentiate" the ability of selenium to inhibit the development of artificially induced mammary cancer in rats.

Because both of these nutrients possess antioxidant properties, either directly or indirectly, this characteristic was explored as a potential mechanism for their combined anticarcinogenic effects. Selenium exerts its antioxidant influence by regulating selenium-dependent glutathione peroxidase enzyme. Increased biosynthesis of this enzyme depends on the availability of its protein constituent.

Providing selenium levels above the enzyme's protein constituent level will not further increase this enzyme's activity. Therefore, the anticarcinogenic properties of selenium in large doses are probably not related to its antioxidant properties in glutathione peroxidase.

Although it has greater activity as an antioxidant than selenium, vitamin E was not capable of inhibiting tumor formation. The authors concluded that "vitamin E might provide a more favorable climate against oxidant stress, thereby potentiating the action of selenium through some other mechanism."[72] (See also pp. 140, 133.)

VITAMIN E: ALPHA TOCOPHEROL VS. GAMMA TOCOPHEROL

Natural vitamin E mixtures contain alpha, beta, gamma and delta forms of tocopherol. Purified concentrates of natural vitamin E are exclusively alpha tocopherol. Whether an antioxidant difference exists between the purified alpha form and the natural mixture of tocopherols has been a topic of debate.

A recent study at the University of California, Davis, found that the alpha-tocopherol form of vitamin E is more effective than gamma tocopherol as an in vivo antioxidant. The study also noted that natural source vitamin E was more effective as an in vivo antioxidant than previously reported. This finding was based on natural E's inhibition of vitamin E deficiency symptoms in animals.[73]

VITAMIN E: NATURAL VS. SYNTHETIC

Natural RRR tocopherol (vitamin E) may have a different effect upon the enzyme phospholipase A_2 from that of the synthetic all-rac tocopherol (dl-tocopherol).

Recent studies indicate that there is a difference in the biochemistry at the cellular level in the potential control of precursors to hormones (such as the prostaglandins) between the natural vitamin and synthetic vitamin E. This may be the result of a difference in stereoisomerism of the various vitamin E substances.[74]

VITAMIN E, PLATELETS AND THROMBUS FORMATION

Vitamin E has an impact upon blood clotting and prevention of thrombus formation, and has been used historically in the treatment of thrombophlebitis. The effect of vitamin E administration on platelet function was examined in a group of normal volunteers.

Platelet aggregation was induced by collagen ADP and epinephrine, and the effect of vitamin E on this activation in twenty men and twenty-seven women divided into three experimental groups was measured in weekly intervals. The vitamin E dose ranged from 400 to 1200 IU per day, with a second treatment group receiving aspirin, 300 mg, every other day, and the third group a combination of vitamin E and aspirin.

Adhesiveness of platelets in response to collagen was not affected by aspirin, but showed a highly significant reduction when vitamin E or vitamin E and aspirin were given together. The authors concluded that vitamin E is not a potent antiaggregatory agent when administered in doses up to 1200 IU per day, but that it is a mild antiaggregating substance. A difference was observed in its impact in men and women, with the impact of vitamin E in women on platelet aggregation being slightly greater than in men.

This study demonstrates that different individuals may have significantly different responses to vitamin E in terms of platelet dynamics, and concludes that a broader trial with varying dose ranges of vitamin E should be initiated to clarify this biochemical individual difference.[75]

VITAMIN E AND MENORRHAGIA

In studies of human subjects and animals, intrauterine contraceptive devices (IUDs) have been associated with increased menstrual blood loss (MBL), also called menorrhagia.

Women with MBL and IUDs in situ have been shown to have levels of H_2O_2 in the endometrium that are substantially higher than is control groups. There appears to be a correlation between MBL and endrometrial H_2O_2 formation at levels greater than can be disposed of by catalase or other homeostatic mechanisms. H_2O_2 seems to be involved in the production of highly reactive free radicals causing lipid peroxidation in cell membranes and possible tissue damage.

Researchers at the Institute of Post Graduate Medical Education and Research in Calcutta, India, have conducted clinical trials of vitamin E as an antioxidant and free-radical-trapping agent that may benefit IUD-fitted women. The fifty-one women who participated in the study were given 100 mg doses of vitamin E orally every other day for two weeks, without regard for where the day fell in their menstrual cycles.

Practically every participant responded positively to the vitamin E treatments, with their MBLs restored to normal limits. The results offer promise for vitamin E as an antioxidant in the management of MBL associated with IUD use. This news may have a far-reaching impact, especially as the governments of underdeveloped countries encourage the widespread use of intrauterine contraceptive devices to control population growth.[76]

VITAMIN E AND CHOLESTEROL

Research from the Department of Chemical Pathology, University of Pretoria, Republic of South Africa, has failed to support claims that alpha-tocopherol supplements can significantly increase serum total HDL levels. This particular study suggests that vitamin E increases LDL cholesterol and HDL_3 cholesterol.

The authors state that "the established lipoprotein risk indices (LDL/HDL and HDL_3/HDL_2 ratios) were unfavorably affected as a result of alpha-tocopherol treatment." On the basis of available evidence, the researchers conclude that there is no reason to believe that alpha-tocopherol plays a role in the prevention and treatment of atherosclerotic disease.

In a related study from the Harvard Medical School, LDL cholesterol was marginally decreased in test subjects after sixteen weeks of vitamin E supplementation at 800 IU daily. The authors concluded that "vitamin E does not alter plasma lipids in normal adults."[77,78]

VITAMIN E AND THE NERVOUS SYSTEM

Many investigators feel that there is no diagnosable deficiency disease symptom seen with vitamin E deficiency in children or adults; however, a number of recent reports have indicated that poor absorption of fats and fat-soluble vitamins in children is associated with certain problems in the nervous system, the symptoms of which resemble those of muscular dystrophy.

A progressive neuromuscular disease was found in children who had gallbladder problems and could not properly emulsify and absorb fats and fat-soluble vitamins efficiently. These children were found to have very low blood vitamin E levels. When they were given injections of vitamin E, symptoms of nervous system degeneration improved markedly. In most of these children oral high dose vitamin E supplementation was not effective, because they were unable to absorb vitamin E properly. This indicates that a diet rich in a nutrient does not necessarily guarantee optimal nourishment.

The major symptoms of these vitamin E deficiency cases were poor balance and equilibrium, eyesight difficulties, loss of delicate sense of touch and hyper reflexes. Most of these symptoms were successfully treated with vitamin E therapy.[79, 80]

VITAMIN E: MISCELLANEOUS NOTES

Vitamin E and Air Pollution. Vitamin E may be the answer for city dwellers seeking protection from air pollution and its damaging effects on exposed and sensitive tissues such as the lung and retina. A recent study showed vitamin E to be protective against the damaging effects of high concentrations of oxidant pollutants commonly found in the air of our cities.[81]

Vitamin E and Infections. Resistance to bacterial diseases and antibody response are enhanced in animals with the use of vitamin E even where no previous deficiency existed.[82]

Vitamin E and Aging. Some of the degenerative problems of aging, such as cramp-like pains and weakness in the legs, are alleviated with high levels of vitamin E.[83]

Vitamin E: Safe Dosages. Twenty-eight subjects were tested with vitamin E doses ranging from 100 IU to 800 IU per day. Evaluation of twenty standard clinical blood tests failed to reveal any disturbance in liver, kidney, muscle, thyroid, erythrocyte, leukocyte and coagulation parameters.[84]

Vitamin E Labeling. Supplements are labeled with an unusually wide variety of hyphenated terms, each term referring to a specific compound of the E family, known as tocopherols. The first part of the complete name of a specific vitamin E compound will be either dl- or d-. The tocopherols that occur in nature are named d-. Those named dl- are synthetics. The d-forms of the vitamin show two to three times more biological activity than dl- forms.[85]

The second part of the name can be alpha, beta, gamma or delta. These four terms name the four different vitamin E compounds found in nature. The alpha form is by far the most active as a nutrient.

The third part of the name will have a -yl ending if the alpha compound has been chemically isolated from the beta, gamma and delta by a special procedure. The -ol ending is used if no such chemical isolation process has taken place.

The fourth part of the name, if there is a fourth part, shows that the vitamin has been combined with another compound to improve its stability. The acetate formulation is used for liquids; the succinate form is used for tablets and dry capsules.

The term ''mixed tocopherols'' indicates that the product contains all four forms of the compound, alpha through delta. The International Units (IU) listed on labels refer only to the alpha form, because that is the accepted standard of measurement.

REFERENCES

1. Bjelke, E. Dietary vitamin A and human lung cancer. *Int.J.Canc.*, 15:561, 1975.

2. Wald, N., Idle, M., Borehan, J. et al. Low serum-vitamin A and subsequent risk of cancer: Preliminary results of a prospective study. *Lancet*, 2:813, 1980.

3. Peto, R., Doll, R., Buckley, J.D., et al. Can dietary beta-carotene materially reduce human cancer rates? Review article. *Nature*, 290:201, 1981.

4. Sporn, M.B. and Newton, L. Chemoprevention of cancer with retinoids. *Fed.Proc.*, 38:2528, 1979.

5. Seifter, E., Rettura, G. and Levenson, S. C3HBA tumor therapy with radiation, b-carotene and vitamin A: A two-year follow-up. *Fed.Proc.*, 42(4):768, 1983.

6. Shekelle, R. Dietary vitamin A and risk of cancer in the Western Electric study. *Lancet*, 1:1185-1190, 1981.

7. Atukorala, S., Basu, T.K., Dickerson, J.W., et al. Vitamin A, zinc and lung cancer. *Br.J.Canc.*, 40:927-931, 1979.

8. Whelan, P., Walker, B.E. and Kelleher, J. Zinc, vitamin A and prostatic cancer. *Br.J.Urol.*, 55:525-528, 1983.

9. Kolonel. L., Hankin, J. and Lee, J. Diet and prostate cancer. *Am.J.Epid.* 118:454, 1983.

10. Rocchi, P., Ferreri, A.M., Capucci, A., et al. Effect of vitamin A acetate on mutagenesis induced by ultraviolet light in human cells. *Eur.J.Canc.Clin.Onc.*, 19:1312, 1983.

11. Camisa, C., Eisenstat, B., Ragaz, A., et al. The effects of retinoids on neutrophil functions in vitro. *J.Am.Acad.Derm.*, 6:620-629, 1982.

12. Kaplan, R.P., Russell, D.H. and Lowe, N.J. Etretinate therapy for psoriasis: clinical responses, remission times, epidermal DNA and polyamine responses. *J.Am.Acad.Derm.*, 8:95-102, 1983.

13. Olson, T.G. Therapy of acne. *Med. Clin. North. Am.* 66(4):851-871, 1982.

14. Grummer, M.A. and Erdman, J.W. Effect of chronic alcohol consumption and moderate fat diet on vitamin A status in rats fed either vitamin A or beta-carotene. *J.Nutr.*, 113:350-364, 1983.

15. Lohle, E., Scholmerich, J., Vuilleumier, J.P., et al. Vitamin A-Konzentration im Plasma und das Horvermogen bei Patientenmit chronischer alkholischer Leberschadigung.'' *HNO*, 30:375-380, 1982.

16. Butturini, U. Vitamins E and A in vascular diseases. *Acta Vit.Enzym.*, 4:15-19, 1982.

17. Palgi, A. Association between dietary changes and mortality rates: Israel 1949 to 1977: A trend-free regression model. *Am.J.Clin.Nutr.*, 34:1569-1583, 1981.

18. Butturini, U. Vitamine E prevenzione delle iper-lipoproteinemia e dell'aterosclerosi. *Acta Vit.Enzym*, 2:135-146, 1980.

19. Congden, P.J., Bruce, G., Rothburn, M.M., et al. Vitamin status in treated patients with cystic fibrosis. *Arch.Dis.Child.*, 56:708-714, 1981.

20. Seifter, E., Rettura, G., Padawer, J., et al. Impaired wound healing in streptozotocin diabetes. Prevention by supplemental vitamin A. *Ann.Surg.*, 194:42-50, 1981.

21. Smolle, J., Wawschin, O., Hayn, H., et al. (GE) Serum levels of vitamin A and carotene in thyroid-disease. *Acta Med.Aust.*, 10:71-73, 1983.

22. Effect of zinc supplementation of plasma levels of vitamin A and retinol-binding protein in malnourished children. *Clin.Chim.Acta*, 93:97, 1979.

23. Richardson, G.G. and Cook, D.A. Effect of dietary fat on B-carotene bioavailability. *Fed.Proc.*, 42:811, 1983.

24. Glover, J. Factors affecting vitamin A transport in animals and man. *Proc.Nutr.Soc.*, 42:95-101, 1983.

25. Brown, L.M., et al. Efficacy of vitamin supplementation in chronic alcoholics undergoing detoxification. *Alc.Alcsm.* 18: 157-166, 1983.

26. Abraham, G. E. Nutritional factors in etiology of the premenstrual tension syndromes. *J.Repr.Med.*, 28:446-461, 1983.

27. Grimm, U., Wulff, K. and Schmidt, W. (GE) On the

supply with vitamin B1, vitamin B2 and vitamin B6 in the case of carcinoma before and after X-ray therapy. *Deut.Gesund.*, 38(40):1563-1566, 1983.

28. Kwee, I.L., and Nakada, T. Wernicke's encephalopathy induced by tolazamide. *N.E.J.Med.*, 309:599, 1983.

29. Arts, W.F.M., Scholte, H.R., Bogaard, J.M., et al. NADH-CoQ reductase deficient myopathy: successful treatment with riboflavin. *Lancet* 2:581, 1983.

30. Ruenwonasa, P. and Pattanavibag, S. Decrease in the activities of thiamine pyrophosphate dependant enzymes in rat brain after prolonged tea consumption. *Nutr.Rep.Int.*, 27: 713-721, 1983.

31. Scheulen, M.E., Schmitt-Graff, A. and Schmidt, C.G. Reduction of adriamycin cardiotoxicity by niacin and isocitrate. *Proc.Am.Assoc. Canc.Res.*, 24:251, 1983.

32. Abou El-Enein, A.M., Hafez, Y.S., Salem, H., et al. The role of nicotinic acid and inositol hexanicotinate as anticholesterolemic and antilipemic agents. *Nutr.Rep.Int.* 28:899-911, 1983.

33. Powers, J.J., Bates, C.J., Prentice, A.M., et al. The relative effectiveness of iron and iron with riboflavin in correcting a microcytic anemia in men and children in rural Gambia. *Hum.Nutr.Clin.Nutr.*, 37:413-425, 1983.

34. Zaslove, M., Silverio, T. and Minenna, R. Severe riboflavin deficiency: A previously undescribed side effect of phenothiazines. *Ortho.Psych*, 12:113-115, 1983.

35. Belko, A.Z. and Roe, D.A. Exercise effects on riboflavin status. *Fed.Proc.*, 42:804, 1983.

36. Varma, R. N., et al. Depressed erythrocyte glutathione reductase activity in sickle cell disease. *Am.J.Clin.Nutri.* 38: 884-887, 1983.

37. Byers, C.M., DeLisa, J.A., Frankel, D.L., et al. Pyridoxine metabolism in carpal tunnel syndrome, with and without peripheral neuropathy. *Arch.Phys.Med.Rehab.*, 64:125, 1983.

38. Leklem, J.E. and Schultz, T.D. Increased plasma pyridoxal 5'-phosphate and vitamin B6 in male adolescents after 4500-meter run. *Am.J.Clin.Nutr.*, 38:541-548, 1983.

39. Russ, C.S., et al. Vitamin B6 status of depressed and obsessive-compulsive patients. *Nutr.Rep.Int.*, 27:867-873, 1983.

40. Temesvari, P., Szilagyi, I., Eck, E., et al. Effects of antenatal load of pyridoxine on the blood oxygen affinity and prolactin levels in newborn infants and their mothers. *Acta Ped.Scan.*, 72:525, 1983.

41. Balcke, P., Schmidt, P., Zazgorni, J., et al. Pyridoxine therapy in patients with renal calcium-oxalate calculi. *Kidney Int.*, 24:419, 1983.

42. Simon, R.A., et al. Sulfite-sensitive asthma. *Research Institute of Scripps Clinic Scientific Report*, 39, 57-58, 1982-83.

43. Dawson, D.W., Sawers, A.H. and Sharma, R.K. Malabsorption of protein-bound vitamin B12. *Br.Med.J.*, 288:675, 1984.

44. Hall, C.A., Begley, J.A. and Green-Colligan, P.D. The availability of therapeutic hydroxocobalamin to cells. *Blood*, 63:335-341, 1984.

45. Bhatt, H.R., Linnell, J.C. and Matthews, D.M. Can faulty B12(cobalamin) metabolism produce diabetic neuropathy? *Lancet*, 2:572, 1983.

46. Check, W.A. Folate for oral contraceptive users may reduce cervical cancer risk. *J.A.M.A.*, 244:633–634, 1980.

47. Reynolds, E.H. and Stramentinoli, G. Folic acid, S-adenosylmethionine and affective disorder (editorial). *Psych.Med.*, 13:705-710, 1983.

48. Janko. A., Dembure, P., Priest, J., et al. The response of human lysyl hydroxylase to ascorbic acid in the biosynthesis of collagen. *Clin.Res.*, 31:897A, 1983.

49. Basu, T.K. Impairment of absorption of ascorbic acid following ingestion of aspirin in guinea pigs. *Bioch.Pharm.*, 31:4035-4038, 1982.

50. Basu, T.K. Vitamin C–aspirin interactions. *Int.J.Vit.Res.*, 23:83-90, 1982.

51. Hughes, R.E. Vitamin C and cholesterol metabolism. *J.Hum.Nutr.*, 30:315, 1976.

52. Kapeghian, J.C., and Verlangieri, A.J. Effect of glucose on C-14-labeled ascorbic acid uptake by endothelial-cells in the presence of insulin. *Fed.Proc.*, 42:795, 1983.

53. Chen, M.S., Hutchinson, M.L., Pecoraro, R.E., et al. Hyperglycemia-induced intracellular depletion of ascorbic acid in human mononuclear leukocytes. *Diabetes*, 32:1078-1081, 1983.

54. Spillant, C.R. Hollinshead, M.E. and Lazaro, E.J. The beneficial effects of ascorbic acid in murine burns. *Clin.Res.*, 31:A690, 1983.

55. Mirza, J. and Amaral, L. The effect of ascorbic acid on the human lymphocyte. *Int.J.Tiss.*, 5:141-143, 1983.

56. Giunta, J.L. Dental erosion resulting from chewable vitamin C tablets. *J.Am.Dent.Ass.*, 107:252-256, 1983.

57. Kallner, A. Influence of vitamin C status on the urinary excretion of catecholamines in stress. *Hum.Nutr.Clin.Nutr.*, 37:405-411, 1983.

58. Schorah, C.J., Morgan, D.B. and Hullin, R.P. Plasma vitamin C concentrations in patients in a psychiatric hospital. *Hum.Nutr.Clin.Nutr.*, 37:447-452, 1983.

59. Gonzalez, E.R. Sperm swim singly after vitamin C therapy. *J.A.M.A.*, 249:2747-2751, 1983.

60. Vinson, J.A. and Bose, P. Comparative bioavailability of synthetic and natural vitamin C in guinea pigs. *Nutr.Rep.Int.*, 27:875-880, 1983.

61. Jones, F.E., Komorowski, R.A. and Condon, R.E. Hydroxyanisole in the chemoprevention of 1, 2–Dimethylhydrazine-induced large bowel neoplasms. *J.Surg.Oncol.*, 25:54-60, 1984.

62. Holmes, R.P. and Kummerow, F.A. The vitamin D status of elderly Americans. *Am.J.Clin.Nutr.*, 38:335-336, 1983.

63. Omdahl, J.J. and Garry, P.J. Reply to letter by Holmes and Kummerow. *Am.J.Clin.Nutr.*, 38:337-338, 1983.

64. Brookes, G.B. Vitamin D deficiency—a new cause of cochlear deafness. *J.Laryng.Otol.*, 97:405-420, 1983.

65. Chow, C.K. Nutritional influence on cellular antioxidant defense systems. *Am.J.Clin.Nutr.*, 23:1066, 1979.

66. Capel, I.D., Leach. D. and Dorell, H.M. Vitamin E retards the lipoperoxidation resulting from anticancer drug administration. *Anticanc.Res.*, 3:59, 1983.

67. Pickering, L.K., et al. Modulation of polymorphonuclear leukocyte function by dioxorubicin (adriamycin) and alpha tocopherol (vitamin E). *J.Clin.Lab.Immun.*, 11:95-100, 1983.

68. Prasad, K.N. and Edwards-Prasad, J. Effects of tocopherol acid succinate on morphological alterations and growth inhibition in melanoma cells in culture. *Canc.Res.*, 42:550-555, 1982.

69. Walker, E.A. *Environmental Aspects of Nitroso Compounds.* IARC Scientific Publications No. 19, Lyon, France: pp. 159-212.

70. Jain, S.K. Vitamin E and stabilization of membrane lipid organization in red blood cells with peroxidative damage. *Biomed.Biochim. Acta*, 42:43-47, 1983.

71. London, R.S., Sundaram, G.S., Murphy, L., et al. The effect of a-tocopherol on premenstrual symptomatology: A double-blind study. *J.Am.Coll.Nutr.*, 2:115, 1983.

72. Horvathe, P.M. and Clement, L.P. Synergistic effect of vitamin E and selenium in chemoprevention of mammary carcinogenesis in rats. *Canc.Res.*, 43:5335-5341, 1983.

73. Dillard, C.J., Gavino, V.C. and Tappel, A.L. Relative antioxidant effectiveness of alpha-tocopherol and gamma-tocopherol in iron-loaded rats. *J.Nutr.*, 113:2266-2273, 1983.

74. Chan, A.C. and Luttinger-Basch, C. Vitamin E inhibits platelet phospholipase A2 in vivo and in vitro: Demonstration of

potency difference between RRR tocopherol and all-rac tocopherol. *Fed. Appl. and Biol. Sci. Abst.*, 3028, 1983.

75. Steiner, M. Effect of alpha-tocopherol administration of platelet function in man. *Thrombosis and Hemeostasis*, 49:73-77, 1983.

76. Dasgupta, P.R., Dutta, S., Banerjee, P., et al. S. Vitamin E in the management of menorrhagia associated with the use of intrauterine contraceptive devices (IUCD). *Int.J.Fert.* 28:55-56, 1983.

77. Serfontein, W.J., Ubbink, J.B., and deVilliers, L.S. Brief scientific reports: Further evidence on the effect of vitamin E on the cholesterol distribution in lipoproteins with special reference to HDL subfractions. *Am.J.Clin.Path.*, 79:604-606, 1983.

78. Stampfer, M.J., et al. Effect of vitamin E on lipids. *Am.J.Clin.Path.*, 79:714-716, 1983.

79. Werlin, S.L., Harb, J.M., Swick, H., et al. Neuromuscular dysfunction and ultrastructural pathology in children with chronic cholestasis and vitamin E deficiency. *Ann.Neur.*, 13:291, 1983.

80. Guggenheim, M., Ringel, S.P., Silverman. A., et al. Progressive neuromuscular disease in children with chronic cholestasis and vitamin E deficiency: diagnosis and treatment with alpha tocopherol. *J.Ped.*, 100:51, 1982.

81. Ehrenkranz, R.A., Bonta, B.W., Albow, R.C., et al. Amelioration of bronchopulmonary dysplasia after vitamin E administration: A preliminary report. *N.E.J.Med.*, 299:564, 1978.

82. Tengerdy, R.L. *Vitamin E: A Comprehensive Treatise* (L.J. Machlin, ed.). New York: Marcel Dekker, 1980.

83. Haeger, K. Long-term treatment of intermittent claudication with vitamin E. *Am.J.Clin.Nutr.*, 28:1179, 1974.

84. Farrell, P.M. and Bieri, J.G. Megavitamin E supplementation in man. *Am.J.Clin.Nutr.*, 28:1381, 1975.

85. Horwitt, M.K. Relative biological values of d-a-tocopheryl acetate and all-rac-a-tocopheryl acetate in man. *Am.J.Clin.Nutr.*, 33:1856-1860, 1980.

6

............MINERAL RESEARCH:..
SELECTED TOPICS

CALCIUM

LOW CALCIUM INTAKE ASSOCIATED WITH HYPERTENSION

CALCIUM and magnesium play important roles in cardiovascular physiology. Both calcium and magnesium are important in the regulation of blood pressure. But of the seventeen nutrients analyzed in the Health and Nutrition Examination Survey I, conducted by the National Center for Health Statistics, only calcium distinguished hypertensives from normotensives in all subgroups. Dietary calcium consumption was 18 percent less in hypertensive persons than in the normotensive.[1]

YOGURT AND CALCIUM SUPPLEMENTATION LOWERS CHOLESTEROL LEVELS

Cultured milk products have been shown to have a beneficial effect on serum cholesterol levels. In the work of Hepner at the North Carolina Agricultural Research Service, North Carolina State University, Raleigh, the use of yogurt and other dairy products in humans resulted in a significant fall in total serum cholesterol within seven days. The mechanism for this cholesterol-lowering effect is not known, but may be attributed to increased calcium intake due to the high calcium content of these dairy products.

To study this hypothesis, the effects of yogurt and calcium supplementation upon total serum and HDL cholesterol were studied in twenty-one human subjects.

The impact of yogurt supplementation on serum cholesterol levels was most significant in females. Total serum cholesterol was reduced and HDL cholesterol was elevated by both yogurt and calcium supplementation. At least some of the effect of dairy products on serum cholesterol is thus attributable to enhanced calcium intake.

The sensitivity difference between males and females in this study was not well understood. The difference may be related to differing calcium metabolism in the two sexes.[2]

CALCIUM, MAGNESIUM, AND HYPERTENSION

Investigators have continued exploring the effect that calcium and magnesium deficiencies may have on increased renin activity and essential hypertension. Serum magnesium levels were inversely related to renin hypertension, while serum calcium levels were lower in patients with low renin hypertension and higher in patients with high renin hypertension.

This relationship indicates that hypertensive disorders could be related in part to a defect in membrane transport of calcium and magnesium. Calcium is high extracellularly and magnesium is high intracellularly. If there is a defect in the pump mechanism whereby calcium is transported out of the cell, or magnesium is transported into the cell, this can set up renin effects that increase the risk to hypertensive disorders.

This would explain why a number of reports have indicated that calcium can be used as a supplement to treat certain forms of human hypertensive conditions, and there are other reports that have indicated that magnesium supplementation may be useful in the treatment of these conditions. Some individuals may be better calcium responders and others magnesium responders, depending upon the defect in their own renin control system.

The authors concluded that the use of ionized serum calcium and magnesium may be very helpful in determining what the defects are, and whether calcium or magnesium is more likely to be the mineral of need in the treatment of hypertension.[3]

ALZHEIMER'S DISEASE: CALCIUM-ALUMINUM RELATIONSHIP EXPLORED

The American food supply, along with medications such as aluminum-containing antacids, contributes to an excessive body burden of aluminum. Moreover, cooking in aluminum cookware has been reported to result in leaching of aluminum into the food. It is disturbing to note that aluminum toxicity is associated with Alzheimer's disease, other neuromuscular disorders, hyperparathyroidism and bone loss.[4]

Recently, Judith Marquis at the Department of Pharmacology, Boston University, found that aluminum concentration can result in inhibition of human serum cholinesterase, which may account for the role that aluminum has in diseases such as Alzheimer's. Her work also supports the hypothesis that serum calcium levels may be a limiting factor for aluminum toxicity and that when an individual is properly calcium-nourished, the difficulty of aluminum accumulation is reduced.

This work does not yet indicate that aluminum is the cause of Alzheimer's disease, but rather points out that there may be an association between aluminum concentration in the nervous system and interruptions in acetylcholine metabolism. This is consistent with the presently accepted mechanism for the production of this neurological disorder.[5] (See "Magnesium, Aluminum and ALS," p. 108.)

CALCIUM AND OSTEOPOROSIS

Osteoporosis is a degenerative bone disease that drastically increases the susceptibility to bone fractures. This disease is the result of dietary imbalances, years of low physical activity and, in women, fairly rapid calcium loss encouraged by the hormonal changes of menopause. Osteoporosis contributes to major orthopedic problems in approximately 25 to 30 percent of postmenopausal women.[6]

There is a constant turnover of calcium within bone, the storage depot for nearly 99 percent of the body's calcium. The remaining 1 percent travels in the bloodstream, maintaining the function of nerves and muscles. If an adequate amount of calcium is not supplied in the diet, calcium will be mobilized from the bones into the bloodstream. This reduces the calcium content of the bones which, in turn, increases their fragility.

At first, bone loss proceeds with no symptoms. Then there may be some persistent pain in the lower spine area. In some people, there may even be deformities of the vertebrae such as "dowager's hump" and loss of weight. In some cases, osteoporosis advances without any apparent sign until a spontaneous fracture occurs. Once bones suffer extensive calcium loss, it is difficult to restore their strength. The best way to handle osteoporosis is to prevent it. Yugoslavian studies have shown that individuals who maintain high calcium intakes throughout life have fewer fractures.[7,7a]

The Recommended Dietary Allowance for calcium is 800 mg/day, except for adolescents between the ages of eleven and eighteen, who need 1200 mg/day, and pregnant or lactating mothers, who need an additional 400 mg/day. Although calcium is abundant in the food supply, inadequate intakes of the mineral are common. It appears that the average woman's diet is relatively deficient in calcium. Women over forty-five typically consume 450–500 mg of calcium a day. At this low level of intake, a loss of 1.5 percent of total bone mass could occur within a year's time.[6,8]

Milk is frequently replaced by soft drinks, a beverage change that may contribute to osteoporosis and deposition of calcium in soft tissue. Soft drinks are generally buffered with phosphoric acid, which can ultimately stimulate the release of calcium from the bones. Other common sources of phosphorus in the American diet include the phosphate preservatives and beef. Before supplementing with calcium, women should be advised to lower their consumption of soft drinks and other dietary sources of phosphorus.

Many researchers have suggested a higher calcium intake for the post-menopausal woman. Studies have shown that 1500 mg of calcium daily will inhibit the age-related bone loss in older women. Supplemental calcium may be necessary to fill the gap between the dietary supply and the 1500 mg recommendation.[9]

LOW CALCIUM INTAKE
MAY CAUSE ECLAMPSIA

Eclampsia is one of the most serious obstetrical complications. Fetal losses from this disease range from 30 to 35 percent. Approximately 10 percent of all maternal mortality is due to eclampsia. This condition is associated with symptoms of high blood pressure, protein in the urine, and edema. The cause of eclampsia remains undetermined, although epidemiological studies have identified certain causative factors. First pregnancy, poor prenatal care, poor nutrition, and geographic variations have been implicated as risk factors for this condition.

A recent study conducted at Johns Hopkins University, Baltimore, and Centro Rosarino de Estudios, Rosario, Argentina, showed that women living in Guatemala have a very low incidence of eclampsia despite the presence of factors that would normally be expected to favor the disease. In Colombia, among women in a similar socioeconomic caste, there were very high incidences of eclampsia. The only difference between the two groups was dietary calcium intake. The women in Guatemala were found to have diets higher in calcium than the women in Colombia. The results of this study support the contention that calcium intake could be a very important factor in the prevention of eclampsia.[10]

HOW MUCH CALCIUM IS AVAILABLE
FROM DAIRY PRODUCTS?

Some researchers have expressed concern that the calcium in homogenized, pasteurized dairy products is not biologically available and does not serve as a good source of calcium. In standard nutrition literature, dairy products have been suggested as the most important source of calcium in the American diet, supplying about 85 percent of total calcium. The calcium content of dairy products ranges from 52 mg/100 g for cottage cheese to 113 mg/100 g for fluid milk and 716 mg/100 g for cheddar cheese.

During the processing of milk, the forms in which calcium occurs can be altered; as a result, a shift in its distribution can occur. For example, the calcium in cheddar cheese is calcium paracaseinate, whereas calcium in high acid products such as yogurt and buttermilk occurs as ionic calcium.

In a study of calcium in dairy products, the pH of the dairy product was found to influence the form of calcium and its relative bioavailability. Calcium appears to be more readily available when it occurs as colloidal calcium phosphate or calcium paracaseinate than as simple ionic calcium.

From these findings, the authors conclude that milk has more bioavailable calcium than yogurt, with cheese being intermediary. For example, dietary calcium as nonfat dry milk was utilized 100 percent as effectively as a calcium carbonate supplement; yogurt, 109 percent; and casein-rich milk protein, 140 percent. Thus, the calcium from dairy products, whether it is homogenized, pasteurized or cultured, is bioavailable. But the most bioavailable forms appear to be in the noncultured products, where protein-bound forms of calcium, rather than just ionized calcium, are present.[11]

CALCIUM AND MAGNESIUM PREVENT
DRUG-INDUCED KIDNEY DAMAGE

Damage to the kidney associated with aminoglycoside antibiotics is known to be a common clinical problem. Investigations to determine the cause of this drug-induced kidney damage have recently revealed that a receptor for these aminoglycoside antibiotics exists on the membrane of the kidney cells. It has also been demonstrated that calcium can act as a competitive inhibitor to the binding of the antibiotic to these receptors.

The Oregon Health Sciences University and Providence Hospital and Medical Center, Portland, have examined the role of dietary calcium supplements on gentamicin-induced kidney damage. Animal diets that were enriched with calcium carbonate provided protection against gentamicin nephrotoxicity. Magnesium supplementation was found to achieve a similar positive outcome.

In a related study by the Veteran's Administration Medical Center and the University of Michigan, Ann Arbor, supplementation with calcium and magnesium greatly reduced the incidence of kidney damage in gentamicin-loaded animals.

These results indicate that high-calcium diets exert a nonspecific salutory effect on the tubular cell integrity of the kidney and help prevent the toxic reactions of these aminoglycoside antibiotics.[12, 13]

MAGNESIUM

MAGNESIUM AND
PREMENSTRUAL SYNDROME

Dr. G. Abraham, a Los Angeles physician, examined the serum and red cells of women with premenstrual syndrome and found magnesium levels to be low. Dr. Abraham demonstrated that women with symptoms of headache, dizziness and craving for sweets responded to magnesium, zinc, niacin and vitamin C supplementation, whereas those who had breast tenderness responded to vitamin E supplementation. Women with symptoms of tension anxiety associated with premenstrual syndrome improve with increased doses of vitamin B6.[14, 15]

MAGNESIUM, DIURETICS AND HYPERTENSION

Magnesium loss often accompanies diuretic therapy but the extent of this drug-induced hypomagnesemia has not been well studied. Preliminary research in this area indicated that chronic low-grade magnesium deficiency from diuretic treatment is more common than published reports suggest.

Patients receiving either short-term vigorous diuretic treatment or moderate-dosage long-term treatment are magnesium deficient. Typical symptoms of poor magnesium status in this study included depression, muscle weakness, refractory hypokalemia and atrial fibrillation refractive to digoxin treatment. When given intramuscular injections of magnesium sulfate, all patients experienced a rapid improvement in their symptoms.[16]

MAGNESIUM AND DIGITALIS

Digitalis may cause fatal arrythmias in patients who are magnesium deficient. Animal studies indicate that in magnesium deficiency, significantly low doses of digitalis are required to elicit a potentially fatal arrythmia.

Magnesium is required to activate Na-K-ATPase, an enzyme needed to transport potassium into the cell. In magnesium deficiency, this enzyme functions poorly, resulting in a disturbance in potassium balance that cannot be effectively treated with potassium supplementation. Potassium supplementation in this situation may perpetuate the cardiac consequences of potassium depletion, including arrythmia.

Digitalis is also an inhibitor of Na-K-ATPase, and heightens the effects of magnesium depletion. Therefore, low doses of this drug are required in magnesium deficiency. In animal studies, administration of magnesium corrected the arrhythmia brought about by the combination of digitalis and hypomagnesemia.[17, 18]

MAGNESIUM, ALUMINUM AND ALS

In Guam, a high percentage of amyotrophic lateral sclerosis symptomatology (ALS or Lou Gehrig's disease) is seen in young men. This disease has been traced to high levels of aluminum and manganese exposure. The impact of this exposure has been evaluated by the Departments of Agronomy and Animal Science at the Louisiana Agricultural Experiment Station. The researchers administered aluminum sulfate and manganese sulfate to animals in varying doses. In the aluminum-treated animals, serum magnesium levels decreased remarkably within twenty-four hours and declined 32 percent within four days. Manganese treatment was found to have no effect on magnesium. Continued administration of aluminum resulted in hypomagnesemic tetany with cramping, gastrointestinal complications and nervous system disorders.

The investigators conclude that aluminum administration depresses serum magnesium and can result in clinical manifestations of magnesium deficiency. Removal of the aluminum resulted in increased magnesium levels and an improvement in the clinical picture of the animals. This confirms earlier work suggesting that calcium and magnesium are competitive inhibitors of the absorption and effects of aluminum, and that a calcium- and magnesium-rich diet offers some protections against aluminum-induced toxicity.[19]

SELENIUM

SELENIUM AND CANCER

The work of Dr. Gerald Schrauzer at the University of California, San Diego, supports the theory that selenium helps prevent cancer. This work has been challenged by some investigators, who claim it is work done with animals who have spontaneous tumors, and not with humans. The challenging investigators suggest that humans are getting adequate selenium in their diets to meet their needs.

Dr. Willet and colleagues studied selenium levels in 111 subjects who developed cancer within five years after their blood samples had been taken. The samples from these cancer patients were compared with blood selenium samples taken from 210 cancer-free subjects who were matched for age, weight, sex and smoking history. They found that the mean blood selenium level of the cancer victims was significantly lower than that of the individuals who did not get cancer (0.129 mcg/ml compared to 0.136 mcg/ml).

Other dietary variables, including levels of various fats, vitamins A and E, and beta-carotene, did not alter the important selenium relationship. The researchers found that the association between low selenium levels and cancer was strongest for cancers of the intestinal tract and prostate gland. Low levels of serum vitamins A and E were found to amplify the effect of low selenium and increase the risk of cancer by almost four times in the selenium, E and A group.[20]

SELENIUM AND HEART DISEASE

A study involving 8,113 men and women randomly selected from two counties in eastern Finland has been reported. Blood samples were collected, frozen and stored. Over the next seven years, the number of hospital admissions for myocardial infarction (MI) and the number of deaths from heart disease were determined for the group and then compared to those of a matched control group. When the serum selenium levels were compared, it was determined that a selenium level of less than 35 mcg/l was associated with a six- to seven-fold increase in risk of death from heart disease and a two-fold increase in risk of MI. At levels of 33–44 mcg/l, there was a two-fold increase in risk for either MI or death from heart disease.[21]

LOW SOIL SELENIUM AND LOW BLOOD SELENIUM

A number of regions in the United States have low soil selenium. One such region producing grain products low in selenium is the grain belt region in eastern Washington. Animals raised on these grains may have compromised selenium status. In New Zealand, where the soil selenium is very low, the residents have very low blood selenium and glutathione peroxidase levels. Populations consuming protein from animals raised on low-selenium soil will probably be at risk for selenium adequacy.[22]

SELENIUM AND ALCOHOLICS

Dr. Klaus Schwartz has demonstrated that selenium deficiency produces fatty liver infiltration. Selenium depletion in humans has been found to result in progressive cardiomyopathy (Keshan's disease). Because these two conditions are often seen in alcoholics, the question was raised as to whether selenium deficiency in the alcoholic plays a role in the appearance of these disorders.

Drs. Dutta and Miller of the Veterans Administration in Maryland looked at the selenium status in alcoholic subjects by collecting blood and urine samples during hospitalization. They found that the plasma and urinary levels of selenium were significantly lower in alcoholic subjects as compared to control subjects. The conclusion: selenium depletion is a result of poor dietary selenium intake and may increase the risk of alcoholics to selenium-deficiency symptoms.[23]

IRON

IRON AND ZINC INTERACTION

Studies by Dr. Meadows (*Lancet*, October 8:1013, 1983) noted that inorganic iron as a supplement reduces the absorption of pharmacological amounts of inorganic zinc. Drs. Mitchell and Watson (Gartnavel General Hospital and West of Scotland Health Boards, Glasgow) have pointed out that the sites of absorption of iron and zinc are not identical in the gastrointestinal tract, with iron being absorbed preferentially from the duodenum and zinc at a more distal site.

It is known that the bioavailability of inorganic zinc is impaired in the presence of inorganic iron. However, administration of organic zinc in the form of Atlantic oysters is unaffected by 100 mg of inorganic iron. This seems to indicate a difference in the antagonism of iron or zinc in the diet versus supplements of each.

The authors of this study conclude that iron does compete with zinc when both are administered as inorganic supplements at high levels. However, iron, given along with the zinc-containing diet or with organically bound zinc, may nullify this antagonism.[24]

IRON, CALCIUM AND MAGNESIUM INTERACTION

Prenatal multivitamin and mineral supplements are widely used to ensure that pregnant women meet their daily iron requirements. The general practice has been to include 60–65 mg of iron in the daily dose to provide at least 3.5 mg of absorbed iron.

The University of Colorado School of Medicine has evaluated four different brands of prenatal supplements for their ability to deliver the required 3.5 mg of absorbed iron. The amount of iron in the supplements ranged from 1.8 to 3.0 mg. Iron absorption from all four brands was insufficient to meet the required 3.5 mg. Since 65 mg of iron, when given by itself, provides 8.1 mg of absorbed iron, the researchers evaluated the prenatal supplements for mineral-mineral interactions.

The authors have demonstrated that the decreased iron absorption was a result of inhibition by calcium carbonate and magnesium oxide. When one of the four brands was reformulated with less calcium carbonate and magnesium oxide, the mean iron absorption increased to 4.5 mg.

The authors thus concluded that prenatal supplements with iron, calcium carbonate and magnesium oxide need to be reformulated.[25]

IRON AND BEHAVIOR

Research using iron-deficient animals has suggested an impairment in dopaminergic neurotransmissions that can affect behavior. It has been suggested that specific attentional control systems are dependent upon dopaminergic pathways that mediate cognitive function in humans. Iron is highly concentrated in the brain's dopamine-pathway regions.

In studies on humans, Tucker and colleagues (Grand Forks Human Nutrition Research Center, University of North Dakota) have evaluated the relationship between iron status and cognitive performance. This is the first type of study to explore the relationship between iron status and brain function using "normally nourished," as opposed to clinically malnourished, individuals.

The researchers followed iron status in sixty-nine healthy university students by charting serum ferritin and iron levels. These levels were then related to cognitive performance and quantitative EEG measurements. Higher levels of serum ferritin were associated with greater activation of the left hemisphere of the brain, the hemisphere related to analytic thought and abstract cognitive performance.

Iron status was significantly related to cognitive performance on two of the tasks assigned to the subjects. Higher ferritin levels were associated with greater verbal fluency.

The investigators concluded that body iron stores are relevant to specific neurophysiological processes supporting attention. In fact, chronic impairment in iron metabolism or nutriture could have dramatic effects on attention span and ability to concentrate.

Dr. Leibel and his colleagues at the University of Colorado have recently demonstrated that there are reversible alterations in cognitive function in mildly iron deficient three- to six-year-old children. The behavior disorders apparently related to iron apathy are impaired attention and low responsiveness.

In another study that investigated anemic versus non-anemic one-year-olds and their behavior, Drs. Johnson and McGowan of the University of Houston were unable to find significant differences between the two groups. The researchers concluded that previous studies were flawed because of either uncontrolled variables or the length of time that the children were anemic.

A comparison of the two studies suggests that the symptoms of iron-deficiency-related behavior may be associated more with children who have undergone long-term chronic iron deprivation, rather than with those who have had only short-term iron deprivation.[26,27,28]

CHROMIUM

CHROMIUM AND CHOLESTEROL

Chromium is an essential trace element in humans. It comprises part of the glucose tolerance factor (GTF) molecule and facilitates insulin receptivity at peripheral cellular binding sites. The use of chromium as a supplement in human diabetes mellitus has met with mixed success. In another role, chromium status could be important in modulating serum lipids in humans.

A study reported in the *American Journal of Clinical Nutrition* indicated that a 200 mcg/day supplement of chromic chloride given to humans resulted in a lower total cholesterol level and an increase in HDL cholesterol.[28]

An oral supplement of chromium-rich brewer's yeast was given to another group of forty-six subjects for eight weeks. The yeast caused a slight reduction in serum cholesterol levels and an increase in HDL levels. The effect was produced using much lower levels of total chromium in the yeast form than were required when using the inorganic chromium supplement.

This study indicated that normal torula and other yeasts do not have levels of GTF chromium sufficient to produce this effect on serum lipids. Apparently, only the chromium-rich brewer's yeast grown under unique conditions can produce the positive effects.[29]

CHROMIUM, GLUCOSE TOLERANCE AND DIABETES

Turner's syndrome is a disease associated with a high prevalency of diabetes. Individuals with Turner's syndrome have been shown to be resistant to insulin and have abnormal carbohydrate metabolism. Because the major physiological role of chromium is that of improved carbohydrate metabolism through facilitation of insulin activity, chromium has been suggested for possible use in the management of Turner's syndrome patients with glucose intolerance.

Oral glucose tolerance tests were performed in fourteen patients age eight to nineteen years. Eight of the fourteen subjects were given 30 grams of brewer's yeast containing 50 micrograms of chromium each day for eight weeks, and the glucose tolerance test was repeated. The studies indicated that, in many individuals, a state of chromium deficiency exists which can be treated effectively by oral chromium supplementation from brewer's yeast. This treatment decreases the pathogenesis of the abnormal glucose tolerance test encountered in the Turner's syndrome patients.

This study is one of the first to demonstrate that supplementation of chromium from brewer's yeast is capable of ameliorating glucose intolerance and improving insulin receptivity. Investigators also found that during chromium supplementation, the serum lipid levels decreased while there was an increase in HDL; this suggests a decreased risk of atherosclerotic disease in these glucose-intolerant patients.

In another double-blind supplementation trial of chromium given to twenty-one ketosis-prone and twenty-two ketosis-resistant diabetic men for four months, the chromium supplementation resulted in a rise in plasma insulin with no decrease in fasting plasma glucose or lipids.

In comparing a yeast chromium supplement to an inorganic chromous chloride supplement, it was found that either form was capable of affecting plasma insulin levels, and may be useful in the amelioration of glucose intolerance when due to chromium deficiency.[30,31]

CHROMIUM AND SUGAR CONSUMPTION

As stated previously, chromium is a vital component of "glucose tolerance factor" (GTF), a substance that promotes the action of insulin.

Long-term ingestion of sugar and other refined carbohydrates is considered a major factor in producing a dietary chromium deficiency which leads to disturbances in the body's handling of sugar. Essentially, the abnormalities in sugar metabolism resemble those seen in maturity-onset diabetes, i.e., high levels of sugar in the blood and urine along with an excessive amount of insulin in the bloodstream.

An adequate supply of chromium enables the insulin to function properly, that is, to transport and deliver sugar from the bloodstream to the cells. In chromium depletion this ability is compromised, even though there may be an abundance of insulin in the bloodstream.

Several studies have shown that supplemental chromium can benefit elderly diabetics. When given chromium-rich brewer's yeast, some older maturity-onset diabetics have shown improvements in blood cholesterol levels, thus lowering the risk of heart disease.[32,33]

CHROMIUM AND THE NEED FOR SUPPLEMENTS

A Canadian study (forty-seven women living in a university community and consuming self-selected diets) indicates that perhaps as many as two-thirds of premenopausal women do not meet the RDAs for iron. Similar findings were reported for the trace element chromium. More than two-thirds of the women studied had daily intakes of chromium below the U.S. Food and Nutrition Board's safe and adequate range.

The authors suggested that there may be cause for concern because of the increasing evidence of chromium depletion during pregnancy.[34]

COPPER

COPPER, EMPHYSEMA AND CARDIOMYOPATHY

Current research has linked lung pathology, similar to that found in emphysema, with copper deficiency. Apparently, copper deficiency impairs the proper crosslinking of elastin for structural integrity in the lung. These structural defects are not readily reversible by dietary copper supplementation. Therefore, copper adequacy during early growth and development appears to be essential.

A second facet of this study noted that in animals chronic copper deficiency can also result in cardiomyopathy. This is interesting because Klevay has suggested that a copper deficiency in low calorie weight loss diets may be responsible for the myocardial degeneration seen in individuals on these diets.[35, 36]

COPPER AND CARDIOVASCULAR DISEASE

Copper is necessary for insulin binding, transport of sugar and breakdown of fats by adipose tissue. In test situations, animals on copper-deficient diets are known to develop anemia, high blood cholesterol and degeneration of the heart muscle. This seems to be particularly aggravated when the copper deficiency comes in conjunction with a diet that is high in sugar.

Reiser and his colleagues from the U.S. Department of Agriculture have found that copper seems to be critically important in the appropriate metabolism of the sugar fructose. Diets now consumed by Americans (in which 22 percent of the calories are in the form of sugar) are high in fructose and marginally low in copper. With the introduction of increasing amounts of fructose as corn sweeteners, we can expect fructose in the United States food supply to increase.

Given these trends, the ever-increasing intake of fructose in conjunction with the marginal depletion of copper may increase the risk to cardiovascular problems or difficulty in managing blood sugar. The interesting part of the Reiser study is that the question of the influence of sugar on metabolism is not an easy question to answer. There are many other nutrients, such as copper, that participate in the body's proper regulation of dietary carbohydrate and simple sugars.

A diet that is high in simple calories and low in supporting micronutrients may, in some clinicians' opinions, be the offender in reducing the body's optimal functioning. With the increasing evidence that numbers of people may suffer from marginal copper deficiency, particularly in the face of a higher fructose or sucrose intake, reevaluation of the need for copper enrichment should be initiated.[37]

COPPER AND CHOLESTEROL

Cholesterol and copper metabolism have been associated in studies conducted with animals and humans. Many of these studies have found elevated cholesterol levels linked to low liver copper. And similarities have been identified between animals with a deficiency of copper and humans with ischemic heart disease.

The cholesterol-lowering agent clofibrate (Atromid-S) can induce copper deficiencies. A recent study at the USDA (ARS Grand Forks Human Nutrition Research Center, Grand Forks, North Dakota) suggests that clofibrate (Atromid-S) exerts its cholesterol-lowering activity by altering copper metabolism.[38,39]

COPPER, ZINC AND HIGH BLOOD PRESSURE

An association has been made in epidemiological studies between mineral intake and the incidence of heart disease: for example, populations living in hard-water areas have a lower incidence of heart disease than those in soft-water areas.

Drs. Medeiros and Brown have studied the relationship between blood pressure and copper/zinc status in young adults. They assessed copper and zinc levels in blood serum, urine, hair and dietary intake. The research team at Mississippi State University found that the association between blood pressure and mineral intake was highest for males. In these cases, elevated blood pressure was associated with increased dietary copper intakes and lower dietary zinc intake. Serum zinc concentrations were found to have an inverse relationship to blood pressure. This work seems inconsistent with Dr. Klevay's hypothesis that low copper levels are associated with an increased risk of cardiovascular disease, but consistent with the findings of the World Health Organization that excess copper may be the problem, particularly in conjunction with low levels of zinc.

Drs. Medeiros and Brown also note that one problem in interpreting the present work is the lack of knowledge concerning the best indicators of copper and zinc status. Until an unequivocal method for ascertaining trace element status is discovered, there will be a continuing debate as to optimal levels of zinc and copper in the prevention of cardiovascular disorders.[40]

COPPER, ZINC AND IMMUNITY

In a study at the University of Medicine and Dentistry at New Jersey, fifty-eight patients with confirmed secondary immunodeficiency syndrome were tested for plasma copper and zinc levels. These patients had depressed cell-mediated immunity and were found to have a low serum zinc and elevated serum copper level.

The authors conclude that zinc and copper homeostasis are significantly altered in many immunodeficiency disorders and may be important factors in host defense.

Cellular immunity is known to be impaired by zinc deficiency, but it is not clear from this study whether the immunodeficiency observed in these patients is caused by the zinc/copper imbalance or whether the imbalance results from the immunodeficiency.

When given zinc supplements, the patients with primary or secondary immunodeficiency conditions apparently improved. This supports the hypothesis that the alteration of zinc and copper metabolism through dietary imbalance contributes to the cause of immunodeficiency.[41]

OTHER MINERALS

SODIUM AND KIDNEY STONES

Kidney stones are often involved when there is poor calcium metabolism and may result from excessive calcium intake or the inappropriate use of calcium by the body. According to a recent study, a high salt diet contributes to an increase of kidney stones. Most kidney stone formers have normal blood calcium but spill excessive amounts of calcium in their urine. One of the reasons for this may be that the individual is consuming excessive dietary protein.

Too much protein in the diet causes an excessive intake of sulfur-containing amino acids, which may lead to a rise in acid excretion and increased calcium excretion. A second reason is that a very low dietary phosphorus intake may stimulate high intestinal calcium absorption but inhibit retention of calcium, thus resulting in increased calcium spill in the urine. Finally, this study suggests that increasing salt consumption in the diet may increase urinary calcium excretion and the risk of kidney stones because of the tendency of sodium to increase urine volume and prevent calcium retention in tissues.[42]

PHOSPHORUS AND BONE

There has been considerable discussion over the past several years as to whether American diets (which are very high in phosphorus, reasonably low in calcium, and contain large amounts of protein) have an adverse impact on calcium metabolism.

A recent study by Drs. Yuen and Draper at the University of Guelph, Canada, has explored the effect of high dietary protein and phosphorus on bone status in animals. The study concluded that high dietary phosphorus (found in soft drinks, phosphorus preservatives and some meats) leads to reduced bone density with calcium loss from the bone, whereas high dietary protein seems to have a lesser effect. The researchers found that there is no interaction between protein and phosphorus, so that these are independent variables in controlling bone status.

In humans, a high protein diet leads to bone loss because of a decrease in the resorption of calcium by the kidney.[43]

FLUORIDE AND BONE

Fluoride is now suggested to be an essential element in the diet of humans, and is thought to be required for normal dental and skeletal growth. The Recommended Dietary Allowance for fluoride is 1 to 4 milligrams per day, which could be obtained from beverages in a normal diet if the fluoride content is 1 part per million.

It has been reported that fluoride has a direct effect on bone cells by increasing proliferation and alkaline phosphatase activity. Fluoride not only increases the proliferation rate of bone cells, but also enhances the growth and mineralization of embryonic bone.[44]

LEAD AND BEHAVIOR

Drs. Marlowe and Errera reported that children who are chronically exposed to dietary or inhaled lead have an increased body burden of lead, and have more behavior and learning problems than children who have not been exposed to lead.

Lead has been removed from gasoline for the past several years, and it has been shown that the general lead levels of children are going down. However, some investigators, such as Dr. Herbert Needleman, are concerned that many children are lead impaired as a result of inhaling lead from dust and pollution, and also from consuming lead in foods. Certain canned food products are known to contain lead, as was reported by Dr. Clair Patterson at California Institute of Technology. The long-term exposure to canned food and inhaled or ingested lead in dust and air may account for an increased body burden of lead which can impair the sensitive nervous system of children, causing them to be easily fatigued and unable to concentrate. Dr. Needleman has even reported decreases in IQ in children who are chronically lead impaired.[45]

LEAD AND SUDDEN INFANT DEATH SYNDROME

Dr. Marilyn Erickson reported that lead levels are significantly higher in infants who die of Sudden Infant Death Syndrome (SIDS) than infants who die of other causes. Dr. Erickson was quick to point out that her findings do not prove a cause and effect relationship. However, the findings could explain reports linking SIDS to environmental toxins.

A previous study by Erickson and her colleagues found that babies born in late summer and early fall had higher levels of lead in umbilical cord blood at birth. The elevated lead could be a result of either pre- or post-natal exposure. At birth, SIDS infants appear to have more than twice the lead in the liver than non-SIDS infants, suggesting that the SIDS infants were exposed to more lead in gestation.

One important observation of this study is that prenatal lead exposure may arise from a release of maternal stored lead. This lead, an estimated 90 percent of which is stored in the mother's bones, would be free to cross the placenta into the fetal circulatory system.[46]

REFERENCES

1. McCarron, D.A. Calcium and magnesium nutrition in human hypertension. *Ann.Int.Med.*, 98:800-805, 1983.

2. Bazzarre, T.L., Shih-min Liu Wu, M.S. and Yuhas, J.A. Total and HDL-cholesterol concentrations following yogurt and calcium supplementation. *Nutr.Rep.Int.*, 28:1225–1232, 1983.

3. Resnick, L., Laragh, J., Sealey, J., et al. Divalent cations in essential hypertension: Relations between serum ionized calcium, magnesium, and plasma renin activity. *N.E.J.Med.*, 309:888-891, 1983.

4. Koning, J. Aluminum pots as a source of dietary aluminum. *N. E. J. Med.*, 304:172, 1981.

5. Marquis, J.K. Aluminum inhibition of human serum cholinesterase. *Bull.Envir.Cont.Tox.*, 31:164-169, 1983.

6. Avioli, L. Postmenopausal osteoporosis: Prevention versus cure. *Fed.Proc.*, 40:2418-2422, 1981.

7. Albanese, A.A. Osteoporosis. *Cont.Nutr.*, 2, #2, 1977.

7A. Matkovic, V. Bone status and fracture rates in two regions of Yugoslavia. *Am.J.Clin.Nutr.* 32:540, 1979.

8. National Research Council. *Recommended Dietary Allowances,* 9th edition. Washington, D.C.: National Academy of Sciences, 1980.

9. Recker, R., Saville, P. and Heaney, R. Effect of estrogens and calcium carbonate on bone loss in postmenopausal women. *Ann.Int.Med.*, 87:649, 1977.

10. Villar, J., Belizah, J.M. and Fischer, P.J. Epidemiologic observations on the relationship between calcium intake and eclampsia. *Int.J.Gyn.Obst.*, 21:271-278, 1983.

11. Wong, N.P. and LaCroix, D.E. Biological availability of calcium in dairy products. *Nutr.Rep.Int.*, 21:673, 1980.

12. Quarum, M.L., Houghton, D.N., Gilbert, D.N., et al. Increasing dietary calcium moderates experimental gentamicin nephrotoxicity. *J.Lab.Clin.Med.*, 103:104, 1984.

13. Humes, H.D., Sastrasinh, M. and Weinberg, J.M. Calcium is a competitive inhibitor of gentamicin-renal membrane binding interactions and dietary calcium supplementation protects against gentamicin nephrotoxicity. *J.Clin.Inv.*, 73:134-147, 1984.

14. Abraham, G.E. and Lubran, M. Serum and red cell magnesium levels in patients with premenstrual tension. *Am.J.Clin. Nutr.*, 34:2364-2366, 1981.

15. Abraham, G.E. Nutritional factors in the etiology of the premenstrual tension syndromes. *J.Repr.Med.*, 28:446-461, 1983.

16. Sheehan, J. and White, A. Diuretic-associated hypomagnesemia. *Br.Med.J.*, 285:1157-1159, 1982.

17. Swales, J.D. Magnesium deficiency and diuretics. *Br.Med.J.*, 285:1377-1378, 1982.

18. Dyckner, T., Wester, P.D. Magnesium in cardiology. *Acta Med.Scand.* (Supp.), 661:27-31, 1982.

19. Allen, V.G., Robinson, D.L. and Hembry, F.G. Effects of ingested aluminum sulfate on serum magnesium and the possible relationship to hypomagnesemic tetany. *Nutr.Rep.Int.*, 29:107, 1984.

20. Willett, W.C., et al. Prediagnostic serum selenium and risk of cancer. *Lancet*, July 16, 1983, 130.

21. Salonen, J.T., Alfthan, G., Huttunen, J.K., et al. Association between cardiovascular death and myocardial infarction and serum selenium in a matched pair longitudinal study. *Lancet*, July 24:175-179, 1982.

22. Selenium deficiency in cattle associated with Heinz bodies and anemia. *Science*, 223:491, 1984.

23. Dutta, S.K., et al. Selenium and acute alcoholism. *Am.J.Clin.Nutr.*, 38:713-718, 1983.

24. Mitchell, K. and Watson, W.S. Oral iron and the bioavailability of zinc. *Br.Med.J.*, 287:1629, 1983.

25. Seligman, P.A., Caskey, J.H., Frazier, J.L., et al. Measurements of iron absorption from prenatal multivitamin-mineral supplements. *Obst.Gyn.*, 61(3):356-362, 1983.

26. Tucker, D.M., Sandstead, H.H., Penland, J.G., et al. Iron status and brain function–serum ferritin levels associated with asymmetrics of cortical electrophysiology and cognitive performance. *Am.J.Clin.Nutr.*, 39:105-113, 1984.

27. Pollitt, E., Leibel, R.L. and Greenfield, D.B. Iron deficiency and cognitive test performance in preschool children. *Nutr.Behav.*, 1:137-146, 1983.

28. Johnson, D.L. and McGowen, R.J. Anemia and infant behavior. *Nutr.Behav.*, 1:185-192, 1983.

29. Chromium status and serum lipids (review). *Nutr.Rev.*, 41:307-310, 1983.

30. Saner, G., Yuzbasiyan, V., Nevzi, O., et al. Alterations of chromium metabolism and effect of chromium supplementation in Turner's Syndrome patients. *Am.J.Clin.Nutr.*, 38:574-578, 1983.

31. Rabinowitz, M.B., et al. Effects of chromium and yeast supplements on carbohydrate and lipid metabolism in diabetic men. *Diabet.Care*, 6:319, 1983.

32. Offenbacher, E.G., et al. Beneficial effect of chromium-rich yeast on glucose tolerance and blood lipids in elderly subjects. *Diabetes*, 29:919-925, 1980.

33. Boyle, E. Mondschein, B. and Dash, H.H. Chromium depletion in the pathogenesis of diabetes and atherosclerosis. *S.Med.J.*, 70:1449, 1970.

34. Gibson, R.S. and Scythes, C.S. Dietary chromium, selenium and other trace element intakes of a sample of Canadian premenopausal women. *Fed.Proc.*, 42(4):816, 1983.

35. Copper deficiency and developmental emphysema (review). *Nutr.Rev.*, 41:318–320, 1983.

36. Kopp, S.J., Klevay, L.M. and Feliksik, J.M. Physiological and metabolic characterization of a cardiomyopathy induced by chronic copper deficiency. *Am.J.Phys.*, 245:H855, 1983.

37. Reiser, S., Ferretti, R.J., Fields, M., et al. Role of dietary fructose in the enhancement of mortality and biochemical changes associated with copper deficiency in rats. *Am.J.Clin.Nutr.*, 38:214-222, 1983.

38. Klevay, L.M. Hypercholesterolemia in rats produced by an increase in the ratio of zinc to copper ingested. *Am.J.Clin.Nutr.*, 26:1060, 1973.

39. Klevay, L.M. Clofibrate hypocholesterolemia associated with increased hepatic copper. *Fed.Proc.*, 42(4):808, 1983.

40. Medeiros, D.M. and Brown, B.J. Blood pressure in young adults as influenced by copper and zinc intake. *Biol.Tr.El.Res.*, 5:165-174, 1983.

41. Oleske, J.M., et al. Plasma zinc and copper in primary and secondary immunodeficiency disorders. *Biol.Tr.El.Res.*, 5:189-194, 1983.

42. Silver, J., Rubinger, D., Friedlaender, M.M., et al. Sodium-dependent idiopathic hypercalciuria in renal stone formers. *Lancet*, II:484, 1983.

43. Yuen, D.E. and Draper, H.H. Long-term effects of excess protein and phosphorus on bone homeostasis in adult mice. *J.Nutr.*, 113:1374, 1983.

44. Farley, J.R., Wergedal, J.E. and Baylink, D.J. Fluoride directly stimulates proliferation and alkaline phosphatase activity of bone-forming cells. *Science*, 222:330-332, 1983.

45. Marlowe, M. and Errera, J. Low lead levels and behavior problems in children. *Behav.Dis.*, 7:163, 1982.

46. Erickson, M.M., Poklis, A., Gantner, G.E., et al. Tissue mineral levels in victims of sudden infant death syndrome: Toxic metals—lead and cadmium. *Ped.Res.*, 17:779, 1983.

7

················ NUTRITIONAL SUPPLEMENTS:························
ARE THEY NECESSARY?

INTRODUCTION

TODAY as many as 40 percent of American adults take vitamin supplements on a regular basis.[1] Some nutrition professionals question whether the use of supplements is justified, since they feel that all essential nutrients are available through the food supply. Indeed, with so many technological advances in growing, processing, preserving and distributing foods, a nourishing and balanced diet is more readily obtained in modern-day America than in any other society throughout history. But new lifestyles and new eating habits such as dieting, meal skipping, between-meal snacking and the consumption of "empty calories" can work against good nutrition. Another modern notion is that very high levels of vitamins or other food substances can promote a state of "super health." This is a special concern among nutritionists who fear that the American penchant for "more is better" could lead to overconsumption of some micronutrients, such as vitamin D and iron, which can be harmful at excessive levels.

What is the proper role of supplementation in this environment? When and for whom can supplementation serve as a useful adjunct to the diet?

In examining this issue, two eminent nutrition authorities with divergent opinions—Dr. Alfred E. Harper of the University of Wisconsin and Dr. Willard A. Krehl of Jefferson Medical College—were invited to give their perspectives on vitamin supplementation. They were asked to respond to the following report, titled "Food, Nutrition and Health," developed by the Vitamin Nutrition Information Service, Nutley, New Jersey. This report describes problem nutrients, risk populations and other factors which, taken together, suggest a rationale for supplementation in certain populations. Drs. Harper and Krehl present their "Perspectives on Vitamin Supplementation" courtesy of the Vitamin Nutrition Information Service. Their perspectives illustrate different interpretations of the same facts.

FOOD, NUTRITION AND HEALTH MICRONUTRIENT STATUS:
Risk Populations and Problem Nutrients

The most widely used guideline for micronutrient requirements is the RDA, or Recommended Dietary Allowances, developed by the Food and Nutrition Board of the National Academy of Sciences/National Research Council (NAS/NRC). Dietary standards such as the RDA do not represent individual requirements; they are "recommendations for the average daily amounts of nutrients *population groups* should consume over a period of time."[2] Thus, in addition to their usefulness in large-scale menu planning, nutrition labeling (as adapted by the Federal Food and Drug Administration into U.S.RDA) and to some degree new product development, the RDA also provide broad guidelines for measuring the adequacy of national dietary intakes and the overall nutritional status of the population. Various researchers have used 80 percent, 70 percent and 66.7 percent of the RDA as levels below which diets may need improvement.[3]

Among the national nutrition surveys conducted periodically by government agencies are the Food Consumption Surveys of the U.S. Department of Agriculture (USDA) and the Health and Nutrition Examination Surveys (HANES) of the Department of Health and Human Services (HHS). USDA surveys analyze dietary intakes by calculating the nutrient levels of foods people say they are eating, as recorded in food diaries. In addition, USDA estimates national dietary intakes by measuring how much total food has been produced and used in the country.

HHS surveys not only assess food intakes, but also gather clinical data about nutritional health from biochemical analyses of body fluids, physical examinations and medical histories.

According to the major nutrition surveys of the past 15 + years, there are significant shortages of the following micronutrients among various population segments:[4-8]

National Survey	Problem Nutrients	
USDA Household Food Consumption Survey, 1965-66	Vitamin A Vitamin C	Calcium
Ten State Nutrition Survey, 1968-69 (lower income groups only)	Vitamin A Vitamin C Riboflavin	Calcium Iron
First Health and Nutrition Examination Survey (HANES I) 1971-72	Vitamin A Vitamin C	Calcium Iron
USDA Nationwide Food Consumption Survey (NFCS) 1977-78	Vitamin B6 Vitamin A Vitamin C	Calcium Iron Magnesium
National Health and Nutrition Examination Survey (N-Hanes II), 1977-78	Vitamin C Thiamin Riboflavin	Iron

Micronutrient shortages are more prevalent among some demographic groups than others. The population segments most often shown to be at risk for selected nutrients include women, the elderly, adolescents, low income groups, ethnic minorities and to a lesser degree, infants/children.[3-8] The nutrients most often lacking among these groups include the following:

Women: Marginal intakes of vitamin A, vitamin C, vitamin B6, calcium, iron and magnesium were found among substantial numbers of American women.[3] Some analysts attribute these shortages to the relatively low average caloric intakes of women.[9] At the 1600-1800 calorie range, food choices must be made with care in order to supply recommended levels of all essential vitamins and minerals.[10]

Teenagers: In the 1977-78 USDA survey, the diets of adolescent girls who consumed less than 70 percent of their energy requirements met the RDA for only one of the twelve nutrients studied—and that was protein, not any of the vitamins or minerals. It has been suggested that micronutrient inadequacies may result from habitual dieting for weight control among female teenagers. Teenage boys, on the other hand, generally averaged higher caloric intakes and correspondingly higher micronutrient intakes, although iron, magnesium and vitamin C were identified as problem nutrients among some 20–40 percent of male teens studied.[3]

Elderly: Problem nutrients identified in recent surveys include calcium and vitamin B6;[3,7] thiamin, riboflavin and niacin;[8] and vitamin C among elderly men[3,7] and low-income elderly groups.[6] Nutritional problems in this age group may occur as a result of decreased caloric intakes, impaired absorption, poor dentition, drug/nutrition interactions or any combination of these and other factors.

Infants/Children: Iron and vitamin C were found to be problem nutrients among infants and youngsters in the USDA-NFCS; vitamins A and C were insufficient among many children aged one to five in HANES-I; children aged one to five were shown to be at greater risk for niacin insufficiency in N-HANES-II. With these exceptions, the majority of micronutrients are generally adequate for most infants and children. [3,6,8]

Low Income Groups: In N-HANES-II, low income has been correlated with shortages of vitamin C, thiamin, riboflavin, niacin and iron.[8] In fact, all surveys have shown that micronutrient inadequacies are generally more prevalent among low income populations. An analysis of food stamp households from USDA-NFCS data found the percentage of households which met the RDA for eleven nutrients studied to be consistently 10 percent to 20 percent lower among food stamp households than non-foodstamp households. Only 12 percent of food stamp allotment households met the RDA for all eleven nutrients studied.[11]

Ethnic Minorities: Vitamin A has been shown to be a problem nutrient among Spanish Americans, apparently because the typical diet in this cultural group lacks sufficient vitamin A food sources. Vitamins A and C, thiamin, riboflavin, niacin and iron have been identified as problem nutrients among lower-income blacks in the Ten State Survey and HANES-I.[5,6]

There is no simple or universal explanation for these vitamin and mineral shortages in a nation where a nourishing, well-balanced diet is available from the food supply and is within the economic reach of most people. Nonetheless, they show up repeatedly in authoritative government surveys. Some of the possible reasons are explored in the following sections.

EATING HABITS: FADS, FOODS AND FALLACIES
Lifestyles and Eating Patterns

Traditional nutrition teaching has relied on the "common pot" theory—the assumption that everyone in the family unit, which was assumed to be most everyone in the country, was eating the same meals together. The homemaker, usually the mother, was also the meal planner, who probably had been taught that a balanced meal included foods from each of the "basic four" food groups—dairy products, fruits/ vegetables, cereals/grains, and protein-rich foods (meat, poultry, fish).

Today the lifestyles, eating patterns and even the structure of the "typical" American family have changed. More than half of adult females are now in the labor force, and of the 46.7 million women now employed, the majority are married.[12] More than half of working married women have children under eighteen.[13] In 1982, 32 million children, or 55 percent of all children under eighteen, had working mothers. Another new non-traditional family arrangement is the single-parent household, increasing at twice the rate of two-parent families.[12]

These sociological changes have an impact on eating habits insofar as they re-prioritize the values governing food selections. Taste and cost have always been significant factors; now convenience also may carry greater weight than a food's nutritional contribution to the diet. Increased demand for convenience foods and the success of the fast food market throughout the past two decades might be interpreted as testimony to the fact that many former homemakers now have less time to spend in the kitchen. Cost is of particular importance in households headed by single working women, since women's salaries average only about 60 percent of those of their male counterparts.[12]

Eating patterns are also changing in households structured along more traditional lines (*i.e.*, fulltime homemaker, wage earner and children). Meal skipping, snacking, away-from-home meals and varied meal schedules among different family members are typical phenomena. According to a nine-year study by the National Center for Health Statistics, more than a quarter (26 percent) of the population say they never eat breakfast. Conversely, 60 percent say they always do, but the breakfast eaters tend to be older.[12] This pattern is also evident in the USDA Nationwide Food Consumption Survey, where breakfast skipping was most prevalent among the nineteen- to twenty-two-year-olds (29 percent) and twenty-three- to thirty-four-year-olds (25 percent) as compared to 14 percent of the population overall. In addition, the USDA survey showed nearly one fourth of the study groups (23 percent) skipping lunch.[14]

Snacking was reported by 61 percent of USDA-NFCS respondents and by 38 percent of the National Center for Health Statistics study population.[12] Away-from-home meals accounted for an overall 18 percent of eating occasions in the USDA-NFCS but were again most frequent among young adults—60 percent of the men and 50 percent of the women aged twenty-three to thirty-four had eaten away from home on the day surveyed.[14]

These data imply that today's eating patterns do not generally conform to traditional concepts such as "three square meals" and the "common pot"; nor does a meal or mini-meal necessarily include a proper variety of foods.

Low-Calorie Diets

Another trend which may be influencing micronutrient status is reduced caloric intake. The 1977–78 USDA survey revealed average energy intakes of 1500-1600 kcal/day among women nineteen to fifty and 2300-2500 kcal/day among men, levels significantly lower than previously thought.[7] Because micronutrient intakes decrease proportionately with calorie content, diets at these low energy levels may not provide recommended amounts of vitamins and minerals.

An analysis of USDA survey data showed that micronutrient inadequacies were, in fact, more widespread among people with reduced energy intakes. "One-fourth of all individuals had energy intakes above the RDA . . . for these diets. . . , mean intakes of nutrients were well above the RDA for most nutrients and at least 80 percent of the RDA for all nutrients . . .

". . . One third of the individuals had intakes with caloric content below 70 percent of the RDA. Included in this group were two-fifths of the women nineteen to fifty . . . For these low-caloric diets, mean intakes of calcium, iron, magnesium and vitamin B6 values for some sex-age groups were in the range of 40-60 percent of the RDA . . . In addition. . . , others [nutrients] are identified here as potential problems for individuals who continue on these low-caloric intakes for long periods. For example, girls fifteen to eighteen met the RDA for only one of the twelve nutrients studied—protein—and most other individuals for only four or five of the nutrients."[3]

In a recent controlled study of dietary intakes, the researchers stated, "If caloric intakes recorded by women are accurate and representative, they may have difficulty in obtaining necessary amounts of calcium, vitamin A and iron without dietary changes or vitamin and mineral supplemtation . . . Recorded intakes of B vitamins are generally adequate, because many foods are now enriched with these vitamins."[15]

Presumably, among those with restricted caloric intakes are people dieting for weight control. An estimated 20 percent of the population or 40 million Americans are dieting at any given time.[16] Among some age groups of women, this figure is higher than 50 percent.[16] Reducing diets must be very well planned and/or supervised in order to supply adequate amounts of vitamins and minerals. Of concern are "fad" diets which often lack balance, variety and/or micronutrient adequacy.

Nutrient Density

In assessing nutritional status one must also look at the quality of diets Americans habitually consume. Data on food trends from the beginning of the century to the present indicate that consumption of such nutrient-dense foods as vegetables, breads and cereals has declined, while the consumption of foods and beverages that are high in calories but low in or devoid of micronutrients has increased. In the latter category are fats/oils, sugars and alcoholic beverages.[17]

The distribution of energy sources in the national diet according to analysis of the USDA 1977-78 survey data is 18.8 percent dairy products; 7.6 percent cereals/grains; 20.8 percent fruits/vegetables; 16 percent meat, fish, poultry and other protein-rich foods; and 36.8 percent "other" foods including sugar, desserts, beverages, condiments, fats and oils.[18]

If in fact average caloric intakes have declined, while at the same time a greater percentage of foods eaten are high in calories but lacking in sufficient micronutrient value, this combination of factors might well contribute to the vitamin and mineral insufficiencies reported in nutrition surveys.

Environmental Factors and Special Demands

Micronutrient status may be influenced by factors other than eating habits, including cigarette smoking, drug interactions, alcohol consumption and physiological stress.[2]

Heavy cigarette smoking has been observed to lower plasma levels of vitamin C by as much as 40 percent.[19] Under acute environmental stress, such as exposure to elevated temperatures, increased intakes of vitamin C are required to maintain normal plasma levels of the vitamin.[2] If the diet is already inadequate in vitamin C—say for example 70 to 80 percent of the RDA—such factors may seriously compromise vitamin C status over time.

Heavy alcohol consumption has been shown to affect adversely levels of folic acid, thiamin, riboflavin, niacin, vitamin C, vitamin B6, vitamin B12, magnesium and zinc.[20] Severe cases of alcoholism may also produce protein calorie malnutrition and iron deficiencies, which in turn can foster anemia and other blood abnormalities. Today an estimated 90 million Americans consume alcoholic beverages, and of these, approximately nine to ten million are alcoholics.[21]

Drug nutrient interactions may be a significant factor among the elderly and other persons suffering from chronic diseases. Daphne Roe, M.D., a leading authority in this field, writes as follows:

> Diverse drug groups, including such widely used medications as anticonvulsants, antimalarials, anti-tuberculous drugs and contraceptive steroids have been shown to increase nutrient requirements. These drugs, as well as certain antibiotics, sedatives and cholesterol-lowering agents, can cause specific vitamin deficiencies, if the increased vitamin requirements imposed by drug intake are not met by diet or by oral and parenteral vitamin supplements . . .
>
> . . . drugs can impair absorption, increase excretion or decrease nutrient utilization. Certain drugs can also lead to decreased nutrient intake because of attendant anorexia. The risk of drug-induced nutritional deficiencies varies, being highest in those on marginal diets, and in those whose nutritional status is compromised by physiological stress such as pregnancy, or by pre-existent disease . . .
>
> . . . it is predictable that for any given population, drugs will have the most effect in chronic drug users. Within this group, the drugs will emphasize pre-existing nutrient lack, incurred by marginal intakes of nutrients or by disease.[20]

It is assumed that most chronic users of medicines are under a physician's care and that appropriate dietary adjustments have been made and/or supplements recommended. However, such items as laxatives and mineral oil (which deplete fat soluble vitamins), oral contraceptives (which deplete folacin, vitamin B6 and vitamin C) and aspirin (which impairs utilization of vitamin C and folacin) may be widely and chronically used without any accompanying medical or nutritional guidance.[20]

Air pollution may be an additional factor with a significant impact, although this is difficult to measure. Animal research has indicated that increased vitamin E may be helpful when certain tissues are exposed to free radicals such as are present in polluted air (ozone and nitrogen dioxide). Free radicals are also present in heavy concentrations in cigarette smoke. Although animal data suggest that increased vitamin E may be advisable in heavily polluted areas,[22] such data may not be obtainable in man since there would be serious ethical questions in designing and conducting definitive experiments to establish a need in humans.

Pregnancy, lactation and acute physiological stress such as surgery, injury or disease can create special nutritional demands. Increased micronutrient requirements are reflected in the RDA for pregnant and nursing women, but "the special nutritional needs arising from metabolic disorders, chronic diseases, injuries, prematurity and many other medical conditions require therapeutic treatment which is not covered by the RDA for healthy persons."[2]

"Infections, even mild ones, increase metabolic losses of a number of vitamins and minerals. In addition, acute or chronic infections of the gastrointestinal tract impair the absorption of nutrients. The period of recuperation following illness, trauma, burns, and surgical procedures, during which body stores are being replenished and tissues restored, is probably comparable to a period of growth."[2] In these cases, as with the treatment of chronic disease and the use of prescription drugs, appropriate dietary adjustment and/or supplementation should be a matter of medical management.

NEW RESEARCH: IMPLICATIONS FOR HEALTH

As research continues to enhance our understanding of micronutrient functions and actions in the body, the importance of maintaining good nutritional status becomes increasingly evident. While the concept of marginal deficiency is not accepted by some, there is research which shows that intermediate stages of depletion can have a decided impact on health. For example, marginal deficiencies of protein, vitamins A, C, E, B6 and folacin have been shown to result in greater vulnerability to a number of viral and bacterial processes.[23] Since these vitamins help to maintain immune function, inadequacies can impair the body's ability to resist disease. Similarly, vitamins C, A, D, K and the B-complex vitamins, plus zinc, iron and copper are critical for proper wound healing.[24]

In recent years, there has been considerable interest in the possible role of diet and nutrition in the fight against cancer. Epidemiological data suggest that foods rich in certain vitamins may have a positive effect in reducing the incidence of certain types of cancer, and new research promises to elucidate this important area over the next decade. The current state of the art has been reported by the National Research Council as follows:[25]

> **Vitamin A.** A growing accumulation of epidemiological evidence indicates that there is an inverse relationship between the risk of cancer and the consumption of foods that contain vitamin A (e.g., liver) or its precursors (e.g., the carotenoids in green and yellow vegetables) . . . In these studies, investigators found an inverse association between estimates of 'vitamin A' intake and carcinoma at several sites, e.g., the lung, the urinary bladder and the larynx.
>
> Studies in laboratory animals indicate that vitamin A deficiency generally increases susceptibility to chemically induced neoplasia and that an increased intake of the vitamin appears to protect against carcinogenesis in most, but not all, cases. Because high doses of vitamin A are toxic, many of these studies have been conducted with its synethetic analogues (retinoids), which . . . have been shown to inhibit chemically induced neoplasia of the breast, urinary bladder, skin and lung in animals.
>
> "The committee concluded that the laboratory evidence shows that vitamin A itself and many of the retinoids are able to suppress chemically induced tumors. . ."
>
> **Vitamin C.** The results of several case-control studies and a few correlation studies suggest that the consumption of vitamin-C-containing foods is associated with a lower risk of certain cancers, particularly gastric and esophageal cancer.
>
> In the laboratory, ascorbic acid can inhibit the formation of carcinogenic N-nitroso compounds (nitrosamines) . . . In recent studies, the addition of ascorbic acid to cells grown in culture prevented the chemically induced transformation of these cells and in some cases caused reversion of transformed cells.
>
> **Vitamin E (alpha tocopherol).** Vitamin E, like ascorbic acid, inhibits the formation of nitrosamines . . . Limited evidence from studies in animals suggests that vitamin E may also inhibit the induction of tumorigenesis by other chemicals. The data are not sufficient to permit any firm conclusion to be drawn about the effect of vitamin E on cancer in humans.

In these and other areas, scientists continue to investigate the impact of diet and nutrition on health and well-being. However, it should be stressed that these data were based on consumption through foods, not supplements, and ultimate conclusions regarding the role of specific micronutrients and/or the advisability of supplementation must await the completion and evaluation of carefully conducted studies.

VITAMIN SUPPLEMENTATION:
A Skeptical View

Alfred E. Harper, Ph.D.

Dr. Alfred E. Harper has been a key participant in the development of the Recommended Dietary Allowances (RDA), as a former Chairman of the RDA Committee, Chairman of the Amino Acids Committee, and member of other RDA subcommittees. Most recently, he served as Chairman of the Food and Nutrition Board (1979-1982) of the NRC/NAS. Dr. Harper is currently a Professor of Biochemistry and Professor of Nutritional Sciences at the University of Wisconsin, Madison.

Vitamin deficiency diseases have not been encountered in the major health and nutrition surveys done recently in the United States; in fact, such diseases occur so rarely now in this country as to be medical curiosities. Large numbers of apparently healthy people, nonetheless, take vitamin supplements. The reasons they give for this are: the belief that they are not getting enough vitamins from their diets and the belief that they will be less healthy without them.[1] There is obviously a widespread popular perception that health is at risk when food is the only source of nutrients and that taking vitamin supplements will ensure a better state of health. Is this popular perception accurate? What type of evidence can be marshalled to support it? Is the available evidence reliable?

Probably the main evidence used to support recommendations for vitamin supplements is that, in health and nutrition surveys, intakes of some vitamins by some segments of the population are found to be below the recommended dietary allowances (RDA). To evaluate evidence of this type critically requires knowledge of how the RDA are established and how dietary surveys are done.

RDA are dietary standards. They were designed to provide food service personnel who procure or prepare food for large groups of people with a set of values for desirable intakes of key essential nutrients and appropriate intakes of calories. They could then compare the quantities of these essential nutrients in the food offered each day with the RDA and thereby determine if the key nutrients were being provided in large enough amounts to prevent any nutritional inadequacy.

Because people differ in size and genetic makeup, their nutrient requirements vary; requirements of individuals for essential nutrients range from about 50 percent below to 50 percent above the population average. The RDA, therefore, were set high enough to ensure that, if the quantities of nutrients in the food being served met this standard, they would meet the needs of individuals with the highest requirements.[2] Thus, the amounts of nutrients required by most people will be below the RDA and about half the population should require less than half the RDA. Obviously a dietary standard of this type cannot be used to determine if the intakes of people who are consuming less than the RDA are inadequate. Using the RDA as standards for evaluating the adequacy of nutrient intakes is like setting the standard for height at seven feet and assuming that all of those under seven feet have suffered growth retardation.

Even then, when the estimates of nutrient intakes obtained during dietary surveys are compared with the RDA, we find that only two vitamins, A and C, are identified consistently as "problem" nutrients. In interpreting these observations, we encounter two additional problems. The RDA for vitamin C is twice as high as that used by the World Health Organization.[26] It is high enough to ensure that a person who is consuming an amount of vitamin C equal to the RDA will have a store of the vitamin sufficient to prevent signs of deficiency from occurring even if he/she consumes no vitamin C for about two months. With a standard such as this, which is disproportionately high, one would expect to find problems of inadequate intake where none exist, and that is exactly what happens. With vitamin A, a different problem is encountered. The main source of vitamin A in the diet are carotenoids in dark green and yellow to orange vegetables. These foods are not usually eaten every day so, when the results of dietary surveys are based on measurements of nutrient intakes for a single day, as they ordinarily are, many people will have low intakes of vitamin A on that day. Others will have unusually high intakes. As vitamin A is stored efficiently in the liver, a surplus of vitamin A consumed on one day will provide a store that will be available on subsequent days. Intakes of vitamin A can probably be estimated accurately only by averaging daily intakes over at least a week.

Because of the nature of the RDA and of dietary surveys, it is not possible to assess nutritional status by comparing estimates of nutrient intakes with the RDA. The only way that vitamin status can be determined reliably is from clinical observations and measurements of blood or tissue concentrations or the rates of metabolic reactions for which the vitamins are needed. When this is done, a very small proportion of the population surveyed is found to have low, but seldom deficient, values.[5] With such a high proportion of the population showing no evidence of inadequate vitamin intakes, the low values cannot be attributed to inadequacies of the food supply.

Estimates of the nutrient content of the food supply indicate that amounts of nutrients available to the consumer have increased during this century.[27] Consumption of fruits, vegetables, cheese, fish, poultry and pork, all excellent sources of essential nutrients, have increased during the past ten years more than enough to compensate for declines in the consumption of beef, dairy products and eggs.[28] Of low income families studied by USDA, 42 percent were consuming a diet that met the RDA for eleven nutrients.[11] This is incontrovertible evidence that the food supply contains adequate amounts of essential nutrients. Families that were dependent on food stamp allotments were consuming less adequate diets, indicating that as income falls, food choices become more limited and intakes of some essential nutrients decrease. In adequate intakes of food, and hence usually of nutrients, occur because of neglect, illness, alcoholism and ignorance. These are not problems that can be solved by the use of vitamin or other dietary supplements.

Another reason given for the use of vitamin supplements is deteriorating or haphazard eating habits. That eating habits have changed is undeniable but whether or not this represents deterioration is certainly debatable. A pattern of eating three or more substantial meals a day is common in agricultural communities and others in which energy expenditure is high. This was accepted as the most desirable pattern when our population was largely rural and when mechanization was much less in both the home and the workplace than it is today. One might well ask if, in a society in which energy expenditure is low, it may not be preferable to eat several small meals throughout the day and to eat when hungry rather than when the clock says it is mealtime. There is much speculation but little evidence that unusual eating patterns result in consumption of inadequate amounts of essential nutrients except when total calorie (food) intake is low.

Even the evidence that many people, especially women, have low caloric intakes, and therefore low intakes of essential nutrients,[7] deserves careful scrutiny. The basis for the RDA for energy (calories) is different from that for essential nutrients. RDA for energy represent average requirements. Half of the population should thus require less than the RDA. Also, with as much as 20 percent of the population, especially women, on weight reduction regimens at any one time, the proportion found to have caloric intakes below the RDA in any dietary survey would be expected to exceed 50 percent. Despite this, underweight is a problem for very few people in this country; hence, the number of dieters who stay on low calorie diets for very long cannot be high. It is notable, furthermore, that in dietary surveys protein intakes are usually found to meet the RDA.[11] As protein tends to make up a relatively constant proportion of calories in most diets, this raises a question as to whether caloric intake has been underestimated. Persons with calorie intakes above the RDA are reported to have intakes of most essential nutrients that are well above the RDA.[3] Hence, if caloric intakes have been underestimated, this could account for some of the low estimates of micronutrient intakes.

There is little evidence that will stand up to scrutiny to suggest that any substantial proportion of the U.S. population is consuming a nutritionally inadequate diet for any length of time. There is thus little reason to assume that vitamin supplements will be beneficial for a substantial portion of the population. Foods contain many nutrients besides those provided in vitamin supplements; they also contain many constituents whose significance for health is unknown. Learning how to select foods properly to meet nutritional needs, regardless of changing eating patterns or changes in the food supply, is the only reliable way to ensure lifelong nutritional health. Encouraging the use of vitamin supplements as a corrective for poor eating habits defeats the entire purpose of nutrition education, i.e., to learn the nutritional principles needed to select a healthful diet instead of accepting nutritional advice on faith.

In recent years there have been suggestions that larger than usual amounts of vitamins are needed to counteract the effects of environmental hazards and practices that increase risk to health. The suggestion that smokers need high doses of vitamin C seems incongruous when one considers that most of the subjects used in the major experiments that served as the basis for present vitamin C allowances were smokers. It would seem much more appropriate to suggest that non-smokers need less. For heavy consumers of alcohol, vitamin supplements may prevent the development of some nutritional inadequacies. They may also encourage further consumption of alcohol to the point where toxicity becomes more severe than it otherwise might. Minor infections or stresses may increase nutritional needs

modestly for a short time. As the human subjects used in experiments which provided the information on which requirements are based were not protected from usual environmental stresses or infections, it is doubtful that vitamin supplements are needed in these conditions. During illness, recovery from illness and during periods of drug therapy, food intake may be so low that it becomes difficult or even impossible to meet nutritional needs from foods. RDA are not therapeutic recommendations. Nutritional supplements are often appropriate under such conditions but as part of a comprehensive program of treatment under the guidance of a physician.

There have been a variety of observations suggesting that certain vitamins, A, E, and C in particular, may have some unique value in preventing or reducing adverse effects from environmental hazards. Some of these observations are tantalizing, e.g., that these vitamins may act in some way to protect against certain cancer-inducing agents; and, that vitamins E and C, as antioxidants, may protect against ill effects from certain chemical contaminants. These studies are suggestive, not conclusive. They are the subject of much current research. They suggest that vitamin deficiencies often increase susceptibility to toxic agents, but the assumption that large doses of nutrients—larger than the usual recommended intakes—are uniquely beneficial is controversial. Promotion of vitamin supplements as therapeutic agents tends to encourage self-medication with large quantities of specific vitamins. Such practices create the risk of people delaying or not accepting appropriate medical treatment for illnesses and taking doses of vitamins that create risks of toxicity. With the advent of the widespread use of large doses of vitamins the incidence of vitamin toxicity has increased.[29]

The most appropriate use of vitamin supplements is in conditions in which caloric intake is low, below 1200 kcal per day, and particularly if, at the same time, requirements are increased, say as the result of illness. An appropriately balanced multivitamin supplement for the pregnant woman and supplements of vitamins A and D of appropriate potency for the young infant can be justified as insurance against nutritional inadequacy. Evaluation of the nutrition literature on vitamin requirements and intakes and claims for the use of vitamins as therapeutic and pharmacologic agents, however, provides no evidence to convince me that the population generally requires vitamin supplements but much to convince me that the nutritional knowledge of the public generally is inadequate and inaccurate. The assumed nutritional problems of most people are best solved by providing them with accurate nutrition information about food and health and countering the nutrition misinformation to which so many of them are constantly exposed.

VITAMIN SUPPLEMENTATION:
A Practical View

Willard A. Krehl, M.D.

Dr. Willard A. Krehl is the President and Medical Director of the Health Maintenance Program at Jefferson Medical College Hospital, Philadelphia. He received his M.D. degree from the Yale School of Medicine, where he was also an Associate Professor of Nutrition for seven years. Prior to his present position, he was Chairman of the Department of Community Health and Preventive Medicine at Jefferson and editor-in-chief of the *American Journal of Clinical Nutrition*.

My own bias on the value of nutrient supplementation has

developed over the years through my experience in clinical practice. One of the standard procedures at our clinic is to take a dietary history of each patient. Reviewing these, I continually see that in spite of the fact that our clients are generally in the executive category and can therefore easily purchase an excellent diet, most of them do not eat properly. For whatever reasons, a large percent either skip breakfast or eat the wrong things for breakfast; they have a fast food lunch high in fat and often low in micronutrients; they consume a good deal of sugar, sweets and alcoholic beverages. In short, my search for the individuals who consistently eat a well-balanced, varied and nutritionally adequate diet has merely impressed me with the fact that millions of people do not.

Thus it comes as no surprise to me that national surveys reflect the nutritional imbalances and micronutrient shortages they do. It's not that the food supply is deficient; the "deficiency" lies in people's ability or motivation to use food properly.

I strongly favor multivitamin supplementation and recommend it to my patients because I believe it is a simple, economical and highly practical way to insure they receive 100 percent of the RDA for essential micronutrients, and because I believe these intakes are important to health and well-being.

Some of the standard arguments against supplementation are that it encourages poor food habits, that marginal vitamin intakes are not really significant, and that people spend too much money on supplements. Let us consider each of these points.

Does supplementation encourage poor eating habits? I know of no evidence to support the notion that the diets of people who take supplements are worse than those of people who do not. In fact, the opposite seems to be true: supplement users tend to be more health- and nutrition-conscious than non-users.[1] Perhaps the reason there is no support for this "logic" is that it is, upon closer examination, illogical. What comes first? Food habits, of course. Eating habits are in place long before people consider supplementation. People consider supplementation when they learn why their eating habits need improvement. Something usually prompts this realization. It may be pregnancy, when supplements are prescribed, or dieting, which requires education about foods, or some medical crisis requiring nutritional support. In any case, supplementation seems to occur as part of the first stage of nutrition "consciousness-raising," when maintaining good nutrition becomes a matter of personal importance. As people attempt to make some positive changes in their habits, supplementation is *one* of the things they may do. Saying that supplementation encourages us to eat poorly is like saying antiseptics encourage us to cut ourselves more frequently.

This argument usually goes on to say that nutrition education can correct poor eating habits and eliminate the need for supplementation. It usually positions supplementation *versus* nutrition education. I think that is a mixture of wishful thinking and misinformation. More in tune with reality and therefore more useful would be nutrition education which encompasses the proper role of supplementation. Eating habits are deeply ingrained and are often a function of lifestyle, divorced from nutritional considerations altogether.[30] This makes them quite difficult to change. Change requires a willingness to undergo some inconvenience (there are no salads in the office candy machine), deprivation (cutting down on favorite sweets, alcohol, snacks, etc.) and rescheduling of activites (setting aside time

for exercise and proper meals). Such changes do not come easily. They require time, patience and commitment, in addition to education/knowledge.

Moreover, even with the best nutrition planning and knowledge, there is no guarantee that all nutritional guidelines and recommendations can be met, notably when caloric intakes fall below about 1600 calories. Consider the menus published by the U.S. Department of Agriculture in "Ideas for Better Eating." Even with thorough and careful nutritional planning by competent professionals, these diets fall short of recommended levels of some essential nutrients at the 1600 calorie level.[10] If nutritionists have trouble devising menus to meet nutrient recommendations at the 1600 calorie level, we should not be surprised at consumers' inability to do so. As it happens, the average caloric intakes of women in the United States hover around this level or lower.[7] Other groups, such as the elderly and dieters, also consume low calorie diets that may put them at risk for some micronutrients.

Preliminary data from the National Health and Nutrition Survey (N-HANES II) indicate the median caloric intake of the general population is 1,831 calories.[8] (For women, the median is even lower, at 1,493 calories.) Median means that 50 percent of the population take in higher amounts and 50 percent take in lower amounts. So these data are telling us that the caloric intakes of half of American women are lower than 1,493 calories—a level where even trained nutritionists have trouble creating meals to provide RDA levels of vitamins and minerals!

This trend was spotted a few years ago in the USDA's Nationwide Consumption Survey. Pondering the data, Dr. Mark Hegsted wrote,

> These low levels of food consumption make it increasingly difficult for many Americans to achieve the rather generous levels of nutrients specified in the RDA. The Food and Nutrition Board has repeatedly warned that consumption of less than the RDA does not mean an individual is deficient in that nutrient, yet we must also assume that this Board does believe that consumption at [RDA] levels is desirable.[9]

Indeed, the data from these surveys have shown shortages of vitamins and minerals among numerous sex-age groups, and the shortages were more prevalent among those who consumed lower calorie diets.[3]

Are these micronutrient shortages significant? Most nutrition professionals agree that intakes below the RDA do not necessarily indicate serious nutritional risk, because the RDA are set higher than average requirements. The *requirement* for a nutrient is the minimum intake needed to prevent failure of a specific function or the development of specific deficiency signs. Because of individual variations, this minimum level will span a certain range among a given group of people. The *allowance* or RDA is set high enough to meet the needs of people with the highest requirements, thereby covering the needs of most people within the group. For this reason, nutritionists generally look at the percent of population groups with intakes lower than 70 to 80 percent of the RDA, rather than the percentages below 100 percent, as indicative of nutritional risk. The Food and Nutrition Board has noted in the 1980 edition of the Recommended Dietary Allowances:

In assessing dietary surveys of populations, if the amounts of nutrients consumed fall below the RDA for a particular age-sex group, some individuals can be assumed to be at nutritional risk. When the proportion of individuals with such low intakes is extensive, the risk of deficiency in the population is increased.[2]

What is "extensive"? Ten percent? Twenty? If one projects the numbers, ten percent of our present population would include more than 23 million people—an "extensive" group by any standards. According to the 1977-78 Nationwide Food Consumption Survey, significant percentages of the population were consuming less than 70 percent of the RDA for the nutrients listed.[3]

Nutrient	Percent of individuals with intakes less than 70 percent RDA
Vitamin B6	51 percent
Calcium	42 percent
Magnesium	39 percent
Iron	32 percent
Vitamin A	31 percent
Vitamin C	26 percent
Thiamin	17 percent
Vitamin B12	15 percent
Riboflavin	12 percent

Since at 70 percent of the RDA or lower we can no longer be certain about an ample margin of safety, these data should alert us to an astonishing prevalence of potential nutritional risk. Furthermore, factors such as smoking, the use of alcohol, oral contraceptives or other drugs may increase risk among individuals whose diets are inadequate.

Among the strongest evidence illustrating widespread nutritional inadequacies are studies of our hospitalized population.[31-33] Marginal or deficient levels of vitamins have been found in at least 30 percent of hospital patients, and protein-calorie malnutrition has been seen in some 44 percent. These individuals are in "double jeopardy," so to speak. Their disease or injury dramatically increases nutritional needs, even to the point of precipitating malnutrition which in turn impairs the immune response and the ability to heal.[34-38]

In healthy people, suboptimal nutrition may result in vague symptoms such as depression, loss of appetite, irritability and so forth. These everyday complaints may be tolerable; however, serious problems can arise when illness, injury and/or surgery are superimposed upon preexisting marginal status.

The wisdom of maintaining the best nutritional health possible is self-evident. From my perspective, it certainly makes sense to err on the side of caution and insure adequate micronutrient intakes with a well-balanced multivitamin supplement, especially among populations known to be at nutritonal risk—dieters, pregnant and lactating women, adolescent girls, smokers, alcoholics, the elderly, low income groups and others. When one considers the number of people potentially involved, the 60 million or so currently taking supplements probably far undershoots the number who could benefit from them.

I think it also makes sense for physicians to make this recommendation, since we can at the same time deter our patients from self-medicating or using supplements irresponsibly. I do not believe anyone should take therapeutic amounts of nutrients without medical supervision, but unless doctors are willing to give strong counsel on the proper use of supplements, I doubt if anyone will listen to our warnings about improper use.

Some people believe Americans are spending huge sums of money on vitamin supplements. Actually the average cost is about 8-9¢ per day, which is within the economic reach of just about everyone.[1] The total vitamin supplement market was under $2 billion last year; I should think that those who are concerned with "unnecessary" expenditures might better target their efforts toward the $40 billion alcoholic beverage market or the $20 billion tobacco market.[39]

One of the areas that concerns me most is the cost of health care in general—some $322 billion in 1982.[40] This cost has been increasing at a rate of 12-15 percent per year, about three times the general rate of inflation. It is breaking the back of American industry, which supplies much of the health care, and it is overwhelming the taxpayer who has to foot the bill for Medicare, Medicaid and other government insurance programs. I believe that improved nutrition, in which vitamin supplementation can play an important role, might help to reduce this problem.

In sum, the high incidence of below-RDA micro-nutrient intakes, resulting from multiple factors including poor food choices, decreased caloric intakes and personal/environmental/lifestyle factors, presents a situation in which multivitamin supplementation is both a rational and beneficial choice. Supplementation provides a practical and economical means of insuring adequate nutrient intakes and is of particular importance for risk groups such as dieters, the elderly, heavy drinkers, chronic drug users and others whose diets are insufficient or whose ability to utilize food is impaired. Therapeutic amounts of micronutrients should not be used without medical supervision. In addition to education about food, consumers need nutrition education that teaches the proper role and value of rational supplementation and cautions against improper use. I see absolutely no reason to tolerate nutrient inadequacies when such a simple and sensible alternative as a multivitamin exists.

REFERENCES

1. Stanton, J.L. *"Vitamin Usage: Rampant or Reasonable?"* Vitamin Issues, No. 1, 1983.

2. *Recommended Dietary Allowances.* Food and Nutrition Board, National Academy of Sciences, Washington, D.C., 1980.

3. Pao, E. and Sharon Mickle. "Problem Nutrients in the United States," *Food Technology,* Sept. 1981.

4. *Dietary Levels of Households in the United States, Spring 1965.* Agriculture Research Service, U.S. Dept. of Agriculture, pp. 12-17, 1968.

5. *Ten State Nutrition Survey*. U.S. Dept. of Health, Education and Welfare, Health Services and Mental Health Administration Center for Disease Control, DHEW Publ. No. (HSM) 72-8130-8134, Atlanta, GA.

6. *First Health and Nutrition Examination Survey*. Public Health Service, Health Resources Administration, U.S. Dept. of Health, 1971-72.

7. *Nationwide Food Consumption Survey, Spring 1980*. U.S. Dept. of Agriculture, Science and Education Administration, Beltsville, MD.

8. *Dietary Intake Source Data: United States 1976-80*. Data from the National Health Survey, Series 11, no. 231, DHHS Publication No. (PHS) 83-1681, March 1983.

9. Hegsted, Mark D., "Nationwide Food Consumption Survey—Implications," *Family Economics Review*, Spring 1980, U.S. Dept. of Agriculture, Science and Education Administration, Beltsville, MD.

10. *Ideas for Better Eating*. Menus and Recipes to Make Use of the Dietary Guidelines, Science and Education Administration/ Human Nutrition, U.S. Dept. of Agriculture, Jan. 1981.

11. Peterkin, B.B., R.L. Kerr and M.Y. Hama. "Nutritional Adequacy of Diets of Low Income Households," *J.Nut.Ed.* 14:102, 1982.

12. Sheils, Merrill. "Portrait of America," *Newsweek* Special Report, Jan. 17, 1983.

13. *Statistical Abstracts of the United States, 1980*. U.S. Dept. of Commerce, Bureau of the Census, Washington, D.C.

14. Pao, Eleanor M. and Sharon J. Mickle. "Nutrients from meals and snacks consumed by individuals," *Family Economics Review*, U.S. Dept. of Agriculture, Science and Education Administration, Beltsville, MD.

15. Hallfrisch, Judith, Priscilla Steele and Lynette Cohen. "Comparison of Seven Day Diet Record with Measured Food intake of Twenty-four Subjects," *Nutrition Research*, 2:262-273, 1982.

16. *Who's Dieting and Why*. A.C. Nielsen Co., 1978.

17. Welsh, Susan O. and Ruth M. Marston. "Review of trends in food use in the United States, 1909 to 1980," *J. Am. Dietetic Assn.*, 81:120-126, 198.

18. Schwerin, Horace S., John L. Stanton, Alvin M. Riley, Jr. and Barbara E. Brett. "How Have the Quantity and Quality of the American Diet Changed During the Past Decade?," *Food Technology*, 50–57, Sept. 1981.

19. Pelletier, O. "Vitamin C and Tobacco," In A. Hanck, and G.G. Ritzel (eds.) *Reevaluation of Vitamin C, Int. J. Vit. Nutr. Res.* 16:147-169, 1977.

20. Roe, Daphne. *Drug-Induced Nutritional Deficiencies*, The AVI Publishing Company Inc., Westport, CT, 1976.

21. Krehl, Williard A. "The Role of Nutrition in Preventing Disease," presented at Davidson Conference Center for Continuing Education, Univ. of Southern California School of Dentistry, Feb. 29, 1981.

22. Menzel, Daniel B. "Protective Effects of Vitamin E Against Environmental Pollutants," presented at *Vitamin E: New Frontiers to Health*, Port St. Lucie, FL, 1981. Presentation summaries available through VNIS.

23. Brin, Myron. "Marginal Deficiency and Immunocompetence," presented at American Chemical Society Symposium, Las Vegas, NV, Aug. 1980.

24. Schumann, I. "Preoperative Measures to Promote Wound Healing," *Nursing Clinics of North America*, Vol. 14, No. 4, Dec. 1979.

25. *Diet, Nutrition and Cancer*. Committee on Diet, Nutrition and Cancer, Assembly of Life Sciences, National Research Council, National Academy Press, Washington, DC, 1982.

26. *World Health Organization Handbook on Human Nutritional Requirements* FAO and WHO, Rome, 1974.

27. Gortner, W.A. "Nutrition in the United States, 1900-1974," *Cancer Res.* 35:3246, 1975.

28. Prescott, R. "Food Consumption, Prices and Expenditures USDA," ERS Stat. Bull. 672, Sept. 1981.

29. Dubick, M.A. & R.B. Rucker. "Dietary Supplements and Health Aids," *J. Nutr. Ed.* 15:47, 1983.

30. "Nutrition: A Study of Consumers Attitudes and Behavior Toward Eating at Home and Out of Home," *First Woman's Day/FMI Family Food Study*, conducted by Yankelovich, Skelly and White Inc., 1978.

31. Bistrian, Bruce et al. "Prevalence of Malnutrition in General Medical Patients," *JAMA*, 235:1567-1570, 1976.

32. Lemoine et al. "Vitamin B1, B2, and B6 and C Status in Hospital Inpatients," *Am. J. Clin. Nutr.* 33:2595-2600, 1980.

33. Leevy et al. "Incidence and Significance of Hypovitaminemia in a Randomly Selected Municipal Hospital Population," *Amer. J. Clin. Nutr.* 17:259-271, 1965.

34. Dreizen, S. "Nutrition and the Immune Response—A Review," *Internat. J. Vit. Nur. Res.* 49, 1979.

35. Beisel et al. "Single-Nutrient Effects on Immunologic Functions," *JAMA*, 245:53-58, 1981.

36. Leevy, C.M. "Vitamin Therapy: It Means More Than Simply Giving Vitamins," *Drug Therapy*, Feb. 1972.

37. Pollack, S.V. "Nutritional Factors Affecting Wound Healing," *J. Dermatol. Surg. Oncol.*, 5:8, Aug. 1979.

38. Kaminski, M.V. and A.L. Windborn. "Nutritional Assessment Guide," *Midwest Nutrition*, Education and Research Foundation, Inc., 1978.

39. Gallo, Anthony F. "Food Spending and Income," *National Food Review*, USDA Economic Research Service, Winter 1982.

40. *Medical Tribune*. 24(19):1, 1983.

Part III
NUTRITION AND CANCER

8

................FAT, FIBER AND CANCER................................

INTRODUCTION

OVER 450,000 people in the U.S. die of cancer each year. Seventy percent to 90 percent of cancers are related to our environment and lifestyles. Approximately 135,000 or 30 percent of these deaths are the result of cigarette smoking. Genetic factors, radiation, air pollution and certain occupational exposures contribute to another 45,000 to 90,000 cancer deaths annually. But in 40 percent to 60 percent of all environmental cancers, diet and nutrition are in some way related.[1,2]

Exposure to cancer-causing agents usually does not create a statistically significant increase in cancer for twenty to thirty years. This makes it extremely difficult to come up with concrete evidence for making dietary recommendations. But there is sufficient information at this time to make dietary recommendations based on epidemiological evidence. This type of evidence is gathered by comparing differences in the incidence of specific types of cancers from one country to another and from one region to another within a country. Although some of the differences may be due to genetic or local environmental factors, dietary factors appear to be the major explanation for differences in cancer and incidence.

When dietary factors and the incidence of cancer are explored, certain foods appear to have a protective effect while others have been identified as containing potential cancer-causing agents. Research also suggests that vitamins A and C along with the trace element selenium play an important role in decreasing the incidence of certain types of cancer. Current research regarding these nutrients, along with key dietary factors as they relate to the incidence of cancer, are discussed in this chapter. Dietary guidelines endorsed by the American Cancer Society are also presented.

PROBLEMS WITH POPULATION STUDIES

Attempting to correlate incidence of cancer with characteristics of groups within a population can lead to erroneous conclusions. For example, Figure 10 has been presented as evidence that there is a strong positive correlation between dietary fat intake and the incidence of breast cancer. This type of correlational study does not take into account other factors that might have caused this effect, such as genetics, cultural patterns, level of economic development and general nutritional status.

Another problem with this type of evidence is that the information is based on food disappearance data and not on the actual dietary habits of individuals. Food disappearance data is acquired by determining the total food production in a country plus food imports and subtracting food exports. This figure is then divided by the population and the resulting figure is then used as the amount consumed by that population. This crude estimate of food intake is not accurate and therefore, findings from this type of study must be incorporated into findings acquired using other research methods before recommendations can be made.

Another research method that is employed and coupled with the type of information produced in Figure 10 is the prospective study. This type of research

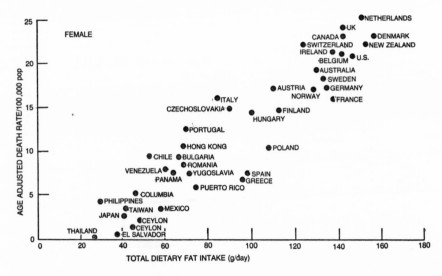

Figure 10

Correlation between per capita consumption of dietary fat and age-adjusted mortality from breast cancer in different countries. The values for dietary fat are averages for 1964 to 1966 and those for cancer mortality are for 1964 to 1965, except in a few cases where data were available only for 1960 to 1961 or 1962 to 1963.

Source: Reddy, B. S., Cohen, L. A., McCoy, G. D., et al. Nutrition and its relationship to cancer. *Adv. Cancer Res.*, 32:237–345, 1980. Reprinted by permission.

operates from a hypothesis that may have been developed from the data gathered in a food disappearance study. The hypothesis might say something like: "Individuals who regularly eat a suspected cancer-causing food will have a higher incidence of cancer than those who do not eat this food." Or the hypothesis might say that individuals who regularly eat foods that are thought to have a protective effect against cancer will have a lower incidence of cancer than those who do not consume these foods.

In order to determine if the hypothesis is correct, a large number of people are requested to complete a survey on dietary habits. The incidence of cancer is tracked for a number of years to determine if there is a relationship between a certain food or nutrient and the disease.

The accuracy of the prospective study is to a large extent dependent upon the design of the questionnaire used to gather the dietary information. In addition, the accuracy of the individuals' ability to recall what foods they have eaten and in what quantity can have a significant impact on the accuracy of the findings.

Once a strong correlation has been established between certain foods or nutrients and cancer, groups of individuals must be studied to determine if the inci-

dence of this disease can be reduced by changing dietary habits. This presents another problem. Generally, eating behavior is difficult to change. When individuals are asked to cooperate in a study that requires them to follow strict dietary guidelines, noncompliance is very high.

Even with all of the problems inherent in studying cancer in human populations, there appears to be sufficient evidence, especially when combined with the evidence from animal research, to warrant a change in the American diet and perhaps a recommendation for specific nutritional supplements, especially in at-risk populations.

Figures 11 and 12 show the American Cancer Society tests for bowel and breast cancer.

FAT, FIBER AND COLON CANCER

The incidence of colon cancer varies significantly from country to country. The differences in incidence are associated with economic development, industrial development and dietary habits. The epidemiologic studies suggest that diets which are high in total fat and low in fiber, vegetables, vitamins and minerals are associated with an increased incidence of cancer.[3–7]

Cancer of the colon is primarily a disease of the

Add up the numbers beside the boxes that apply to you and place the total on the score panel for each cancer. The color darkens as the risk increases.

BOWEL

My age is:
[1] under 50   [3] between 50–59   [12] 60 or over

I have close relatives who have had:
[5] colon cancer   [2] polyps of the colon
[1] neither

I have had:
[12] colon cancer   [5] polyps of the colon
[4] ulcerative colitis   [1] none of these

I have bleeding from the rectum
(not obviously hemorrhoids or piles):
[10] yes   [1] no

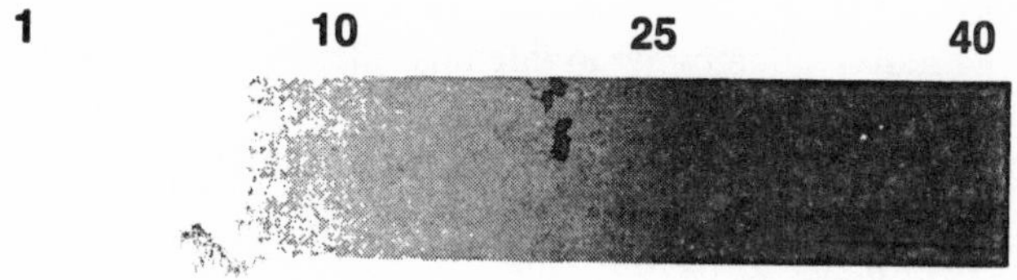

1   10   25   40

Figure 11

Bowel cancer. With early detection, 80 percent of all bowel cancers can be cured. These cancers grow slowly, and they can be detected with three tests during a regular cancer checkup. The **stool blood test, digital rectal exam,** and the **procto test** can save many lives. Talk with your doctor about how often you should have these tests.

BREAST

My age is:
[1] under 40   [3] 40–49   [6] 50 and over

My ethnic group is:
[1] Hispanic   [2] Oriental   [2] Black   [3] White

My family medical history includes:
[1] no breast cancer   [3] mother, sister, aunt or grandmother who has had breast cancer

I have had:
[1] no breast disease   [3] previous breast cancer

My history of pregnancies is:
[1] first live birth before age 18
[2] first live birth at age 18–34
[4] first live birth age 35 or older   [3] no live births

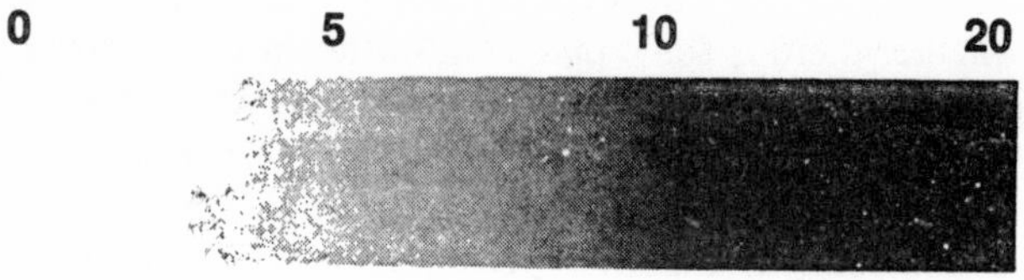

0   5   10   20

Figure 12

Breast cancer. Finding breast cancer early is the best safeguard. All women over the age of 20 should do a monthly **breast self-exam.** Women between the ages of 20 and 40 also should have a doctor examine their breasts every three years. After the age of 40 women should have an examination annually and a **mammogram (breast X-ray)** every one to two years. Women over 50 should have an **annual mammogram.** Some people are at higher risk than others, so talk to your physician about how often you should have these tests.

economically developed countries.[3,5,8] The highest incidence rates for colon cancer are found in North America, New Zealand, Australia, and western Europe (except Finland, which has one of the lowest rates). Developed countries that have the lowest incidence rates of colon cancer include eastern Europe, Asia, Africa, and South America (except Uruguay and Argentina, which are close to the incidence seen in North America).[9] Is the difference in incidence of colon cancer between these countries due to dietary factors, or is it primarily due to genetics?

One method for determining whether the difference in incidence of this disease is genetics or diet is to observe the frequency of colon cancer in populations who move from a country with a low incidence to a country that has a high incidence. If colon cancer is primarily genetic, then moving from one country to another would not be expected to change the incidence of this type of cancer.

Studies conducted in the early 70s, along with more recent research, have demonstrated that the incidence of colon cancer can be significantly altered in migrant populations. For example, Japan has a low incidence of colon cancer compared to the U.S. But when Japanese immigrate to the U.S., the first and second generations have a significantly higher incidence of colon cancer than occurs in Japan. The same results are observed when the Polish immigrate to Australia or the U.S.[10–12] The next question that might be asked is whether there is some protective factor in the Japanese or Polish homeland diet, or whether there is some cancer-causing dietary factors in the U.S. and Australian diet. Since the increased incidence of colon cancer is observed in the first generation of Japanese and Polish immigrants, scientists believe that there is something about the U.S. and Australian diet that is responsible for this disease. Additional support for this conclusion is provided by the fact that as Japanese food habits within Japan have become more westernized, the incidence of colon cancer in that country has increased.[12]

Additional support for implicating either dietary factors or lifestyle factors comes from studies comparing the incidence of colon cancer between certain groups that have different dietary preferences but are living in the same geographical area. For example, the incidence of colon cancer among Seventh-Day Adventists living in the U.S. is significantly lower than that of the rest of the population. This religious group maintains a vegetarian diet. The dietary habits of Mormons also lend weight to the theory that dietary factors are responsible for colon cancer. In fact, studies of the Mormon diet suggest that consumption of a specific dietary component—fat—is related to colon cancer.[13]

In the late 1960s, accumulating research suggested that dietary fat intake might be the cause of colon cancer. A number of other studies throughout the 1970s supported this theory and current research continues to point toward dietary fat as a primary culprit.

By 1975 a worldwide correlation between total fat consumption and colon cancer had been established.[14] But during the same period when the fat theory of colon cancer was gaining prominence, other dietary factors were being implicated. A correlation between animal protein and colon cancer deaths was established on both national and international levels.[15–18]

In addition to dietary fat and animal protein, a third dietary factor has been shown to have a significant relationship to the incidence of colon cancer—dietary fiber. Studies have shown that people in countries such as Africa who consume a diet rich in fiber have a low incidence of colon cancer.[4] Other studies have pointed out that in countries where people consume a high-fat diet but have a low incidence of colon cancer—Finland, for example—they also consume diets high in fiber.[19–23]

Studies attempting to identify dietary factors that might have a preventive or protective effect for cancer continue to present a positive role for high-fiber foods. In addition, certain vegetables high in fiber appear to have a more cancer-protective or preventive role than other foods with high fiber content. In particular, brussels sprouts, broccoli and cabbage may have certain characteristics beyond their fiber content that can confer a cancer-protective effect on the colon.[23,24,6]

Once sufficient correlational and epidemiological data had been gathered to support the theory of the cancer-promoting effect of a high-fat/low-fiber diet, researchers began investigating the mechanism whereby this type of diet might promote colon cancer. The evidence to date indicates that this mechanism involves the alteration of bile acids by dietary fat and the ability of fiber to bind toxic compounds.

High-fat diets stimulate the excretion of bile acids into the gut. In addition, this type of diet alters the activity of microflora in the gut. The altered microflora activity creates compounds from the bile acids that promote colon cancer.[25,26] Dietary fiber can bind these cancer-promoting compounds and also dilute these

TABLE 10
Modifying Factors in Colon Cancer

Dietary Fat*	Dietary Fibers*†	Micronutrients
1. Increases bile acid secretion into gut	1. Certain fibers increase fecal bulk and dilute carcinogens and promoters	(include vitamins, minerals, anti-oxidants, etc.)
2. Increases metabolic activity of gut bacteria	2. Modify metabolic activity of gut bacteria	1. Modify carcinogenesis at activation and detoxification level
3. Increases secondary bile acids in colon.	3. Modify the metabolism of carcinogens and/or promoters	2. Act also at promotional phase of carcinogenesis
4. Alters immune system	4. Bind the carcinogens and/or promoters and excrete them	
5. Stimulation of mixed function oxidase system		

*Dietary factors, particularly high total dietary fat and a relative lack of certain dietary fibers and vegetables, have a role.
†High dietary fiber or fibrous foods may be a protective factor even in the high dietary fat intake.

Source: Wynder, E. L. and Reddy, B. S. Dietary fat and fiber and colon cancer. *Seminars in Oncology*, 10 (3): 264–272, 1983. Reprinted by permission.

substances by virtue of its bulking properties, thereby providing a protective effect.[27]

High-fiber foods such as fruits and vegetables also contain other factors that have been demonstrated to have an inhibitory action on various types of cancer. These compounds include plant sterols, aromatic isothiocyanates, phenols, indoles, and vitamin and minerals such as carotenes, vitamin C, vitamin E and selenium.[28] Thus, there is a strong rationale for recommending that Americans increase their consumption of fresh fruits and vegetables and decrease their intake of fatty foods, especially animal fat. Table 10 lists those factors that have been demonstrated to have a modulating role in colon cancer.[29] When coupled with animal studies, the epidemiological and case-control human studies create a very strong case for the etiology of colon cancer. Populations living in countries such as the U.S. where the incidence of this type of cancer is great should be instructed on how to increase dietary fiber while decreasing total fat intake.

FAT AND BREAST CANCER

Studies have shown that Japan and other Far Eastern countries as well as most undeveloped nations have rates of breast cancer that are as low as one-fifth those of the United States and northern Europe.[30] Since there is a very strong correlation between national per capita consumption of fat and age-adjusted rates of breast cancer in these studies, fat is frequently cited as a possible cause of this type of cancer. But other studies make this relationship between fat intake and cancer less convincing. In England, certain regions have a positive correlation between per capita consumption of dairy fat and breast cancer but an inverse correlation with other types of dietary fats.[31] Some studies have demonstrated that the low consumption of fat by Seventh-Day Adventists explains the low incidence of breast cancer in this population.[32] But more current studies of Seventh-Day Adventists have explained the low incidence of breast cancer by differences in socioeconomic status.[33]

Fat consumption has increased in Japan and Iceland, but the expected increase in breast cancer incidence has been significant only in the Icelandic population. With these conflicting reports, a few American researchers have attempted to relate the consumption of different types of fats to the incidence of breast cancer.[34] To date, the strongest association appears to be with the consumption of trans-fatty acids. These are fatty acids that are created in the process of converting liquid vegetable oils to margarine and solid vegetable

TABLE 11
Comparison of High- and Low-Risk Dietary Factors for Cancer in Specific Organs

| Organ | Lower Risk | | High Risk | |
	Population	Dietary Factors	Population	Dietary Factors
Esophagus	USA—Utah; rural Norway	Less alcohol and tobacco use	France—Calvados, Normandy	Extensive alcohol and tobacco use
			USA—lower socioeconomic groups	Alcohol, smoking
			Eastern Iran	Low intake of vitamin C, A; opium use?
			Central China	Dietary carcinogen? Low vitamin C and E
Stomach	USA	Fresh fruit, salads, vitamins C and E.	Japan, Chile, Columbia	Salted, pickled food; nitrate in soil and water; low vitamins C, E
Colon	Japan	Low fat	USA, Western Europe, New Zealand, Australia, Scandinavia	High fat, low fiber, fried food
	Mormons	Higher fiber	USA in general	High fat, low fiber, fried food
	Seventh-Day Adventists	Low or no fried food, higher fiber	USA in general	High fat, low fiber, fried food
	Finland	Higher fiber, lower fried food	USA in general, Denmark	High fat, low fiber, fried food
Breast	Japan	Low fat	USA, Western Europe, New Zealand, Australia	High fat
Prostate	Japan	Low fat	USA, Scandinavia, Western Europe	High fat

Source: Weisburger, J. H., Horn, C. L. and Barnes, W. S. Possible genotoxic carcinogens in food in relation to cancer causation. *Seminars in Oncology*, 10(3):330–341, 1983. Reprinted by permission.

shortening. But studies attempting to relate margarine and shortening consumption over the past two decades to incidence of breast cancer are confounded by the incidence of this disease that would be expected on the basis of a trend toward later and fewer pregnancies during the same period.

In the U.S., the consumption of eggs is inversely related to breast cancer rates whereas the consumption of milk, a major fat source, is positively associated with rates of breast cancer.[35] Most of these and the other epidemiologic studies look at entire groups within populations and do not address the fat/cancer relationship in individual women. But even in the few studies that have explored the relationship between individual women, the findings are inconclusive.

Studies on the relationship between fat consumption, estrogen levels, and breast-cancer risk have not been conclusive. Most of the human studies have limitations

and design problems that must be overcome before it can be determined if a clear relationship exists between dietary fat, sex hormones and breast cancer. Well-controlled animal studies consistently support the hypothesis that higher dietary fat intake leads to an increased incidence of mammary tumors.

It appears, though, that total fat intake is not the only factor implicated. Without at least a small amount of polyunsaturated fat in the diet, the correlation between dietary fat and increased incidence of mammary tumors is not found.[36]

Some researchers have suggested that dietary fat increases the risk for breast cancer by virtue of its high caloric content and its contribution to excess fat stores and obesity. But a positive relationship between obesity and breast cancer has been demonstrated only in older women and obesity has actually been associated with a decreased risk in premenopausal women.[37]

Perhaps the strongest hypotheses for a mechanism whereby dietary fat might increase the incidence of breast cancer is the one that implicates polyunsaturated fatty acids (PUFA) rather than total dietary fat. PUFA are subject to peroxidation and, when damaged in this manner, can initiate a chain of events that may lead to cancer. The antioxidants vitamin E and selenium play a major role in protecting PUFA from peroxidation and therefore have received considerable attention lately with regard to their cancer-protective role.[38,39]

Because of inconclusive evidence, some health professionals may be reluctant to recommend the reduction of dietary fat as a measure to decrease the risk of breast cancer. In addition, some practitioners may believe that there is a risk associated with a low-fat diet. There may be a risk in making such recommendations for children, especially children in low-income populations. This population may already be at risk for vitamin A, a fat-soluble vitamin. Unless a well-planned, affordable dietary regimen is provided, it has been advised that a recommendation to cut back on fat intake should not be made in this particular population.

But the adult female has little risk in reducing dietary fat intake to 20 percent to 25 percent of total energy. The decreased consumption of preformed vitamin A could be offset by an increase in the carotene precursors found in many vegetables. The requirement for vitamin E, another fat-soluble vitamin, is proportional to the dietary fat intake and therefore decreases in proportion to dietary fat reduction. The other fat-soluble vitamins, D and K, are synthesized in the healthy adult and dietary intake is not significant in this population.

Since dietary fat intake is associated with other types of cancer, heart disease and weight problems, and since there does not appear to be a risk in recommending a moderate reduction in fat intake, there does not appear to be any good rationale for not recommending a low-fat, high-complex-carbohydrate diet for women concerned with the risk of breast cancer. This type of diet will also help women avoid other dietary constituents such as sucrose that have been implicated in breast cancer.[40,41,42] Table 11 compares high-and high- and low-risk dietary factors for cancer in specific organs.[43]

REFERENCES

1. Wynder, E.L. and Gori, G.B. Contribution of the environment to cancer incidence: An epidemiologic exercise. *Natl. Canc. Inst.*, 58: 825–832, 1977.

2. Reddy, B.S., Cohen, L.A., McCoy, G.D., et al. Nutrition and its relationship to cancer. *Adv. Cancer. Res.* 32: 237–345, 1980.

3. Jensen, O.M. Colon cancer epidemiology, in Autrup and Williams (eds.): *Experimental Colon Carcinogenesis*. Boca Raton, Fla.: CRC Press, 1983, pp. 3–23.

4. Burkitt, D.P. Fiber in the etiology of colorectal cancer, in Winawer, Schottenfeld, Sherlock (eds.): *Colorectal Cancer: Prevention Epidemiology and Screening*. New York: Raven Press, 1980, pp. 13–18.

5. Correa, P. and Haenszel, W. The epidemiology of large bowel cancer. *Adv. Cancer. Res.*, 26: 1–141, 1978.

6. Graham, S., Dayal, H., Swanson, M., et al. Diet in the epidemiology of cancer of the colon and rectum. *J. Natl. Canc. Inst.*, 61: 709–714, 1978.

7. Wynder, E.L., Kajitani, T., Ishekawa, S., et al. Environmental factors of cancer of the colon and rectum. II. Japanese epidemiological data. *Cancer*, 23: 1210–1220, 1969.

8. Wynder, E.L. The epidemiology of large bowel cancer. *Canc. Res*, 35:3388–3394, 1975.

9. Teppo, L. and Saxen, E. Epidemiology of colon cancer in Scandinavia. *Isr. J. Med. Sci.*, 15: 322–328, 1979.

10. Haenszel, W., Berg, J.W., Segi, M., et al. Large bowel cancer in Hawaiian Japanese. *J. Natl. Canc. Inst.*, 51: 1765–1799, 1973.

11. Staszewski, J., McCall, M.G. and Stenhouse, N.S. Cancer mortality in 1962–66 among Polish migrants to Australia. *Br. J. Canc.*, 25: 599–618, 1971.

12. Hirayama, T. Diet and cancer. *Nutr. Canc.*, 1: 67–81, 1979.

13. West, D.W., Lyon, J.L., Gardner, J.W., et al. Epidemiology of colon cancer in Utah, in: *1983 Workshop: A Decade of Achievements and Challenges in Large Bowel Carcinogenesis*. Houston, Tex,: National Large Bowel Cancer Project, 1983, 3–5.

14. Carroll, K.K. and Kohr, H.T. Dietary fat in relation to tumorigenesis. *Prog. Biochem. Pharm.*, 10: 308–353, 1975.

15. Gregor, O., Toma, R. and Prasova, F. Gastrointestinal cancer and nutrition. *Gut*, 10: 1031–1034, 1969.

16. Armstrong, B. and Doll, R. Environmental factors and cancer incidence and mortality in different countries with special reference to dietary practices. *Int. J. Canc.*, 15: 617–631, 1975.

17. Drasar, B.S. and Irving, D. Environmental factors and cancer of the colon and breast. *Br. J. Canc.*, 32: 167–172, 1973.

18. Howell, M.A. Diet as an etiological factor in the development of cancers of the colon and rectum. *J. Chron. Dis.*, 28: 67–80, 1975.

19. Reddy, B.S., Hedges, A.R., Laakso, K., et al. Metabolic epidemiology of large bowel cancer. Fecal bulk and constituents of high-risk North American and low-risk Finnish population. *Cancer*, 42: 2382–2388, 1978.

20. Jensen, O.M., MacLennan, R. and Wahrendorf, J. Diet, bowel function, fecal characteristics and large bowel cancer in Denmark and Finland. *Nutr. Canc.*, 4: 5–19, 1982.

21. Domellof, L., Daraby, L., Hanson, D., et al. Fecal sterols and bacterial beta-glucuronidase activity: A preliminary study of healthy volunteers from Umea, Sweden, and metropolitan New York. *Nutr. Canc.*, 4: 120–127, 1982.

22. Reddy, B.S., Ekelund, G., Bohe, M., et al. Metabolic epidemiology of colon cancer: Dietary pattern and fecal sterol concentration of three populations. *Nutr. Canc.*, 5: 34–40, 1983.

23. Dales, L.G., Friedman, G.D., Wry, H.K., et al. Case-control study of relationships of diet and other traits to colorectal cancer in American blacks. *Am. J. Epidemiol.*, 109: 132–144, 1979.

24. Bjelke, E. Epidemiological studies of cancer of the stomach, colon and rectum. *Scand. J. Gastr.*, 9: 1–253 (suppl 31), 1974.

25. Aries, V., Crowther, J.S., Drasar, B.S., et al. Bacteria and etiology of cancer of the large bowel. *Gut*, 10: 334–335, 1969.

26. Reddy, B.S. Dietary fat and its relationship to large bowel cancer. *Canc. Res.*, 41: 3700–3705, 1981.

27. Reddy, B.S. Dietary fiber and colon carcinogenesis: A critical review in Vahouny and Kritchevsky (eds.): *Dietary Fiber in Health and Disease*. New York, Plenum Press, 1982, pp. 265–285.

28. Diamond, L., O'Brien, T. G. and Baird, W.M. Tumor promoters and the mechanisms of tumor promotion. *Adv. Canc. Res.*, 32: 1–74, 1980.

29. Wynder, E. L. and Reddy, B. Dietary fat and fiber and colon cancer. *Seminars in Oncology*, 10:266, 1983.

30. Waterhouse, J., Muir, C., Correa, P., et al. *Cancer Incidence on Five Continents*. Vol. 3. Lyon: International Agency for Research on Cancer, 1976.

31. Stocks, P. Breast cancer anomalies. *Br. J. Canc.*, 24: 633–643, 1979.

32. Phillips, R.L. Role of life-style and dietary habits in risk of cancer among Seventh-Day Adventists. *Canc. Res.*, 35: 2313–2322, 1975.

33. Phillips, R.L., Garfinkel, L., Kuzma, J.W., et al. Mortality among California Seventh-Day Adventists for selected cancer sites. *JNCI*, 65: 1097–1107, 1980.

34. Enig, M.G., Munn, R.J. and Keeney, M.G. Dietary fat and cancer trends: A critique. *Fed. Proc.*, 37: 2215–2220, 1978.

35. Gaskill, S.P., McGuire, W.L., Osborne, C.K., et al. Breast mortality and diet in the United States. *Canc. Res.*, 9: 3628–3637, 1979.

36. Carroll, K.K. and Hopkins, G.J. Dietary polyunsaturated fat versus saturated fat in relation to mammary carcinogenesis. *Lipids*, 14: 155–158, 1979.

37. de Waard, F., Baanders-van Halewijn, E.A. and Huizinga, J. The bimodal age distribution of patients with mammary carcinoma: Evidence for the existence of two types of human breast cancer. *Cancer*, 17: 141–151, 1964.

38. Tappel, A.L. Vitamin E and selenium protection from in vivo lipid peroxidation. *Ann. NY Acad. Sci.*, 355: 18–31, 1980.

39. Ames, B.N. Dietary carcinogens and anticarcinogens. *Science*, 221: 1256–1266, 1983.

40. Hems, G. The contribution of diet and childbearing to breast-cancer rates. *Br. J. Canc.*, 37: 974–982, 1978.

41. Lubin, J.H., Burns, P.E., Blot, W.J., et al. Dietary factors and breast cancer risk. *Int. J. Canc.*, 28: 685, 1981.

42. Wynder, E.L. Tumor enhancers: Underestimated factors in the epidemiology of lifestyle-associated cancers. *Env. Hlth. Perspec.*, 50: 15–21, 1983.

43. Weisburger, J.H., Horn, C.L. and Barnes, S. Possible genotoxic carcinogens in foods in relation to cancer causation. *Seminars in Oncology*, 10:338, 1983.

9

······ALCOHOL, TOBACCO AND······
FOOD CARCINOGENS

THE INTAKE of alcoholic beverages is related to a variety of cancers, according to some studies.[1-5] But researchers have found it difficult to pinpoint alcohol as the causative agent in these beverages.[6-8] Other factors such as cigarette smoking and deficiencies of certain vitamins, minerals or both—deficiencies that are alcohol-induced—can play a significant role in the cancer process. Epidemiologic studies are conflicting and inaccurate as a result of the underrating of alcohol consumption in self-assessment surveys.

A number of mechanisms have been suggested to explain the possible carcinogenic role of alcohol. For example, alcohol or other ingredients in alcoholic beverages may be carcinogenic or work with other agents to promote cancer. Another factor may be the solvent property of alcohol. As an organic solvent, alcohol may facilitate the absorption of carcinogens. Other factors include a modulating role for alcohol in the activation of carcinogens in biological systems, a suppressed immune function from alcohol abuse, and alcohol-induced nutritional deficiencies.[3,9-13]

The strongest relationship between cancer and alcohol occurs when alcohol is consumed excessively. Alcohol abuse is associated with cancers of the oral cavity and esophagus.[9,14-23] But it has also been shown that alcohol abusers are usually smokers.[24] The well-established cancer-causing action of tobacco is probably heightened by alcohol usage and is actually promoted by alcohol abuse. It is estimated that 76 percent of digestive tract cancers could be eliminated by abstention from tobacco and alcohol.[14]

It has been difficult to establish a cause and effect relationship between alcohol itself and cancer. But studies on human lymphocytes have demonstrated a genotoxic effect of acetaldehyde, an alcohol metabolite. A substance that is genotoxic alters the genetic integrity of cells and can be the initiating step in a number of diseases, including cancer. In addition to the genotoxic effect of acetaldehyde that is formed in the body, alcoholic beverages are frequently contaminated with a substance that is genotoxic. Small amounts of methanol occur in alcoholic beverages. This methanol contaminant can be converted to formaldehyde, a substance that has been shown to have a toxic effect on the genetic material within human lymphocytes.[25,26]

Genotoxic compounds are not necessarily carcinogenic, but there is a strong association between genotoxic substances and the carcinogenic process. Other contaminants found in alcoholic beverages that have been shown to be carcinogenic, not just genotoxic, include asbestos,[27-30] benzo (a) pyrene, benzanthracene,[31] fusel oils[32] and nitrosamines.[33]

Although tobacco is generally not considered a topic in nutrition the present authors feel that whenever and wherever there is an opportunity, a statement should be made to reinforce the health risks of smoking. The surgeon general, Dr. C. Everett Koop, was recently quoted in *USA Today* as follows: "We can say today, with greater certainty than ever before, that cigarettes are the most important individual health risk in this country, responsible for more premature deaths and disability than any other known agent." And evidence continues to accumulate demonstrating the serious health threat of second-hand smoke. Parents who smoke and

Add up the numbers beside the boxes that apply to you and place the total on the score panel. The color darkens as the risk increases.

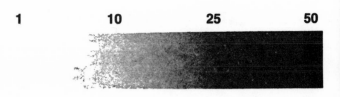

LUNG

My age is:
[1] under 40   [3] between 40–59   [7] 60 or over

The number of cigarettes I smoke per day is:
[1] none   [5] 1–10   [9] 10–19
[15] 20–39   [20] 40 or more

I have been smoking for:
[3] under 15 years   [6] 15–25 years
[12] 25 or more years

My type of cigarette is:
[10] high tar/nicotine   [9] medium tar/nicotine
[7] low tar/nicotine

Figure 13

Lung cancer. Smoking causes 75 percent of lung cancers and 25 percent of all forms of cancer. There is no safe cigarette. The longer and heavier you smoke, the greater the risk. As soon as you **stop smoking** your body starts to repair itself, and your lungs will return to normal as long as no disease is already present.

have young children should be warned as frequently as possible that they are exposing their children to an increased risk of respiratory problems, bronchitis, pneumonia and probably heart disease and cancer. Taxpayers' dollars would be well spent in support of research to find an industrial use for tobacco, thereby offering the tobacco growers an opportunity to make money in a way that does not promote lung cancer, heart disease, emphysema and birth defects.

CARCINOGENS IN FOOD

As discussed previously, dietary fat can promote certain types of cancer, while dietary fiber can play an inhibitory role in the development of this disease. But these are not the only dietary substances that can increase or decrease the risk of cancer. The processing and preparation of some foods may actually create carcinogens. Other foods have protective constituents, such as certain vitamins and trace elements, that have been demonstrated to decrease the risk of cancer.

Research was presented in 1982 that demonstrated the presence of mutagenic compounds on the surface of fried or broiled fish and meat.[34] A mutagenic compound is one that can cause a genetic mutation. While it does not necessarily follow that a genetic mutation

caused by a mutagenic compound will develop into cancer, it is generally believed that mutagens increase the risk of cancer. In addition, many carcinogens are mutagens and many mutagens that have been studied for a significant period of time after their discovery have been proven to be carcinogenic.

The formation of mutagens during the cooking of foods appears to be a function of cooking time and temperature.[35,36] Fried hamburgers contain mutagens whereas broiling appears to produce fewer mutagenic compounds.[37–39] Some studies have shown that meat can be cooked without the formation of mutagens if the cooking temperatures are kept low or if the food is cooked in a microwave.[36,39] In addition to fried or broiled beef and fish, mutagens have been isolated from broiled or grilled chicken and grilled mushrooms.[40] Foods that have a high sugar or starch content can also form mutagenic substances, although to a much lesser extent than meats or fish.[35]

Excessive consumption of salted and pickled foods can result in cancer of the stomach, oral cavity and esophagus.[41–44] The cancer-causing agents from these foods are formed from the nitrates, nitrites and other compounds that are either contained in the food or created during the digestive process. It is important to note that cancer formation from these type of foods may be blocked by vitamin C or vitamin E, or foods that contain these nutrients.[45] And there are probably other cancer-protective substances in food that have not yet been identified.

Many foods contain natural carcinogens, yet these foods have not been associated with an increased risk of cancer. A number of herbal teas, celery, parsnips, figs, parsley, honey, fava beans, cottonseed oil and cottonseed meal may all contain naturally occurring carcinogens.[46] But these foods may not necessarily be implicated as cancer-causing agents. Perhaps these foods do not cause cancer because of the simultaneous ingestion of foods that contain natural anti-carcinogens such as vitamin C in citrus and green leafy vegetables, vitamin E in whole grains and seeds, beta-carotene in orange and yellow vegetables and selenium in muscle meats and whole grains.

Some researchers have also suggested that there is a cancer-protective quality in a vegetable protein-based diet because this type of diet is high in linoleic acid and low in arachidonic acid. The basis for this theory is that the fatty acid linoleic acid can be converted in normal human cells to other essential fatty acids such as gamma-linolenic acid. But in cancer cells, linoleic acid cannot be converted to these necessary fatty acids. It has been suggested that a diet, such as a vegetarian diet, that is high in linoleic acid but low in arachidonic acid will selectively promote the proper metabolism of normal cells at the expense of cancer cells. In addition, the vegetarian diet high in linoleic acid may alter the integrity of the lipid membrane surrounding cancer cells, thereby suppressing the ability of these cells to proliferate.[47]

REFERENCES

1. Breslow, N.E. and Enstrom, J.E. Geographic correlations between cancer mortality rates and alcohol-tobacco consumption in the United States. *J. Natl. Cancer Inst.* 53:631-639, 1974.

2. Enstrom, J.E. Colorectal cancer and beer drinking. *Br. J. Cancer* 35:674-683, 1977.

3. Vitale, J.I., Broitman, S.A. and Gottlieb, L.S. Alcohol and carcinogenesis, in Newell G., Ellison, N.M. (eds.): *Nutrition and Cancer*. New York: Raven Press, 1981, 291-301.

4. Stocks, P. Report on cancer in North Wales and Liverpool region. *Br. Emp. Cancer Res. Camp. 35th Annual Report,* Supplement to Part II, 1957.

5. Bjelke, E. *Epidemiologic Studies of Cancer of the Stomach, Colon, and Rectum, with Special Emphasis on the Role of Diet.* vol. I-IV. Ph.D. thesis, University of Minnesota, 1973.

6. Pernu, J. An epidemiological study on cancer of the digestive organs and respiratory tract. *Ann.Med.Intern.Fenn.49 (suppl 33)* :1-117, 1960.

7. Higginson, J. Etiological factors in gastrointestinal cancer in man. *J. Natl. Cancer. Inst,* 37:527-545, 1966.

8. Bjelke, E. Case-control study of the stomach, colon, and rectum, in Clark, R.L., Cumley, R.C., McCoy, J.E., et al. (eds.): *Oncology 1970. PfOC Tenth Internat Cancer Congress,* Chicago: Yearbook Medical Publishers, 1971, 320-334.

9. Schottenfeld, D. Alcohol as a co-factor in the etiology of cancer. *Cancer,* 43:1962-1966, 1979.

10. McCoy, E.D. and Wynder, E.L. Etiological and preventive implications in alcohol carcinogenesis. *Cancer Res.,* 39:2844-2850, 1979.

11. Lieber, C.S., Seitz, H.K., Garro, A.J., et al. Alcohol-related diseases and carcinogenesis. *Cancer Res.,* 39:2863-2886, 1979.

12. Vitale, J.J., Gottlieb, L.S. Alcohol and alcohol-related deficiencies as carcinogens. *Cancer Res.,* 35:3336-3338, 1975.

13. Committee on Diet, Nutrition and Cancer, Assembly of Life Sciences, National Research Council, Diet, Nutrition and Cancer. Washington, D.C.: National Academic Press, 1982.

14. Wynder, E.L., Bross, I.I., Feldman, R.M.: A study of the etiological factors in cancer of the mouth. *Cancer,* 10:1300-1323, 1957.

15. Vincent, R.G. and Marchetta, F. The relationship of the use of tobacco and alcohol to cancer of the oral cavity, pharynx, or larynx. *Am.J.Surg.,* 106:501-505, 1963.

16. Keller, A.Z. and Terris, M. The association of alcohol and tobacco with cancer of the mouth and pharynx. *Am.J.Public Health,* 55:1578-1585, 1965.

17. Rothman K.J. and Keller, A. The effect of joint exposure to alcohol and tobacco on risk of cancer of the mouth and pharynx. *J. Chronic Dis.,* 25:711-716, 1972.

18. Some consequences of alcohol use. I. Alcohol and cancer, in Keller, M. (ed.) *Alcohol and Health, Second Special Report to the U.S. Congress.* Rockville, Md.: United States Department of Health, Education, and Welfare, National Institute on Alcohol and Alcoholism, 1974.

19. Bross I.J. and Coombs, J. Early onset of oral cancer among women who drink and smoke. *Oncology,* 33:136-139, 1976.

20. Wynder E.L. and Bross, I.J. A study of etiological factors in cancer of the esophagus. *Cancer,* 14:389-413, 1961.

21. Moore, C. Cigarette smoking and cancer of the mouth, pharynx and larynx. *JAMA,* 191:104-110, 1965.

22. Schottenfeld, D., Gant, R.C., Ywnder, E.L. The role of alcoholic and tabacco in multiple primary cancers of the upper digestive system, larynx and lung: A prospective study. *Prev. Med.*, 3:277–293, 1974.

23. Kamionkowski, M.D. and Flesher, B. The role of alcoholic intake in esophageal carcinoma. *Am. J. Med. Sci.*, 249:696-699, 1965.

24. Flamant, R., Lasserre, O., Lazar, P., et al. Differences in sex ratio according to cancer site and possible relationship with use of tobacco and alcohol: Review of 65,000 cases. *J. Natl, Cancer Inst.*, 32:1309-1316, 1964.

25. Ristow, H. and Obe, G. Acetaldehyde induces crosslinks in DNA and causes sister chromatid exchanges in human cells. *Mutat. Res.*, 58:115-119, 1978.

26. Obe, G. and Beck, B. Mutagenic activity of aldehydes. *Drug and Alc. Dep.*, 4:91-94, 1979.

27. Biles, B. and Emerson, T. Examination of fibers in beer. *Nature*, 219:93-94, 1968.

28. Bignon, J., Bientz, M., Bonnaud, G., et al. Evaluation numérique des fibres d'amiente dans des échantillons de vins. *Nouv. Presse Med.*, 6:1148-1149, 1977.

29. Wehman, H.J., Plantholt, B.A. Asbestos fibrils in beverages 1. Gin. *Bull. Environ. Contam. Toxicol.*, 11:267-272, 1974.

30. Gaudichet, A., Sebastien. P., Dufour, G., et al. Asbestos fibers in wines: Relation to filtration process. *J. Environ. Pathol. Toxicol.*, 2:417-425, 1978.

31. Goff, E.U. and Fine, D.H., Analysis of volatile N-nitrosamines in alcoholic beverages. *Food Cosmet. Toxicol.*, 17:569-573, 1979.

32. Gibel, W., Wildner. G.P., Lohs, K. Untersuchungen zur Frage einer kanzer ogenen und hepatotoxischen Wirkung von Fuselol. *Arch. Geschwulstforsch*, 32:115-125, 1968.

33. Lijinsky, U. and Epstein, S.S. Nitrosamines as environmental carcinogens. *Nature*, 225:21-23, 1970.

34. Sugimura, T. Mutagens, carcinogens, and tumor promoters in our daily food. *Cancer*, 49:1970-1984, 1982.

35. Barnes, W.S., Spingarn, N.E., Garvie-Gould, C., et al. Mutagens in cooked foods: Possible consequences of the Maillard reaction in foods and nutrition, in Waller, G.R., Feather, M.S. (eds.): *The Maillard Reaction in Foods and Nutrition*, ACS Symposium Series 215. Washington, D.C., American Chem. Soc., 1983, 485, 492.

36. Pariza, M.W., et al. Mutagens and modulators of mutagenesis in fried ground beef. *Cancer Res.*, 43:2444s-2446s, 1983.

37. Commoner, B., Vithayathil, A.J., Dolara, P., et al. Formation of mutagens in beef and beef extract during cooking. *Science*, 201:913-916, 1978.

38. Weisburger, J.H. and Spingarm, N.E. Mutagens as a function of mode of cooking of meats, in Hirono, I., et al. (eds.): *Naturally Occurring Carcinogens-Mutagens and Modulators of Carcinogenesis*. Tokyo, Japan Sci. Soc. Press,1979, 177.

39. Nadar, C.J., Spencer, L.K., Weller R.J. Mutagens as a function of mode of cooking of meats in Hirono, I., et al. (eds.): *Naturally Occurring Carcinogens, Mutagens and Modulators of Carcinogenesis*, Tokyo: Sci. Soc. Press, 1979, 177.

40. Matsumoto, T., Yoshida, D., and Tomita, H. Determination of mutagens, amino-alpha-carbolines in grilled foods and cigarette smoke condensate. *Cancer Letts.*, 12:105-110, 1981.

41. Magee, R.N. (ed.): *Banburg Rept 12: Nitrosamines and Human Cancer*. Cold Spring Harbor, N.Y.: Cold Spring Harbor Laboratories, 1982.

42. Joossens, J.V. and Geboers, J. Epidemiology of gastric cancer: A clue to etiology, in Sherlock, P., et al. (eds.): *Precancerous Lesions of the Gastrointestinal Tract*. New York: Raven Press, 1983, 97.

43. Tomita, I., Kinae, N., Nakamura, Y., et al. Mutagenicity of various Japanese foodstuffs treated with nitrite (II) direct-acting mutagens produced from N-containing compounds in foodstuffs. *Proc 8th Internatl Meeting on N-Nitroso Compounds, Occurrence and Biological Effects*. Banff, Alberta, Canada, IARC Sci. Publ. (in press).

44. Kawabata, T., Matsui, M., Ishibashi, T., et al. Analysis and occurrence of total N-nitroso compounds in Japanese diet. *Proc 8th Internatl Meetingon N-Nitroso Compounds, Occurrence and Biological Effects*. Banff, Alberta, Canada, IARC Sci. Publ. (in press).

45. Weisburger, J.H., Horn, C.L. and Barnes S. Possible genotoxic carcinogens in foods in relation to cancer causation. *Seminars in Oncology*, 10:330-341, 1983.

46. Ames, B. Dietary carcinogens and anticarcinogens. *Science*, 221:1256, 1983.

47. Siguel, E. Cancerostatic effect of vegetarian diets. *Nutr. and Cancer*, 4:285-291, 1983.

10
............NUTRIENTS AND DIET............................
IN THE PREVENTION OF CANCER

VITAMIN A AND CANCER

THE CONNECTION between vitamin A and cancer was first made in the 1920s, just a few years after the discovery of this fat-soluble vitamin. A vitamin A-deficient diet in laboratory animals was determined to be the cause of gastric carcinoma.[1] Since then, vitamin A and related compounds have been studied extensively with regard to their ability to modulate the development of various types of cancer.

The two-step model of carcinogenesis suggests that there is first an initiation of the process, then a promotion of the cancer. Vitamin A or the plant-derived provitamin A, the carotenes, can affect both phases of this cancer process. A number of mechanisms of action have been proposed, as shown below.

THEORETICAL MECHANISMS OF ACTION FOR VITAMIN A IN CANCER

Inhibits initiation of cancer process (carotenes)

Inhibits promotion of cancer process
- by inhibiting ornithine decarboxylase
- by direct effect
- by inhibiting transforming growth factor

Alters immune function
- by altering humoral immune function
- by altering cellular immune function

Alters of cellular membrane

Alters protein synthesis and cellular differentiation

Adapted from Kummet, T., and Meyskens, F.L., Jr. Vitamin A: A potential inhibitor of human cancer. *Seminars in Oncology*, 10(3):282, Sept. 1983.

In reviewing epidemiological studies, one may conclude that vitamin A appears to have a protective effect for most sites of cancer. Three major prospective dietary studies have compared the incidence of various types of cancer and vitamin A or beta-carotene intake. The largest of these studies was conducted in Japan and involved the monitoring of diets for over 250,000 people for a period of ten years. The findings from this study showed that the daily consumption of vegetables with high levels of beta-carotene reduced the risk of lung, colon, stomach, prostate and cervical cancers.[2] Other prospective studies have shown that the incidence of lung cancer in smokers in inversely associated with vitamin A intake.[3]

The first retrospective study associating vitamin A with cancer was published in 1974. In this study, decreased vitamin A intake was associated with an increased risk of colon cancer.[4] Numerous other studies have confirmed a strong relationship between increased vitamin A and beta-carotene intake and a decreased risk of lung, bladder, oral cavity, larynx, breast, cervical and esophageal cancer.[5] These studies from various countries suggest an anticancer effect of vitamin A and beta-carotene or an increased tendency for cancer in persons with relatively low intakes of these nutrients.

Kummet and Meyskens of the Cancer Center Division, University of Arizona, suggest that the recommended dietary allowances for Vitamin A, based on the amount necessary to prevent night blindness, "may not be appropriate for malignant disease prevention."[5] They suggest that a daily intake of 10,000 to 25,000 IU of vitamin A is a more reasonable level necessary to decrease the risk of cancer. Additional studies will need to be conducted in order to determine if the RDAs for vitamin A should be increased.

VITAMIN C AND CANCER

Humans are exposed to a variety of foods that contain preformed nitrosamines, compounds that have been demonstrated to cause cancer in animals. Cigarette smoking is also a source of nitrosamines.[10] Although vitamin C is not effective in preventing cancer from these sources of preformed nitrosamines, animal studies have demonstrated that this nutrient is effective in blocking the formation of nitrosamines, and therefore cancer, from nitrosamine precursors.[6-9] It has not yet been demonstrated that nitrosamines will cause cancer in humans, but the animal studies present a strong case for these agents as risk factors in human cancers.

Nitrosamines can be formed in the digestive tract from the nitrates and nitrites that are commonly used as food preservatives. Vitamin C has been found to be effective in inhibiting nitrosamine formation from these precursors.[11-16]

In reviewing dietary habits of large populations, there appears to be a cancer-protective effect of foods rich in vitamin C.[17-21] But these foods are also good sources of dietary fiber, and in many cases are good sources of vitamin A and folic acid as well. All of these nutrients, along with dietary fiber, have been shown to offer some protection from cancer.[22]

Vitamin C may be useful for patients with recurrent bladder cancer. In bladder infections, N-nitroso compounds are converted to carcinogens. Vitamin C is helpful in blocking the formation of these carcinogens, thereby decreasing the risk of bladder cancer.[23,24]

Vitamin C may also be useful in preventing stomach cancer. Patients with achlorhydria, including patients on cimetidine therapy, may be at risk for the formation of nitrosamines which in turn can cause cancer.[25-27] In addition, vitamin C, along with vitamin E, has been shown to reduce the production of mutagens in human feces.[28] These mutagens are closely related to carcinogens and may cause changes in the large intestine that could lead to colon cancer. Therefore, the ability of vitamin C and vitamin E to decrease the risk of colon cancer is being explored.

SELENIUM AND CANCER

Selenium is an essential nutrient that is present in human and animal systems as the selenoenzyme glutathione peroxidase.[29] In addition to fat, fiber and vitamins A, E and C, this trace element has been identified as an important factor in the process of carcinogenesis.

Early animal studies exploring the relationship of selenium to cancer suggested that this nutrient may increase the risk of cancer.[30] But the tumor-promoting activity of selenium in these studies may have been due to the form of selenium used in the test animals.[31,32] More recent studies have found that selenium can play a significant role in decreasing the incidence of tumors in experimental animals. The type of tumor and the experimental results of selenium on the reduction of tumor incidence in test animals are listed in Table 12.

Evidence for the cancer-protecting role of selenium in humans is provided primarily by epidemiologic studies. In the United States and other countries, the soil and forage crops in certain regions are deficient in selenium. The incident of death from cancer of the digestive organs, lung, breast and lymph in low-selenium areas is greater than in those areas that have a high-selenium content of forage crops.[33] In comparing the evidence collected from twenty-seven countries, the incidence of cancer is significantly lower in populations with high dietary selenium intake from foods rich in this nutrient.[34]

A number of case-control studies have been conducted on cancer patients to determine if their selenium status differed from that of a control group. Significantly lower selenium levels have been identified in patients with cancer of the breast, gastrointestinal cancers, Hodgkin's disease, lymphocytic leukemia, pulmonary carcinoma, otolaryngeal carcinoma, gastrointestinal carcinoma, genitourinary carcinoma and colon and skin cancer.[35-41] Studies to determine if the low selenium levels actually contributed to the carcinogenesis process are now under way.

Selenium's mechanism of action in preventing cancer is most likely associated with its biochemical function in protecting cells from peroxide-induced oxidation.[44] Selenium supplements have also been demonstrated to be an immune stimulant which, in turn, may play a protective role in the cancer process.[45] Other possible mechanisms of selenium's anti-cancer role are under investigation.

Selenium exists in both inorganic and organic forms. These different forms are metabolized differently and may therefore have different effects on the cancer process. The methylated and selenoamino acids such as dimethyl selenide, selenocysteine, selenomethionine and selenocystine are the organic forms of most importance in health and nutrition.[42] The organic forms of selenium are available in yeast and whole grains and as supplements. Inorganic forms of selenium supplements,

TABLE 12
Effects of Selenium (Se) on Tumor Incidence in Animals

Animal Model	Carcinogenic Factor	Form/Dose Se	% Tumor Incidence Reduction
Liver, rats	Azo dye	5 ppm Na selenite in diet	45%
			50%
Liver, rats	AAF	4 ppm Na selenite in water	58%
Liver, rats	3'-MeDAB	6 ppm Na selenite in water	50%
		6 ppm organic Se (Se yeast) in diet	30%
Mammary, rats	MNU	5 mg/kg Na selenite in diet	43%
Hepatic or Mammary, rats	FAA	2.5 ppm Na selenite	100%
		0.5 ppm Na selenite in diet	83%
Mammary, rats	DMBA	5 ppm selenite fed in diet	
		−2 to +12 wk	65.8%
		−2 to +24 wk	47.4%
		+2 to +24 wk	41.4%
Mammary, rats	DMBA	SeO_2 in water	
		2 mg/L	21%
		4 mg/L	32% to 41%
		(effective both during and after DMBA administration)	(2 series)
Colon, rats	DMH	4 ppm Na selenite in water	54%
	MAM	4 ppm Na selenite in water	7%
Mammary, mouse	DMBA	6 mg/L Na selenite in water	6 mg DMBA 42%
			2 mg DMBA 61%
Mammary, mouse BALB/cfC3H (MuMTV-S position)	Virus	2 ppm Na selenite	41%
		6 ppm in water	85%
Mammary, mouse	Virus	2 ppm SeO_2 in water	88%
Mammary, mouse	Virus	1 ppm organic Se in diet	65%
Skin, mice	a DMBA	1.0 ppm Na selenite in diet	45%
	b benzopyrene		48%

Source: Helzlsouer, K. J. Selenium and cancer prevention. Seminars in Oncology, 10(3): 307, Sept. 1983. Reprinted by permission.

as well as artificially selenized yeasts, should be avoided because of potential mutagenicity.[43] The National Research Council's Recommended Dietary Allowances suggests an adequate and safe range for adults of 50 to 200 mcg of selenium daily.[44]

VITAMIN E AND CANCER

The theoretical role for vitamin E in decreasing the risk of cancer is based upon this nutrient's ability to act as an antioxidant. In this capacity, vitamin E protects the unsaturated fatty membranes throughout the body. In animal studies, vitamin E has been shown to decrease the formation of lipoperoxides, substances that are believed to be carcinogens themselves or to enhance the activation of other carcinogens. Vitamin E has been used successfully in animal studies along with other chemotherapeutic agents to decrease the formation of lipoperoxides during cancer therapy.[46] The ability of vitamin E to inhibit tumor growth in animals is currently being studied. Preliminary findings suggest a potential role for vitamin E in inhibiting the cancer growth process.[47]

Although vitamin E has not been demonstrated to

TABLE 13
Dietary Recommendations to the American Public, 1977–1982

	Limit or Reduce Total Fat (% Calories)	Reduce Saturated Fat (% Calories)	Increase Polyunsaturated Fat (% Calories)	Limit Cholesterol (mg/d)	Limit Simple Sugars	Increase Complex Carbohydrates	Increase Fiber	Restrict Sodium Chloride (g/d)	Moderation in Alcohol	Maintain Ideal Body Weight, Exercise	Other Recommendations
Dietary goals, 1977: general	27% to 33%	Yes, to 10%	Yes, to 10%	250–350	Yes	Yes, to 55-60%	Yes	<5g	NC	Yes	Reduce additives and processed foods
Surgeon general 1979: general	Yes	Yes	NS†	Yes	Yes	Yes	NS	Yes	Yes	Yes	More fish, poultry, and legumes; less red meat
AMA 1979: general	No	No	No	No	Yes	NC‡	NC	12	Yes	Yes	Consider high-risk groups
NCI, 1979: cancer	Yes	NC	No	NC	NC	NS	Yes	NC	Yes	Yes	Variety in diet
USDA DHEW, 1980; general	Yes	Yes	No	Yes	Yes	Yes	Yes	Yes	Yes	Yes	Variety in diet, consider high-risk groups
NAS/FNB, 1980: general	For weight reduction only	No	No	No	For weight reduction only	No	No	3–8	Yes	Yes	Variety in diet, consider high-risk groups
AHA, 1982: heart disease	–30%	To-10%	To-10%	–300	Yes	To-50% calories	NS	Yes	NS	Yes	Public education
NAS/DNC, 1982: cancer	–30%	As total fat only	No	NC	NC	Through whole grains, fruits, and vegetables	NS	Through salt-cured, pickled, smoked foods	Yes	NC	Emphasize fruits and vegetables; avoid high doses of supplements

†NS = not specifically.
‡NC = no comment.
Source: Palmer, S. Diet, nutrition and cancer: the future dietary policy. *Cancer Research*, 43(suppl):2509s, 1983. Reprinted by permission.

prevent cancer in humans, animal studies suggest that this nutrient has a modulating role in cancer. Animal studies have demonstrated that vitamin E can potentiate the ability of selenium to inhibit the development of artificially induced breast cancer in rats.[48] Additional research is necessary before any definitive statement can be made regarding the ability of vitamin E to prevent cancer in humans.

DIETARY RECOMMENDATIONS FOR DECREASING THE RISK OF CANCER

There has been considerable debate over the past seven to eight years regarding what specific dietary recommendations should be made to the American public in order to decrease the risk of cancer. Because it takes twenty to thirty years before a statistically significant increase in cancer can be detected, and then additional years of research to identify a specific cause, dietary recommendations in regard to cancer are usually based on suggestive and correlational evidence. The various recommendations that have been made through 1982 are listed in Table 13.

The most recent dietary recommendations (prior to publishing date of this volume) for decreasing the risk of cancer are contained in a February, 1984, report by the American Cancer Society's Medical and Scientific Committee.[49] The following recommendations and comments are excerpted primarily from this report.

1. Avoid obesity.
2. Cut down on total fat intake.
3. Eat more high-fiber foods, such as wholegrain cereals, fruits and vegetables.

4. Include foods rich in vitamins A and C in the daily diet.
5. Include cruciferous vegetables, such as cabbage, broccoli, brussels sprouts, kohlrabi and cauliflower in the diet.
6. Be moderate in consumption of alcoholic beverages.
7. Be moderate in consumption of salt-cured, smoked and nitrite-cured foods.

These recommendations may be elaborated as follows:

1. Avoid obesity.

Weight reduction can reduce the risk of cancer in obese people. A twelve-year study conducted by the American Cancer Society demonstrated that obese people have an increased risk for cancers of the uterus, gallbladder, kidney, stomach, colon and breast. This study showed that if a man is 40 percent or more overweight he has a 33 percent greater risk of developing cancer than a man who is not overweight. If a woman is 40 percent or more overweight, she has a 55 percent greater risk of developing cancer than a woman of normal weight. Animal experiments corroborate the findings of this study.

2. Cut down on total fat intake.

Animal and human studies suggest that excessive dietary fat increases the risk of developing cancers of the breast, colon and prostate. Both saturated and unsaturated fat, when consumed excessively, have been found to promote cancer. The recommendation is to cut back on fat-rich foods, fats and oils. Since fats are the major contributors to excess calories, a lowering of fat intake will also help most people to maintain proper weight. (See suggestions for decreasing dietary fat, pp. 196-199.)

3. Eat more high-fiber foods, such as wholegrain cereals, fruits and vegetables.

The scientific community has not been able to state unequivocally that dietary fiber will decrease the risk of cancer. But there is sufficient evidence to make the recommendation to increase fiber intake, especially since the high-fiber foods are generally nutrient-rich, low in calories and low in fat. Increasing fiber intake does not mean simply to add bran to the diet. Bran is only one type of fiber among the many different dietary fibers that occur in fresh fruit, vegetables and whole grains. Eating a variety of these fiber-rich foods will provide the best source of vitamins and minerals as well as a variety of different fibrous substances, each with different properties that may have an effect on the carcinogenic process. (See guide to increasing dietary fiber and list of fiber in foods; pp. 189-191.)

4. Include foods rich in vitamin A (and/or carotene) and vitamin C in the daily diet.

Foods such as carrots, tomatoes, spinach, apricots, peaches and cantaloupes are rich in beta-carotene, a precursor of active vitamin A that has been associated with a decreased risk of cancers of the larynx, esophagus and lung. In addition to beta-carotene, preformed vitamin A has also been associated with a decreased risk of cancer. Vitamin C can inhibit the formation of nitrosamines and may therefore be able to decrease the risk of cancer. Vitamin C-rich foods have been associated with a decreased risk of cancers of the stomach and esophagus. It is not yet known if the vitamin C content of these foods is the cancer-preventing agent. But when all of the evidence is presented, it makes good sense to recommend an increase in the consumption of fresh fruit and vegetables.

5. Include cruciferous vegetables, such as cabbage, broccoli, brussels sprouts, kohlrabi and cauliflower, in the diet.

Certain components of these vegetables appear to have a cancer-protective effect. The type of cancers that seem to be reduced in individuals consuming these foods include cancers of the gastrointestinal and respiratory tract.

6. Be moderate in consumption of alcoholic beverages.

In addition to cirrhosis, which can lead to liver cancer, alcohol abuse increases the risk for cancers of the oral cavity, larynx and esophagus. This risk is potentiated in alcohol abusers who are also cigarette smokers.

7. Be moderate in consumption of salt-cured, smoked and nitrite-cured foods.

Nitrates and nitrites are common preservatives used in meats. They are also used to cure or pickle foods. These chemicals can form nitrosamines which in turn can cause cancer.

The smoking of foods can also increase the risk of cancer. Cooking fatty cuts of meat over an open fire or barbeque can result in the formation of carcinogens or procarcinogenic substances in the meat. This results from the fact that fats, as they drip down into the flame, are converted into polycyclic aromatic hydrocarbons (PAH). The PAH are then brought back into the meat through the vapors. One of these pro-carcinogenic PAH materials is called benzo(a)pyrene. Benzo(a)pyrene and related compounds occur in grilled foods primarily from the incomplete combustion of the fuel and secondarily from contact with smoke that is formed when fat is dripped into the fire. Leaner cuts of meat cooked on a fire that prevents considerable smoke production will result in lower procarcinogen production.[50]

REFERENCES

1. Fujimaki, Y. Formation of carcinoma in albino rats fed on deficient diets. *J. Cancer. Res,* 10: 469–477, 1926.

2. Hirayama, T. Diet and cancer. *Nutr. Cancer,* 1: 67–81, 1979.

3. Kvale, G., Bjelke, E. and Gart, J.J. Dietary habits and lung cancer risk, in *Proceedings of the Thirteenth International Cancer Congress.* Seattle: International Union Against Cancer, 1982, 175.

4. Bjelke, E. Epidemiologic studies of cancer of the stomach, colon, and rectum; with special emphasis on the role of diet. *Scand. J. Gastr.* 9: 1–53, 1974.

5. Kummet, T. and Meyskens, F.L., Jr. Vitamin A: A potential inhibitor of human cancer. *Seminars in Oncology,* 10: 281, 1983.

6. Archer, M.C. Hazards of nitrate, nitrite, and N-nitroso compounds in human nutrition. in Hathcock, J.N. (ed.): *Nutritional Toxicol,* vol. 1. New York: Academic Press, 1982, 327–381.

7. Tannenbaum, S.R. Reaction of nitrite with vitamin C and E. *Ann. NY Acad. Sci.,* 355: 277–279, 1980.

8. Lijinsky, W. Structure-activity relationships among N-nitroso compounds, in Scalan and Tannenbaum (eds): *N-nitroso Compounds.* Washington, D.C.: American Chemical Society, 1981, 89–99.

9. Bright-See, E. and Newmark, H.L. Potential and probable role of vitamins C and E in the prevention of human cancer, in *Modulation and Mediation of Cancer by Vitamins.* First Int. Conf., Tucson, Ariz. (in press).

10. Committee on Nitrite and Alternative Curing Agents in Foods, National Academy of Science-National Research Council. *The Health Effects of Nitrate, Nitrite and N-Nitroso Compounds.* Washington, D.C.: National Academy Press, 1981.

11. Fiddler, W., Densabene, J. and Wasserman, J. The role of lean and adipose tissue in the formation of nitrosopyrolidine in fried bacon. *J. Food Sci.,* 59: 1070, 1974.

12. Bharucha, K.R., Cross, C.K. and Rubin, L.J. Long-chain acetals of ascorbic and erythorbic acids as antinitrosomine agents for bacon. *J. Agric. Food. Chem,* 28: 1274–1281, 1980.

13. Newmark, H.L. and Mergens, W.J. Application of ascorbic acid and tocopherols as inhibitors of nitrosamine formation and oxidation in foods, in Solms and Hall (eds): *Criteria of Food Acceptance.* Zurich: Forster Publ. Ltd., 1981, 379–390.

14. Reddy, S.K. Inhibition of N-nitrosopyrolidine in dry cured bacon by alpha-tocopherol-coated salt systems. *J. Food Sci.,* 47: 1598–1602, 1982.

15. Rice, K.N. and Pierson, M.D. Inhibition of Salmonella by sodium nitrite and potassium sorbate in frankfurters. *J. Food Sci.,* 47: 1615–1617, 1982.

16. Wesley, R.L., Marion, W.W. and Sebranek, J.G. Effect of sodium nitrite concentrations, sodium erythorbate and storage time on quality of franks manufactured from mechanically deboned turkey. *J. Food. Sci.,* 47: 1626–1630, 1982.

17. Meinsma, L. Voeding en Kanker. *Voeding,* 25: 357–365, 1964.

18. Graham, S., Lilienfeld, A.M. and Tidings, J.E. Dietary and purgation factors in the epidemiology of gastric cancer. *Cancer,* 20: 2224–2234, 1967.

19. Graham, S., Schotz, W. and Martino, P. Alimentary factors in the epidemiology of gastric cancer. *Cancer,* 30: 927–938, 1972.

20. Haenszel, W. Stomach cancer among Japanese in Hawaii. *J. Nat. Cancer Inst.* 49: 969–988, 1972.

21. Higginson, J. Etiology of gastrointestinal cancer in man. *Natl. Cancer Inst. Monogr.* 25: 191–198, 1967.

22. National Academy of Science Committee on Diet, Nutrition and Cancer. *Diet, Nutrition and Cancer.* Washington, D.C.: National Academy Press, 1982.

23. Schlegel, J.U. Proposed uses of ascorbic acid in the prevention of bladder carcinoma. *Ann. NY Acad. Sci.* 258: 432–437, 1975.

24. Hicks, R.M., Gough, T.A. and Walters, C.L. Demonstration of the presence of nitrosamines in human urine: Preliminary observations of the possible etiology for the bladder cancer in association with chronic urinary tract infaction. in Walker, E.A., et al. (eds.): *Environmental Aspects of N-Nitroso Compounds.* Lyon, International Agency for Research on Cancer, 1978, pp. 465–475.

25. Schlag, P., Bockler, R., Peter, M. Nitrite and nitrosamines in gastric juice: Risk factors for gastric cancer. *Scand. J. Gastr.*, 17: 145–150, 1982.

26. Blackburn. E.K. Possible association between pernicious anemia and leukemia: A prospective study of 1625 patients with a note on the very high incidence of stomach cancer. *Int. J. Cancer,* 3: 163–170, 1968.

27. Bartholomew, B.A., Hill, M.J. and Hudson, M.J. Gastric bacteria, nitrate, nitrite and nitrosamines in patients with pernicious anemia and in patients treated with cimetidine, in Walker, E.A., et al. (eds.): *N-nitroso Compounds: Analysis, Formation and Occurrence.* IARC Publ 31:595–600, 1980.

28. Dion, P.W. The effect of dietary ascorbic acid and alpha-tocopherol on fecal mutagenicity. *Mutat.Res.* 102: 27–37, 1982.

29. Hoekstra, W.G. Biochemical function of selenium and its relation to vitamin E. *Fed. Proc.,* 32: 2083, 1975.

30. Tscherkes, L.A., Volgarev, M.N. and Aptehar, S.G. Selenium-caused tumors. *Acta Univ. Intern. Contra. Cancrum.* 19: 632–633, 1963.

31. Sufler, J.W. Thyroid adenomas in rats receiving selenium. *Science,* 103: 762, 1946.

32. Innes, J.R.M. Bioassay of pesticides and industrial chemicals for tumor genicity in mice: A preliminary note. *JNCI* 42: 1101–1114, 1969.

33. Shamberger, R.J. and Willis, C.E. Selenium distribution and human cancer mortality. *CRC Crit. Rev. Clin. Lab. Sci.,* 2: 211–221, 1971.

34. Schrauzer, G.N., White, D.A. and Schneider, C.J. Cancer mortality correlation studies. III. Statistical associates with dietary selenium intakes. *Bioniorg. Chem.,* 7: 23–34, 1977.

35. Allaway, W.H., Kubota, J., Losee, F., et al. Selenium, molybdenum, and vanadium in human blood. *Arch. Environ. Health.* 16: 342–348, 1968.

36. McConnell, K.P., Jayer, R.M., Bland, K.I., et al. The relationship of dietary selenium and breast cancer. *J. Surg. Onc.,* 15: 67–70, 1980.

37. Shamberger, R.J., Rukovena, E., Longfield, A.K., et al. Antioxidants and cancer. I. Selenium in the blood of normals and cancer patients. *JNCI,* 50: 867–870, 1973.

38. Calautti, P., Mochini, G., Stievano, B.M., et al. Serum selenium levels in malignant lymphoproliferative diseases. *Scand. J. Haematol.,* 24: 63–66, 1980.

39. Brogramhamer, W.L., McConnell, K.P. and Blocky, W.P. Relationship between serum selenium levels and patients with carcinoma. *Cancer* 37: 1384–1388, 1976.

40. Robinson, M.F., Godfrey, P.J., Thomson, C.D., et al. Blood selenium and glutathione peroxidase activity in normal subjects and in surgical patients with and without cancer in New Zealand. *Am. J. Clin. Nutr.,* 32: 1477–1485, 1979.

41. Willett, W., Polk, B.F., Hames, C., et al. Prediagnostic serum selenium and risk of cancer. *Lancet* II: 130-133, 1983.

42. Helzlsouer, K.J. Selenium and cancer prevention. *Seminars in Oncology,* 10: 308, 1983.

43. Noda, M., Takano, T., and Sakurai, H. Effects of selenium on chemical carcinogens. *Mut. Res.* 66: 175, 1979.

44. Griffin, A.B. Role of selenium in the chemoprevention of cancer. *Adv. Canc. Res.,* 29: 419–442, 1979.

45. Spallholz, J.E., Martin, J.L., Gerlach, M.L., et al. Injectable selenium: Effect in the primary immune response of mice. *Proc. Soc. Exp. Bio. Med.,* 148: 37–40, 1975.

46. Capel, I.D., Leach, D. and Dorrell, H.M. Vitamin E retards the lipoperidoxation resulting from anticancer drug administration. *Anticanc. Res.* 3: 59–62, 1983.

47. Prasad, D.N., and Edwards-Prasad, J. Effects of tocopherol (vitamin E) acid succinate or morphological alterations and growth inhibition in melanoma cells in culture. *Canc. Res.* 42: 550–555, 1983.

48. Horvath, P.M. and Clement, L.P. Synergistic effect of vitamin E and selenium in the chemoprevention of mammary carcinogenesis in rats. *Canc. Res.* 43: 5335–5341, 1983.

49. Nutrition and Cancer: Cause and Prevention. *CA-A Canc. J. Clin.,* 34(2): 121, 1984.

50. Larsson, B.K., Sahlberg, G.P., Eriksson, A.T., et al. Polycyclic aromatic hydrocarbons in grilled food. *J. Agric. Food Chem.,* 31: 867–873, 1983.

Part IV
NUTRITION AND
CARDIOVASCULAR DISEASE

11

AN INTRODUCTION

THE UNITED STATES has one of the highest heart disease rates in the world. Since 1940 cardiovascular disease (CVD) has been the leading cause of mortality and morbidity in this country. Although the mortality rate from CVD has declined since the mid-1960s, the disease still affects 42,750,000 Americans, with 550,000 dying each year from heart attack alone.[1]

Diseases due to infection and poor sanitation have diminished since the turn of the century, while the changing American lifestyle has brought with it an increase in lifestyle-related disorders. Death from acute infectious diseases dropped from 580 for every 100,000 people in 1900 to a mere 30 for every 100,000 in 1979. During the same time, deaths from chronic diseases such as cancer, heart disease and stroke escalated by 250 percent. Today, half of all deaths are due to CVD; every fifth man and every seventh woman under the age of sixty suffer from this disease.

The impact of heart disease on Americans is not confined to fatal heart attacks. Its victims, mainly men in their 40s and 50s, are in their prime productive years. To cripple or diminish the working capacity of this group results in enormous social and economic loss. Heart disease is the greatest contributor to permanent disability in workers under sixty-five and it is the reason for more hospitalization days than any other illness. According to the National Heart, Lung, and Blood Institute, heart attacks cost Americans $60 billion in medical bills a year. Lost wages and productivity exceed the total Medicare budget.

The answer to reducing the incidence of cardiovascular disease is not only to develop costly complex technology for possible treatment and cure of these debilitating and slowly progressing diseases, but to focus attention on prevention and individual responsibility for health. As stated in the Surgeon General's report, *Healthy People*, ''We are killing ourselves by our own careless habits.''[2]

The likelihood of a person's developing CVD depends on the individual's decision to avoid or embrace certain risks. Risk factors are any characteristics associated with an above average incidence of a disease. A risk factor, whether a dietary pattern, a habit or an age group, is a warning signal. If not heeded, a risk factor will predispose the individual to a greater chance, now or in the future, of developing the disease(s) that others with the same characteristics have developed.

The Framingham study, initiated in 1948, first identified the three primary health habits considered risk factors in the development of CVD as: 1) high blood pressure (hypertension); 2) cigarette smoking; and 3) elevated serum cholesterol. Since then, the type of cholesterol in the blood has been recognized as increasing or decreasing the risk of CVD, and elevated low-density lipoprotein-cholesterol is now recognized as the fourth primary risk factor. Secondary risk factors are: obesity (a body weight 20 percent or more above ideal), diabetes, stress, lack of cardiovascular (aerobic) exercise, a family history of heart or blood vessel disease, male sex, stress-prone personality type, high serum triglycerides and increasing age.

If an individual has three of the risk factors, the chances of developing heart disease are six times greater than if only one risk factor is present. A person has no control over some risk factors, such as age, genetics, race and sex. Other risk factors are controllable and

THE CARDIOVASCULAR DISEASES

Cardiovascular disease is a group of disorders characterized by an abnormality of the heart or vascular system. The following are forms of CVD:

Atherosclerosis: a form of arteriosclerosis. Fat accumulates in the arterial wall, reducing vascular wall elasticity and blood flow.

Coronary artery disease (CAD): atherosclerosis of the arteries that supply blood and oxygen to the heart muscle.

Heart attack: damage to heart tissue as a result of diminished blood supply and, consequently, a diminished supply of oxygen and nutrients. Metabolic waste products are not removed and accumulate in the affected area. The amount of tissue damage determines the severity of the heart attack.

Stroke: damage to brain tissue as a result of diminished blood supply. It may result from 1) atherosclerosis of the arteries supplying the brain and neck; 2) a blood clot (thrombus) which closes off one of these arteries; 3) a traveling blood clot (embolus) which lodges in an artery; or 4) a cerebral hemorrhage. A cerebral aneurism (a weakened artery in the brain which bursts) can precede the latter event.

Hypertension: elevated blood pressure which reduces arterial wall elasticity, increases the work load on the heart and vasculature and increases the likelihood of heart attack and stroke.

Peripheral vascular disease: a variety of disorders including varicose veins, thrombophlebitis, venous thrombosis, atherosclerosis of the extremities, Raynaud's disease and Buerger's disease.

Congestive heart failure: an abnormal pumping by a weakened heart which results in diminished blood flow and pooling of fluid in the ankles and feet (edema). The lungs may also accumulate excess fluid.

controlling them can reduce the likelihood of contracting the disease. (See Figure 14.) A change in diet alone is no guarantee that heart disease will be prevented. Risk factors are based on population studies and represent the likelihood—not the inevitability—of the occurrence of a certain condition in any one person. Altering one or several risk factors will reduce the probability of developing the associated disease, but it is not a guarantee that a specific individual will be immune to it. Diet does play a critical role in several of the primary and secondary risk factors, however, and can contribute to the prevention and treatment of CVD.

ATHEROSCLEROSIS: THE UNDERLYING CAUSE

The initial link between heart disease and diet was hypothesized when the arteries of heart attack victims were inspected. Instead of finding normal arteries which are smooth, elastic and bright pink in color, researchers found arteries that were hard, inflexible, and clogged with hardened yellowish cholesterol growths—a condition commonly called atherosclerosis.

Atherosclerosis or "hardening of the arteries" is the process that eventually gives rise to the cardiovascular disease conditions of heart attack and stroke. Atherosclerosis begins as fatty streaks along the inner lining of medium and large arteries. These streaks are composed primarily of cholesterol. The endothelial lining becomes roughened and the blood clots more readily in reaction to the irregular surface. At a later stage, these streaks develop into plaques formed by an overgrowth of muscle cells engorged with cholesterol. The plaque protrudes into the lumen (opening) of the artery. As the plaques spread and enlarge, they eventually cause the artery wall to become rigid, reducing its ability to expand and contract in accordance with blood pressure needs. (See Figure 15.) Blood flow is restricted and, in some cases, totally obstructed. Damage or death to the tissue relying on that blood supply results. If the occluded artery is one which supplies the brain with oxygen and nutrients, stroke results. If the artery feeds the coronary muscle, heart attack is the likely outcome. The severity of these events will depend on the amount of tissue affected and the speed with which medical care and first aid are administered.

Two harmful constituents associated with the development of this degenerative process are platelets and low-density lipoprotein-cholesterol.

THE ROLE OF PLATELETS IN ATHEROSCLEROSIS

Platelets are cell fragments important to blood clotting. There are 200,000 to 400,000 of them in a

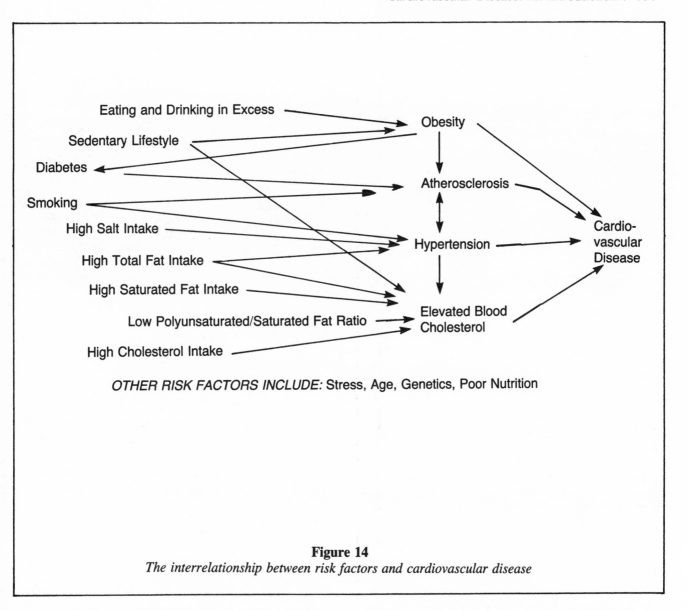

Figure 14
The interrelationship between risk factors and cardiovascular disease

cubic millimeter of blood. Although they have no nucleus, they do contain mitochondria and have the capacity for energy production. They contain lipids (including cholesterol and phospholipids), protein and numerous trace elements such as copper, magnesium, potassium, sodium, calcium, iron and manganese. Their enzyme composition includes catalase, amylase, phosphomonoesterase, cholesterase, lactic and glutamic dehydrogenases, lecithinase, histaminase and many others. This assortment of enzymes reflects the versatility and range of metabolic functions in which platelets are potentially involved. The agglutinogens found in

platelets are similar to those found in red blood cells and are responsible for the clotting ability of platelets.

Platelets are the initiators of blood coagulation. They do not stick to each other or the artery walls unless the endothelium has been damaged and roughened. When there is damage, platelets aggregate, obstructing blood flow to the wounded area and facilitating hemostasis. They release serotonin, a vasoconstrictor important in hemostasis and clot retraction. Once attached to the injured area, platelets release thromboxane, which further stimulates platelet aggregation. They also release a factor which stimulates muscle cell proliferation.

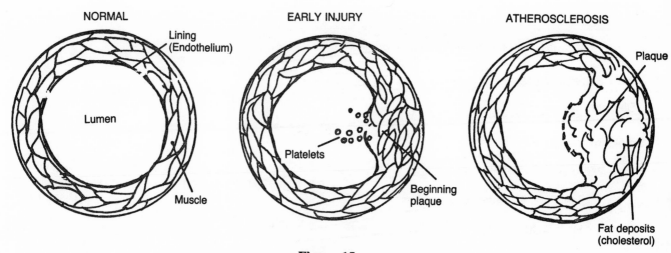

Figure 15

*A cross-section of an artery showing the progression
of atherosclerosis*

THE ROLE OF LOW-DENSITY LIPOPROTEIN-CHOLESTEROL IN ATHEROSCLEROSIS

Low-density lipoprotein-cholesterol (LDL-cholesterol) keeps cholesterol dissolved in the blood and, when modified by platelet by-products, releases its cholesterol into otherwise resistant arterial lining cells. These cells have no efficient way of eliminating the accumulated cholesterol and so enlarge under the burden. The greater the LDL-cholesterol concentration in the blood, the faster this process occurs. So, while platelets encourage cell proliferation, LDL-cholesterol simultaneously stimulates these cells to engorge with cholesterol. The end product is plaque.

THE INITIATION OF ATHEROSCLEROSIS

Fatty streaks along the arterial endothelium mark the beginning stages of atherosclerosis. This condition is observed in infants' arteries and may or may not develop into cardiovascular disease later in life. The origin and reasons for atherosclerotic degeneration of arteries is still a mystery, although several theories have been developed and researched. The encrustation theory states that atherosclerosis is initiated by blood

components deposited onto the artery wall, forming a thrombus that later becomes enmeshed with cells. The imbibition hypothesis states that blood constituents invade the artery lining and cause a reaction which results in plaque. Atherosclerosis has also been theorized to be a tumor-like growth of smooth muscle cells instigated by circulating carcinogens such as cholesterol and components of cigarette smoke.[3]

Another theory involves the possible role of phagocytotic cells in the pathogenesis of atherosclerosis. These cells, including white blood cells, monocytes, macrophages and neutrophils, are capable of ingesting large particulate matter and are found at damaged arterial sites. The foam cells (cells containing fats) found in atherosclerotic lesions are similar to those found in other body sites of fat absorption and necrosis. They are derived from tissue macrophages, products of circulating monocytes.[4] These monocytes migrate into endothial tissue in experimental hypercholesterolemia and hypertension.[5] This phagocytotic cell theory has been observed in animals. Aortas from hypercholesterolemic rats are filled with white blood cells attached focally to the endothelium. The endothelium remains intact while macrophages (converted monocytes) are found below the endothelium and in the intima. Those below the intima accumulate fat. The condition resembles the preliminary atherosclerotic stage (fatty streaks) found in humans[6] and develops in rats within one week on a high cholesterol diet. If these rats are maintained on a high cholesterol diet, smooth muscle cells migrate into the developing plaque and some accumulate fat.

As the attachment and migration of monocytes continues, muscle cells could continue to multiply, producing collagen, elastin and mucopolysaccharides. The fat-filled cells at the heart of the plaque die, releasing their fatty constituents. Since the tissue has no way of removing the necrotic cells, this fat-laden debris continues to accumulate. This hypothetical process of cell proliferation, macrophage migration and accumulation of fats and dead tissue could cause the plaque to swell, ballooning into the arterial lumen and eventually closing off blood flow. The phagocytotic cell theory may be a piece in a puzzle which attempts to explain the initiation and process of atherosclerosis.

The abundance of platelets found in the vicinity of atherosclerotic tissue and the chemical composition and aggregation characteristics of these cell fragments have led to a platelet-derived growth factor theory for cell proliferation in the development of atherosclerosis.[7] According to this theory, the process is set into action by a platelet-induced thrombus resulting from mechanical injury to the artery wall. Rapid or turbulent blood flow would degrade the lining, especially where the artery forks or forms a junction. Hypertension could play its role here by increasing pressure on the linings of blood vessels. In research studies, when endothelial cells are removed, the surrounding smooth muscle cells multiply only in the presence of normal circulating platelets, thus supporting the platelet theory. When blood cholesterol levels are high the damage remains or worsens.

Even though platelet-induced muscle cell proliferation has been observed, the initial endothelial cell loss has not been proven, thus shedding doubt, at least at this time, on the total accuracy of this theory. Lesions and plaque accumulation may be retarded or prevented if arterial smooth muscle cell proliferation and fat deposition can be prevented. The mechanisms responsible for platelet action and the ultimate involvement of platelets in the degenerative process of atherosclerosis are yet to be fully understood.

CHOLESTEROL: THE COMMON THREAD IN ATHEROSCLEROSIS

The ultimate explanation for the genesis of atherosclerosis may not be any single one of these theories but may rest in a synchronizing of several theories into one. One common thread does pervade the literature. In all the theories and research findings it has been verified that atherosclerosis is a process closely related to as well as the result of abnormal lipid metabolism.[8] And in spite of the controversy regarding the mechanisms of atherosclerosis development, two important points are worth noting: 1) as blood fat levels, especially cholesterol, rise, so does the risk of atherosclerosis, and 2) dietary cholesterol and saturated fats increase blood cholesterol. How circulating carcinogens, white blood cells, monocytes, macrophages, or platelets affect or are affected by abnormal lipid metabolism is still being investigated.

REFERENCES

1. American Heart Association. *Heart Facts 1984*, publication 55-005-H.

2. *Healthy People: The Surgeon General's Report on Health Promotion and Disease Prevention*. U.S. Department of Health, Education, and Welfare/Public Health Service. Publication No. 79-55071. 1979.

3. Benditt, E. and Benditt, J. Evidence of a monoclonal origin of human atherosclerotic plaques. *Proc. Natl. Acad. Sci. U.S.A.*, 70: 1753, 1973.

4. Ryan, G. and Majno, G. *Inflammation*. Kalamazoo, Mich.: Upjohn Company, 1977.

5. Gerrity, R. The role of the monocyte in atherosclerosis. I: Transition of blood-borne monocytes into foam cells in fatty lesions. *Am. J. Pathol.*, 103: 181, 1981.

6. Majno, G., Znd, T., Nunnare, J., and Joris, I. The diet/atherosclerosis connection: New insights. *J. Cardio Med.*, Jan., 1984, 21–30.

7. Ross, R. and Harker, L. Hyperlipidemia and atherosclerosis. Chronic hyperlipidemia initiates and maintains lesions by endothelial cell desquamation and lipid accumulation. *Science*, 193: 1904, 1976.

8. McMillan, G. *The Thrombotic Process in Atherogenesis*. New York: Plenum Press, 1978.

Additional Reading

American Heart Association Steering Committee for Medical and Community Programs: Risk factors and coronary disease. *Circulation,* 62, 449A–455A, 1980.

Keys, A. Coronary heart disease in seven countries. *Circulation.* 41: Supple 1., April 1970.

Multiple Risk Factor Intervention Trial Research Group: Multi-ple Risk Factor Intervention Trial: Risk factor changes and mortality results. *JAMA,* 248: 1465–1477, 1982.

Ross, R., et al. A platelet-dependent serum factor that stimulates the proliferation of arterial smooth muscle cells in vitro. *Proc. Natl. Acad. Sci. U.S.A.,* 71:1207, 1974.

Stamler, J. Primary prevention of coronary heart disease: The last 20 years. *Am. J. Cardiol.,* 47: 722–735, 1981.

12

............HYPERTENSION, SMOKING, CHOLESTEROL:.....
THE PRIMARY RISK FACTORS

HYPERTENSION

HYPERTENSION is abnormal and excessive blood pressure against the walls of the arteries. The escalation in pressure may originate from 1) the heart's pumping action; 2) a narrowing of the artery, causing an equal amount of blood to be forced through a smaller canal; or 3) increases in the amount of blood being pumped through an artery of normal dimensions.

Over 37 million Americans had hypertension in 1984; 25 million were borderline, and nearly 32,000 died from the disorder.[1] Two in five do not know they have the disorder and of the 60 percent who do know, only one-third are adequately controlled, while the other two-thirds seek no treatment or have inadequate treatment. In other words, four out of five hypertensives are either not aware of or not successful in handling their condition.

Hypertension is dangerous because it accelerates plaque formation in atherosclerosis and encourages the formation of blood clots which, if stationary (a thrombus), or if dislodged and floating free in the blood (an embolus), can close off an artery. The elevated arterial pressure weakens the blood vessel walls, encouraging aneurisms that diminish cardiovascular function and that, when ruptured, can cause heart attack, stroke, internal bleeding and a host of life-threatening conditions. Congestive heart failure and damage to the kidneys are common in hypertension, too.

Hypertension is one of the primary risk factors in the development of cardiovascular disease (CVD). In the Framingham study, men with blood pressures above 160/95 had a two to three times greater chance of developing heart disease and a three times greater chance of developing stroke than those with blood pressure below this level. Elevated diastolic pressure is the most common sign of hypertension, since it signals excessive pressure within the cardiovascular system even during times of rest. Even seemingly moderate changes in diastolic pressure can drastically influence an individual's risks. If diastolic pressure is between 80 and 90, chances of dying within the next eight years are doubled.

BLOOD PRESSURE VALUES

	Systolic/Diastolic
Normal	120/80 or less
Borderline	140/90–160/95
Hypertension	160/95

What makes hypertension so serious is its lack of symptoms; it is a silent killer. Anxiety, heart poundings, increased pulse rate, or feeling "all wound up" are not indicators of high blood pressure. The only way to detect abnormal pressure is to have a blood pressure check.

Other than the knowledge that certain populations, such as blacks, have a higher incidence of hypertension, no accurate procedure exists to predict who will develop the condition and who will not. Essential hypertension, cause unknown, comprises over 90 percent of the cases. It is known that blood pressure is dependent on several factors including body weight, certain dietary factors, genetic predisposition, cigarette

155

THE BLOOD PRESSURE TEST

Blood pressure is the force applied by the blood against the artery walls. The force is a product of the heart's pumping action against arterial wall resistance. When the heart muscle contracts, the blood pressure increases, creating systolic pressure, the greatest amount of pressure exerted against the walls of the arteries at any one time. Between contractions the heart has a relaxation phase, where the diastolic pressure reflects the lowest amount of pressure.

Blood pressure can be monitored with a stethescope and an instrument called a sphygmomanometer, which includes an airbag or cuff and a column of mercury (Hg) marked in millimeters. When the cuff is wrapped around the upper arm and inflated it restricts the brachial artery, thus halting blood flow to the lower arm and hand. Air pressure supports the column of mercury and as air is released from the cuff, the mercury falls.

As the cuff is deflated, the examiner will hear the initial pumping of blood back through the brachial artery. The level of mercury at this point corresponds to the systolic pressure, the greatest exertion of pressure from the heart's contractions, which is capable of forcing blood through the semi-constricted artery. As the cuff is further loosened, eventually no sound can be heard through the stethescope; at this point the level of mercury reflects the least amount of pressure in the artery, or diastolic pressure. The final reading consists of the systolic pressure over the diastolic pressure, for example, 120 mm Hg/ 80 mm Hg. Several readings taken over a period of time give a more accurate reading of blood pressure than one or even two readings taken together.

smoking, stress, exercise, and percent body fat. Endocrine disorders, including adult-onset diabetes associated with obesity, contribute to hypertension as well.[2]

MAINTAINING OR REGAINING IDEAL BODY WEIGHT

Body weight is of considerable importance, since studies show a direct correlation between increases in body weight and elevation of blood pressure. The loss of excess weight is proportionate to reductions in blood pressure, and epidemiological studies show that as weight increases the risk of developing hypertension increases as well.[3] This reduction is independent of sodium intake.[4] With a drop in body weight, mean arterial pressure declines;[5] blood volume, cardiac output and venous return are reduced; and circulating norepinephrine decreases. The last condition may be related to the drop in weight and arterial pressure.

Although maintaining ideal body weight can help prevent hypertension, it does not guarantee immunity. In one study, overweight subjects were four times more likely to develop high blood pressure than matched lean subjects.[6] However, lean hypertensives are more likely to gain weight, although the reason for this is unknown. Many suffer from the condition regardless of weight loss. Besides, only 5 percent to 25 percent of those who go on weight loss regimens actually lose the weight and keep it off. A combination of fewer calories and attention to sodium and other nutrients may provide a more comprehensive tactic for controlling hypertension.

DIET AND HYPERTENSION: SODIUM

Hundreds of epidemiological, animal and human studies have linked salt (sodium) with hypertension, yet the strength of this connection still remains controversial. The controversy results from evidence that sodium consumption is similar in hypertensive and normotensive subjects and sodium restriction does not always result in normalization of high blood pressure.

Increased dietary sodium increases blood volume.[7–9] Since the 1940s it has been known that the opposite is true as well: a low-sodium diet decreases blood volume, with a resultant reduction in blood pressure.[10] "Where sodium goes, water follows" is a correct statement. The explanation for this association with hypertension is founded on one of the three causes of elevated blood pressure: increases in the amount of blood pumped through an artery of normal dimensions force the blood pressure to rise.

In the 1960s Louis Dahl discovered that salt caused high blood pressure in about three-quarters of salt-fed rats,[11] whereas those fed a diet devoid of added salt did not develop the disorder. By breeding the two sets of rats separately he developed a salt-sensitive and a salt-resistant strain. Dahl concluded that 1) hypertension due to excessive salt intake was inherited and 2) normal blood pressure could be maintained in the sensitive group if a salt-restricted diet were followed.

Obviously, the high intake of salt in the United States does not cause hypertension in the majority of people, but for some, a correlation does exist between salt consumption and risk of hypertension. Restriction of sodium can reduce high blood pressure in some patients[12] but has no effect on others,[13] which suggests salt-sensitivity in humans similar to that which Dahl observed in rats. In 33⅓ percent to 50 percent of patients who are salt sensitive, a reduction in sodium reduces blood pressure,[14] and some researchers postulate that a sodium threshold may exist above which those predisposed to hypertension develop the disorder. Unfortunately, pre-screening for those with salt-sensitivity is difficult.

A level of sodium restriction necessary to lower blood pressure significantly has not been determined. Marked restriction of sodium intake to levels of .2–.5 grams (there are 2.3 grams of sodium in one teaspoon of salt) often reduces blood pressure. The severity of this dietary restriction may not be necessary since an 18 percent reduction in sodium (from 11 grams to 9 grams) has been shown to normalize blood pressure in hypertensives.[15] Mildly hypertensive subjects reduce blood pressure on diets of four to five grams of sodium.[16] This suggests that sodium restriction may prove beneficial for those with less severe hypertension.

Studies have not proven that a low-salt diet will prevent hypertension although low-salt consuming cultures, such as the Alaskan Eskimos, the Melanesian tribes in New Guinea, the Polynesian groups of the Cook Islands, and tribes in Eastern Africa, exhibit little or no hypertension. In these societies blood pressure does not rise with age, as is common in "civilized" Western cultures. Tribes on the Solomon Islands also show a distinct association between salt consumption and incidence of high blood pressure. Those residing in the hills differ from those living on the shores of the lagoons only in their consumption of salt. The lagoon residents boil their food in salt water and show a significant incidence of hypertension. Those living in the salt-free hills are relatively hypertension-free. In areas of northern Japan where salt intake is high, hypertension is endemic. Many groups, however, have a low incidence of hypertension in spite of high sodium intake. So the controversy rages on.

Blacks, relatives of hypertensives, and people over forty-five may be slow in excreting sodium,[17] which may explain the prevalence of hypertension in these three groups. Reduced production of aldosterone (the sodium-retaining hormone produced by the adrenal cortex) after age fifty may affect sodium metabolism in older hypertensive patients.[18]

Despite the ambiguity surrounding sodium's role in the development of hypertension, several publications, including the Surgeon General's report "Healthy People, Toward Healthful Diets," and the U.S. Senate Select Committee's Dietary Goals for the United States, recommend reduction in sodium consumption regardless of intake or blood pressure. If a person is hypertensive or susceptible to the disorder (i.e., has a family history of hypertension, is overweight, is black, is over forty-five years of age, or is borderline hypertensive) restricting dietary sodium becomes even more important. In spite of the lack of definitive proof that consuming less sodium will prevent or cure hypertension, doing so poses no health risks and moderate salt restriction may be of value as one of the factors in the management and prevention of hypertension. There is no reason not to reduce America's salt intake.

DIET AND HYPERTENSION: OTHER ELECTROLYTES

Table salt is a combination of sodium and chloride. Although sodium has attracted the most attention in the control and prevention of hypertension, some research suggests that chloride may play a role as well. Levels of plasma renin (a hormone produced by the kidneys, responsible for water and salt retention) are depressed when rats are fed sodium chloride; this effect is not seen when equal amounts of nonchloride-containing sodium are administered. Dahl rats respond to sodium chloride, but not to nonchloride-containing sodium, with an increase in blood pressure.[19] Chloride may affect hormonal regulation of fluid and salt retention and thus contribute to hypertension.

Potassium and the sodium-potassium ratio are important issues in hypertension control. Potassium has been shown to have a protective effect in rats and a blood-pressure-lowering effect in humans.[20] In groups consuming relatively high amounts of potassium, blood pressures are low.[21] Meneely and Battarbee note that for millions of years the human species existed on less than 0.6 grams of sodium daily.[22] Current processing has artificially increased this intake to 6–18 grams a day and depleted the potassium content. This drastic upset in a preexisting sodium-potassium balance might contribute to electrolyte and fluid imbalances and ultimately to altered blood pressure.

DIET AND HYPERTENSION: CALCIUM

Calcium deficiency may contribute to hypertension. Reduced calcium intake increases blood pressure in rats, and subsequent calcium supplementation lowers the elevated blood pressure.[23] Data from the Health and Nutrition Examination Survey I done by the National Center for Health Statistics showed that hypertensives consume 18 percent less dietary calcium (572 ± 17 mg) than normotensives (695 ± 7 mg). Of the seventeen nutrients analyzed, only calcium showed a correlation.[24]

Whereas calcium levels are positively related to renin levels in hypertensives, serum magnesium may be inversely related.[25] This may suggest abnormal membrane transport of calcium and magnesium. Normally, calcium concentration is high extracellularly and magnesium is high intracellularly. If the pumping mechanism that allows for these differences in concentrations were defective, this could disturb renin functioning and increase the risk of hypertension. Depending on where the abnormality lies in the renin control system, some individuals would respond to magnesium supplementation while others would respond to calcium. Americans are consuming less calcium, and calcium intake is especially low in some segments of the population, such as blacks and the elderly. These groups also exhibit a high incidence of hypertension.

Although the results suggest that calcium intake or metabolism is associated with hypertension, the findings are too scarce at this point to verify a causal link. If low serum calcium is due to inadequate dietary intake or imbalances in the calcium-magnesium intake, then diet and supplementation may play a role in hypertension control. If low serum calcium is a result, rather than a cause, of hypertension, consuming more dietary calcium would have little impact on lowering blood pressure.

DIET AND HYPERTENSION: FATS

Hypertension is responsive to a reduction in dietary fat.[26] When dietary fats are reduced to 25 percent of total calories (average fat consumption in America is 42 percent) or when the ratio of polyunsaturated to saturated fat is increased from 0.3 to 1.0, blood pressure declines up to 10 percent in hypertensives. It has been theorized that with dietary fat restricted to 10 percent of calories, along with salt restriction and maintenance of ideal weight, hypertension might be controlled or eliminated in 85 percent of patients.[27]

A link may exist between sodium and fat. Researchers have found that when daily sodium intake is increased from 4 grams to 24 grams (2 teaspoons to 12 teaspoons), humans show a reduced capacity to clear intravenously administered fat from the blood.

Essential free fatty acids, supplied by polyunsaturated fats (PUFA), may have a protective effect on blood pressure by mediating prostaglandin response.[28] Prostaglandins are important in blood pressure regulation. They are vasodilators and enhance the kidney's excretion of sodium and water, thus reducing blood volume and blood pressure.

The blood pressure of vegetarians is usually lower than that of meat eaters. In addition, when meat eaters switch to a diet of plant foods, their blood pressure declines. Vegetarian diets are high in PUFA and essential fatty acids. It has been postulated that an association exists between vegetarians' increased intake of essential fatty acids and micronutrients (those responsible for the production of vasodilatory and natriuretic prostaglandins) and their reduced blood pressure. No significant difference in urinary excretion of prostaglandin E2 and other hormones has been found, however. This suggests that the effect of the plant diet is more than just its impact on prostaglandin synthesis and regulation.[29] Other food factors in vegetarian diets, such as fibers (see pp. 169–170), saponins (see p. 169), or the type of protein (see below), may enhance the essential fatty acid effect or have an independent effect on blood pressure.

DIET AND HYPERTENSION: PROTEIN

Excessive protein intake, similar to that in the U.S., may speed the progress of vascular disease, especially in the kidney, and contribute to the development of hypertension. Protein consumed in excess also increases calcium excretion. This would coincide with findings that high urinary calcium is positively correlated with incidence of hypertension.[30]

DIET AND HYPERTENSION: OTHER MINERALS:

Dietary intake of copper and zinc may contribute to the hypertension puzzle. A research study at Mississippi State University found high blood pressure to be associated with increased intake of dietary copper and reduced dietary zinc. Serum zinc was inversely related to blood pressure. The copper/zinc association with blood pressure was strongest in males. This finding is in conflict with Dr. Klevay's hypothesis that reduced copper is correlated with increased risk of cardiovascular disease. The finding is in agreement, however, with reports from the World Health Organization that elevated copper, especially in conjunction with reduced zinc, can exacerbate cardiovascular problems. Current indices for determining copper and zinc status are meager and thus interfere with interpretation of results. This may explain the disagreement among various research findings.[31]

IN SUMMARY

Hypertension is a multifaceted disorder and it is not wise to focus on one dietary component when reviewing its prevention, control and elimination. For instance, several trace minerals including copper, zinc, chromium, cobalt, vanadium, molybdenum, manganese and selenium, are cofactors in enzymatic reactions crucial to normal cardiovascular function; coffee consumption has been positively correlated with diastolic pressure (the resting blood pressure increases with each refill[32]); and dietary carbohydrate intake stimulates insulin, temporarily reduces urinary excretion of sodium and moderately reduces blood pressure.[33]

Alcohol has also been linked with hypertension. Industrial studies show that heavy drinkers have the highest blood pressure.[34] Kaiser-Permanente's hypertension study of 87,000 persons found a correlation between alcohol consumption and hypertension. The data suggested that 5 percent of hypertension in the American population could be attributed to the consumption of three or more alcoholic beverages a day.[35] The "to be's or not to be's" of hypertension appear to reflect total nutritional status, ratios among nutrients, individual susceptibility to certain nutrients, and such factors as coffee and alcohol consumption. Other lifestyle choices, such as exercise and smoking, can modify or enhance these risk factors.

CIGARETTE SMOKING

Of the three primary risk factors, eliminating smoking creates the least controversy. Heart and artery disease constitute the largest proportion of the 325,000 deaths related to smoking each year. All smokers are at risk of heart disease and the risk increases substantially if the smoker also has hypertension, elevated blood fats or both. The risk increases with the number of cigarettes smoked; people who smoke a pack a day have more than twice the risk of heart attack as those who have never smoked. Smokers who suffer a heart attack are less likely to survive the attack than non-smokers.

The mechanisms by which cigarette smoking contributes to heart disease and hypertension are poorly understood. It is known that nicotine elevates the heartbeat, thus increasing the heart's oxygen demand, while the carbon monoxide content of tobacco concurrently reduces the blood's oxygen-carrying capacity. The heart is forced to work harder with less oxygen. At the same time smoking constricts arteries, further restricting blood supply to the oxygen-impoverished heart muscle. Any or all of these factors could contribute to angina pectoris, or chest pains, resulting from diminished blood supply to the heart.

Smokers have a higher incidence and severity of atherosclerosis. Peripheral vascular disease is also more common in smokers. If there is no permanent damage, symptoms diminish with cessation of smoking. Diabetics who smoke are at an even greater risk.

There is no way to avoid the deleterious effects of cigarette smoke. Low tar and nicotine cigarettes are not the answer. Smokers tend to smoke these cigarettes longer, inhale the smoke deeper into the lungs and smoke more often, thus eliminating any possible benefits. Non-smokers—whether they are co-workers, roommates, partners, children or those sitting near by—exposed to chronic cigarette smoke are not immune to the hazards. Sidestream smoke has as much as twice the tar and nicotine and five times the carbon monoxide as the secondary smoke that enters the smoker's lungs. Secondary smoke passes through the tobacco and filtered end before entering the lungs, while sidestream smoke has no filter and is more potent to the smoker and those in the vicinity. Seven cigarettes in an hour can raise a room's carbon monoxide level to 20 ppm. The person sitting next to the smoker may be inhaling 90 ppm, twice the maximum limit set for industry. Non-smokers inhaling this sidestream smoke double and quadruple their blood carbon monoxide levels in 1 to 2 hours. Because of poor removal mechanisms, this toxic gas may linger in the body for several hours before it is eliminated.

To reduce the risk of cardiovascular disease the recommendation is obvious: stop smoking, stop exposing others to smoke and stop being exposed to others' smoke.

SERUM CHOLESTEROL

Cholesterol is the culprit of the day. Advertisements

for vegetable oils and butter substitutes proclaim their dissociation from this villain. Diet experts shake their finger at cholesterol-containing foods and scientists clash over dietary recommendations. In the midst of this turmoil, the average American continues to consume 165.2 pounds of meat (30 pounds more than in 1910), 276 eggs, 16.9 pounds of margarine and butter, and 18.1 pounds of ice cream annually,[36] while the heart struggles to pump blood through arteries accumulating cholesterol deposits at a rate of 1–2 percent per year.

In 1912 and 1913 Anitschkow fed cholesterol dissolved in vegetable oil to rabbits that subsequently developed arterial lesions similar to those found in atherosclerosis. The dietary fat and heart disease issue was born. In 1948, the Framingham study popularized Anitschkow's findings by showing that elevated cholesterol levels were closely associated with increased risk of atherosclerosis and cardiovascular disease.

ELEVATED SERUM CHOLESTEROL AND CARDIOVASCULAR DISEASE

It is well established that the risk of developing cardiovascular disease (CVD) is directly related to serum cholesterol levels.[37–38] As cholesterol rises above 200 mg/dl, CVD climbs proportionally. The average serum cholesterol level for middle-aged American men is 230–240 milligrams per one hundred deciliters of blood. This is not an optimal level but is an average

TABLE 14
The Relationship of Serum Cholesterol to the Coronary Death Rate

Serum Cholesterol Level (mg/100 dl blood)	Coronary Death Rate (age adjusted)
140 – 159	0.8%
160 – 179	2.1
180 – 199	2.1
200 – 219	2.5
220 – 239	3.1
240 – 259	3.6
260 – 279	3.1
280 – 299	6.4
300 – 319	7.2
>320	14.4

value for a population in which 50 percent of the deaths are due to heart disease. In populations where the serum cholesterol levels are below 190 mg/dl and in countries where it is below 160 mg/dl, CVD is non-existent.[39–40]

According to the American Heart Association the ideal serum cholesterol level for adults is between 130 and 190 mg/dl.[41] The relationship between serum cholesterol and cardiovascular disease is curvilinear, rather than linear, with a threshold above which risk increases with rising cholesterol. The Pooling Project identified this threshold to be around 200 mg/dl.[42] Over half of American males exceed this limit. Individual variation and additional risk factors such as smoking or obesity would require modification of this desirable range since the more risk factors present, the lower the serum cholesterol should be to counteract the elevated risk.

THE EFFECT OF DIETARY CHOLESTEROL ON SERUM CHOLESTEROL

Serum cholesterol and lipoprotein levels are affected by several of the previously mentioned risk factors, but no lifestyle habit has been more strongly correlated with elevated blood fats than diet, especially dietary saturated fats and cholesterol.[43–44] The effect of diet has been well researched through epidemiological studies comparing population groups, as well as clinically controlled dietary studies on individuals.[45–48]

The coronary heart disease rate has been studied in the predominantly vegetarian Seventh-Day Adventist population. This group exhibits consistently low levels of serum cholesterol and incidence of heart disease.[49–50] The low-fat diet of this group, in conjunction with a reduction in other risk factors, such as smoking, has been identified as the causative factor. Other food components in this group's diet, including fiber (see pp. 169–170, saponins (see p. 169) and essential fatty acids (see pp. 166–168), may also have contributed to the positive results.

A direct correlation exists between the incidence of CVD in a particular group, blood cholesterol levels and the amount of fatty animal foods in the diet. The Finns are the largest consumers of fat and hold first place in incidence of heart disease. Americans consume slightly less than the Finns and come in second. The Japanese, with their low saturated fat intake, are last in the race and have one quarter the heart disease rate of Americans. When these heart disease-resistant people emigrate to the United States and switch to the higher fat diet, heart disease escalates to the same level as that of their American peers.

Atherosclerosis is a multifactorial disease, with cholesterol only one contributor. Serum cholesterol levels will vary among individuals placed on the same diet because of variances in exercise, weight, age, genetics, smoking and other risk factors. In addition, cholesterol biosynthesis, excretion, and regulatory mechanisms are variable and are inconsistent within and among individuals, so that dietary cholesterol may appear to elevate serum levels in some and not substantially affect serum levels in others. One man may eat two eggs a day, smoke cigarettes, engage only in spectator sports and carry an extra roll of fat around the middle yet live a disease-free life; another man with the same behaviors will die of a heart attack. This may be partially due to the body's ability to adjust biosynthesis of cholesterol in response to consumption. The amount of cholesterol synthesized by the body is a function of dietary intake; as intake increases, biosynthesis declines. When intake is excessive, some individuals experience a failure of this homeostatic control, which results in hypercholesterolemia. Extensive research supports the theory that, in spite of individual variation, diet does affect plasma cholesterol, and elevated plasma cholesterol is directly related to development of atherosclerosis in the majority of people.

It is no wonder that the American diet is suspect. The average American consumes the daily equivalent of a full stick of butter in fat and cholesterol. Males eat enough animal foods in one day to total a cholesterol intake of 500–600 mg; even with excessive dieting, women consume an ample 350 mg. These intakes are well above the 300 mg recommended by the American Heart Association and the United States Dietary Goals, and are a third more than they were sixty years ago. This fat consumption is three times that of the Japanese and other groups in Africa and Latin America.

THE EFFECTS OF DIETARY CHOLESTEROL ON ATHEROSCLEROSIS

The issues of dietary lowering of serum cholesterol, and ultimately the ability to prevent, delay or even reverse atherosclerosis, have created controversy in the scientific community. Until recently, lowering serum cholesterol by reducing dietary fats had not been proven conclusively to reduce the risk of CVD.

Recently, dietary modification, drug therapy or both have been shown to be not only effective in lowering serum cholesterol but also beneficial in the prevention or reduction of CVD. The Lipid Research Clinics Coronary Primary Prevention Trial was a ten-year study which followed 3,806 middle-aged men, all of whom had serum cholesterol above 265 mg/dl.[51] This study found that for every 1 percent reduction in serum cholesterol there was a 2 percent reduction in risk of heart disease. The research used a cholesterol-lowering drug, cholestyramine, and a diet moderately reduced in fat. A 19 percent reduction in the rate of CVD in cholestyramine-treated men was preceded by an 8 percent and a 12 percent reduction in total plasma cholesterol and LDL cholesterol as compared to placebo-treated controls. The researchers stated that even without the drug, a low-fat diet alone would be beneficial; if serum cholesterol were reduced 10 percent to 15 percent through diet manipulation, the heart attack incidence would decline 20 percent to 30 percent.

CHOLESTEROL OXIDES AND ATHEROSCLEROSIS

The controversy over the dietary cholesterol-heart disease link is far from settled, and with time and further research additional factors will continue to be identified. Whereas earlier studies showed that dietary cholesterol raised blood cholesterol, later ones showed that the cholesterol-raising effect was encouraged by cholesterol oxides, not cholesterol itself. Of the several cholesterol oxides that exist, 25-hydroxycholesterol is the most atherogenic.[52] Cholesterol is oxidized when exposed to air, oxygen or heat; this suggests a possible atherogenic link to faulty food preparation and storage.[53] Animal studies support this theory by showing a greater rise in serum cholesterol when eggs are fried or hard boiled than if they are eaten raw or softly scrambled.[54] Oxidized cholesterol can be found in any fat that has been used to fry meat. Potatoes and other vegetables fried in animal fat are a potential source of these angiotoxic substances. A 100-gram sample of french fries has been found to contain 12 mg of cholesterol.[55] The 1 to 3 grams of endogenously derived cholesterol is minimally atherogenic, perhaps because of influence of the body's naturally occurring antioxidants—glutathione, vitamin E and vitamin C. The 250 mg to 300 mg of cholesterol found in egg yolks may not be as atherogenic if the eggs are fresh and refrigerated. The glutathione, vitamin C and vitamin E content of eggs are depleted after four to six months of unrefrigerated storage, which may contribute to cholesterol oxide formation. Dried and powdered cholesterol-containing foods that are exposed to air during storage; smoked fish and meats; and egg-containing foods are sources of these cholesterol derivatives.[56]

THE LIPOPROTEINS AND CARDIOVASCULAR DISEASE

After cholesterol is manufactured by the liver or absorbed through the intestinal lining, it travels through the circulatory system in combination with a protein carrier. The proportion, or ratio, of the different cholesterol-bound carriers to the total circulating cholesterol, and thus the type of cholesterol in the blood, is a better indicator of risk for cardiovascular disease (CVD) than total cholesterol alone.

The major lipids—cholesterol, triglycerides and phospholipids—are not soluble in the fluid medium of the blood and so are incorporated into carriers called lipoproteins. These lipoproteins vary in size, weight, and composition and are classified as high-density lipoproteins (HDL), low-density lipoproteins (LDL), very low-density lipoproteins (VLDL) and chylomicrons. VLDL and chylomicrons are the main carriers of triglycerides; LDL and HDL are the main carriers of cholesterol.

High-density lipoproteins are the heaviest lipoproteins and contain the most protein. As these relatively large and dense "strings" of fat-like proteins sweep through the body, they collect cholesterol and transport it to the liver for processing and removal. They are termed "scavengers" since they tend to clean up excess cholesterol lingering in the nooks and crannies of arteries. A larger proportion of total serum cholesterol carried in this lipoprotein is associated with a reduced risk of atherosclerosis and CVD.

HDL-cholesterol can be raised by reducing dietary fat and cholesterol, increasing cardiovascular or aerobic exercise, not smoking, and maintaining ideal body weight. Concentrations of HDL are higher after puberty in females and estrogens may be responsible for this protective effect, since they raise HDL-cholesterol even in males. The major causes of reduced HDL-cholesterol are obesity and sedentary lifestyles. HDL levels are increased in middle-aged men engaged in long-distance running, and Canadian studies at the University of Toronto showed HDL-cholesterol levels to rise substantially in myocardial infarction patients as a result of aerobic exercise. A minimum of 20 km/week was required to induce the serum lipid changes.[57] If ideal weight is maintained, a regular exercise program is developed and followed and dietary saturated fat and cholesterol are restricted, HDL concentration should rise.

Low-density lipoproteins are the primary means by which cholesterol is transported from the liver, where it is produced, to the body's cells for synthesis into hormones and constituents of cell membranes, or deposition into arterial wall plaque. In contrast to HDLs, which return cholesterol to the liver, LDLs transport it out to the tissues. Elevated LDL-cholesterol is associated with atherosclerosis and is the major source of cholesterol and cholesterol esters in plaque. Deposition of cholesterol into the lining of arterial walls is accelerated when LDL-cholesterol is high,[58] and the risk and severity of atherosclerosis increases when LDL-cholesterol is high or when HDL-cholesterol is low.[59-60] In the absence of high LDL-cholesterol, moderately low HDL-cholesterol is not as dangerous.[61] A sedentary lifestyle combined with a diet containing excess calories, saturated fats and cholesterol is correlated with elevated LDL-cholesterol and CVD.

Dietary factors undoubtedly elevate serum cholesterol; however, in people with plasma LDL-cholesterol concentrations above the 90th–95th percentile, genetic factors predominate. Familial hypercholesterolemia, depressed HDL-cholesterol, insufficient LDL-cholesterol clearance and early development of CVD are found in one out of 500 persons.[62-64] For those in the 50th to 90th percentile, genetics may play a role in CVD risk but, for this group, diet alone may be sufficient to reduce and maintain serum cholesterol within the desirable range.

IN SUMMARY

Elevated serum cholesterol levels are unequivocally related to increased incidence of cardiovascular disease. The "rich man's diet"—consisting of fatty meats, gravies and sauces, sautéed and fried foods, desserts and sweets, whole milk dairy products, butter, oils and salty delights—is a primary factor in raising these serum levels and encouraging increases in the carriers of cholesterol associated with atherosclerosis and heart disease. Americans have much to be thankful for. The variety of foods available far exceeds that of any other culture in the history of the world. This is coupled with leisure time, the diversity of recreational activities and the freedom to choose. The challenge is to eat the proper portions of the most healthful foods, engage in regular aerobic exercise, reduce sugar-salt-fat-alcohol-cholesterol intake and continue to keep abreast of accurate information about health and nutrition.

REFERENCES

1. American Heart Association. *Heart Facts 1984*, publication 55-055-H.

2. Sims, E. Mechanisms of hypertension in the syndromes of obesity. *Inter. J. of Obesity*, 5 (Supp. 1): 9, 1981.

3. Berchtold, P., et al. Obesity and hypertension: Conclusions and recommendations. *Inter. J. of Obesity*, 5 (Supp. 1): 183, 1981.

4. Hubert, H., Feinleib, M., McNamara, P., et al. Obesity as an independent risk factor for cardiovascular disease: A 26-year follow-up of participants in the Framingham Heart Study. *Circulation*, 67: 968–977, 1983.

5. Reisin, E., Frohlich, E., Messerli, F., et al. Cardiovascular changes after weight reduction in obesity hypertension. *Ann. Intern. Med.*, 98: 315–319, 1983.

6. Paul, O. (ed.) *Epidemiology and Control of Hypertension*, New York: Stratton, 1975, p. 175.

7. Ledingham, J. Distribution of water, sodium, and potassium in heart and skeletal muscle in experimental renal hypertension in rats. *Clin. Sci.*, 12: 337, 1953.

8. Selkurt, E. Effects of pulse pressure and mean arterial pressure modifications on renal hemodynamics and electrolyte water excretion. *Circulation*, 4: 541, 1951.

9. Tobian, L. A viewpoint concerning the enigma of hypertension. *Am. J. Med.*, 52: 595-609, 1972.

10. Murphy, R. The effect of "rice diet" on plasma volume and extracellular fluid space in hypertensive subjects. *J. Clin. Invest.*, 29:912, 1950.

11. Dahl, L. Salt and hypertension. *Am. J. Clin. Nutr.*, 25: 231, 1972.

12. Kempner, W. and Carolina, N. Treatment of kidney disease and hypertensive vascular disease with rice diet. *N. Med. J.*, 5: 125, 1945.

13. Flanagan, P., Logan, A., Haynes, R., et al. Dietary-sodium restriction alone in the treatment of mild hypertension. *Clin. Res.*, 31: 329A, 1983.

14. MacGregor, G. A. et al. Double-blind, randomized crossover trial of moderate sodium restriction in essential hypertension. *Lancet*, 1:351-354, 1982.

15. Morgan, R., Gillies, A., Morgan, G., et al. Hypertension treated by salt restriction. *Lancet*, 1: 227, 1978.

16. MacGregor, G. A. *Op cit.*

17. Luft, F., et al. Sodium sensitivity and resistance in normotensive humans. *Am. J. Med.*, 72: 726, 1982.

18. Hegsted, R., Brown, R., Jiang, N., et al. Aging and aldosterone. *Am. J. Med.*, 74: 442–448, 1983.

19. Meneely, G. and Battarbee, H. High sodium-low potassium environment and hypertension. *Am. J. Cardiol*, 38: 768, 1976.

20. Parfrey, P., et al. Blood pressure and hormonal changes following alteration in dietary sodium and potassium in mild essential hypertension. *Lancet*, 1: 59, 1981.

21. Tobian, L. On lactose-hydrolyzed milk. *Am. J. Clin. Nutri.*, 32: 2739, 1979.

22. Meneely, G. and Battarbee, H. *Op. cit.*

23. McCarron, D. Disturbances of calcium metabolism in the spontaneously hypertensive rat. *Hypertension*, 3 (Supp. I): I–162, 1981.

24. McCarron, D. Calcium and magnesium nutrition in human hypertension. *Ann. Int. Med.*, 98: 800–805, 1983.

25. Resnick, L. Divalent cations in essential hypertension—relations between serum ionized calcium, magnesium, and plasma renin activity. *New Eng. J. Med.*, 309: 888–891, 1983.

26. Iacono, J., Puska, P., Dougherty, R., et al. Effect of dietary fat on blood pressure in a rural Finnish population. *Am. J. Clin. Nutr.*, 38: 860–869, 1983.

27. Basta, L. Regression of atherosclerotic stenosing lesions of the renal arteries and spontaneous cure of systemic hypertension through control of hyperlipidemia. *Am. J. Med.*, 61:420-421, 1976.

28. Resnick, L. *Op. cit.*

29. Rouse, I., et al. Vegetarian diet and blood pressure. *Lancet* II: 742-743, 1983.

30. Kesteloot, H., and Goboers, J. Calcium and blood pressure. *Lancet*, 1:813–815, 1982.

31. Medeiros, D. and Brown, B. Blood pressure in young adults as influenced by copper and zinc intake. *Biological Trace Element Research*, 5: 165–174, 1983.

32. Lang, T., Bureau, J., Degoulet, P., et al. Blood pressure, coffee, tea, and tobacco consumption—an epidemiological study in Algiers. *Eur. Heart. J.*, 4: 602–607, 1983.

33. Affarah, H., Hall, W., Wells, J., et al. Effect of dietary carbohydrate on serum-insulin, urinary sodium-excretion, plasma-aldosterone and blood-pressure in normotensive males. *Clin. Res*, 31: A842, 1983.

34. Paul, O. *Op. cit.*

35. Freidman, G., Klatsky, A., and Siegelaub, A. Alcohol tobacco, and hypertension. *Hypertension*, Sept.–Oct. 4 III:143-150, 1982.

36. Brewster, L. and Jacobson, M. *The Changing American Diet: A Chronicle of American Eating Habits from 1910 to 1980*. Washington, D.C.: Center for Science in the Public Interest, 1983.

37. Gordon, R. and Verter, J. *The Framingham Study: An epidemiological investigation of cardiovascular disease*. Section 23. Serum cholesterol systolic blood pressure and Framingham relative weight as discriminators of cardiovascular disease. Bethesda, Md.: Natl. Inst. of Health, 1969.

38. Scott, R. et al. Animal models in atherosclerosis, in *The Pathogenesis of Atherosclerosis*, ed. R.W. Wissler and J. C. Geer. Baltimore: Williams and Wilkins, 1972.

39. Blackburn, H. The public view of diet and mass hyperlipidemia. *Card. Rev. and Rep.*, 1(5): 361–369, 1980.

40. Wissler, R. Conference on the health effects of blood lipids: Optimal distributions for populations. Workshop Report: Laboratory Experimental Section. American Health Foundation. *Prev. Med.*, 8: 715–732, 1979.

41. Report of the AHA Nutrition Committee. Rationale of the diet-heart statement of the American Heart Association. *Arteriosclerosis*, 4: 177–191, 1982.

42. Pooling Project Research Group. Relationship of blood pressure, serum cholesterol, smoking habit, relative weight and ECG abnormalities to incidence of major coronary events: Final report of the Pooling Project. *J. Chronic Dis.*, 31: 201, 1978.

43. Keys, A. *Seven Counties—Death and Coronary Heart Disease in 10 Years*. Cambridge, Mass.: Harvard University, 1970.

44. Leren, P. The effect of plasma cholesterol-lowering diet in male survivors of myocardial infarction. A controlled clinical trial. *Acta Med. Scand.*, 466(Supp.):1–92, 1966.

45. Stamler, J. Lifestyles, major risk factors, proof and public policy. *Circulation*, 58: 3-19, 1978.

46. Zannis, E., Third, J., Blum, A., et al. Response of Type III hyperlipoproteinemia (HLP) patients to a cholesterol-free polyunsaturated fat diet. *Arteriosclerosis*, 3: A488, 1983.

47. Hegsted, D., McGandy, R., Myers, M., et al. Quantitative effects of dietary fat on serum cholesterol in man. *Am. J. Clin. Nutr.*, 17: 281, 1965.

48. Shekell, R., Shryrock, A., Leppar, M., et al. Diet, serum cholesterol, and death from coronary heart disease. The Western Electric Study. *N. Engl. J. Med.*, 304: 65, 1981.

49. Taylor, C., Allen, E., Mikkelson, B., et al. Serum cholesterol levels of Seventh-Day Adventists.'' *Paroi Arterielle*, 3: 175, 1976.

50. Walden, R., Schaefer, L., Lemon, F., et al. E. Effect of environment on the serum cholesterol-triglyceride distribution among Seventh-Day Adventists. *Am. J. Med.*, 36: 269, 1964.

51. Lipid Research Clinics Program, The Lipid Research Clinics Coronary Primary Prevention Trial results: The relationship of reduction in incidence of coronary heart disease to cholesterol lowering. *JAMA*, 251: 365–373, 1984.

52. Taylor, C., Peng, S., and Werthessen, N. Spontaneously occuring angiotoxic derivatives of cholesterol. *Am. J. Clin. Nutr.*, 32: 1051–1057, 1979.

53. Smith, L. Mathews, W., Price, J., et al. Thin-layer chromatographic examination of cholesterol autooxidation. *J. Chromaton.*, 27: 187, 1967.

54. Pollack, O. Serum cholesterol levels resulting from various egg diets: Experimental studies with clinical implications. *J. Am. Ger. Soc.*, 6: 614, 1958.

55. WARF Institute, Inc. Nutritional analysis of food served at McDonald's restaurants. Madison, Wis.: McDonalds Systems, Inc. 1977.

56. Taylor, C., Peng, S. and N. Werthessen. Spontaneously occurring angiotoxin derivatives of cholesterol. *Am. J. Clin. Nutr.*, 32: 1051–1057, 1979.

57. Kavanagh, T., et al. Influences of exercise and lifestyle variables upon high density lipoprotein cholesterol after myocardial infarction. *Arteriosclerosis*, 3: 249–259, 1983.

58. Henriksen, T., Evensen, S. and Carlander, B. Injury of endothelial cells in culture induced by low density lipoproteins. *Europe. J. Clin. Invest.*, 7:243, 1977.

59. Lees, R. and Lees, M. High-density lipoproteins and the risk of atherosclerosis. *New. Eng. J. Med.*, 306: 1546–1547, 1982.

60. Hjermann, I., Enger, S. and Helgeland, A. The effect of dietary changes on high density lipoprotein cholesterol. *Am. J. Med.*, 66: 105–109, 1979.

61. Connor, W., Cerqueira, M., Connor, R., et al. The plasma lipids, lipoproteins, and the diet of the Tarahumara Indians of Mexico. *Am. J. Clin. Nutr.*, 31:1131, 1978.

62. Goldstein, J., Albers, J., Schrott, H., et al. Plasma lipid levels and coronary heart disease in adult relatives of newborns with normal and elevated cord blood lipids. *Am. J. Hum. Genet*, 26: 727, 1974.

63. Goldstein, J., Schrott, H., Hazard, W., et al. Hyperlipidemia in coronary heart disease. II: Genetic analysis of lipid levels in 176 families and delineation of a new inherited disorder, combined hyperlipidemia. *J. Clin. Invest.*, 52: 1544, 1973.

64. Greten, H., Wagner, M. and Schettler, G. Early diagnosis and incidence of familial type II hyperlipoproteinemia. Analysis of umbilical cord blood from 1323 newborns. *Dtsch. Med. Wochenschr.*, 99: 2553, 1974.

Additional Reading

Anitschkow, N. Uber organveranderungen, bei ablagerung von anistoropen lipoiden. *Ber. Ges. Russ. Arzte Petersburg*, 80: 1, 1912.

Frohlich, E. Physiological observations in essential hypertension. *J. Am. Dietetic. Assoc.*, 80: 18–20, 1982.

Keys, A., Anderson, J., and Grande, F. Serum cholesterol response to changes in the diet. II: The effect of cholesterol in the diet. *Metabolism*, 14: 759, 1965.

National Diet-Heart Study Final Report. *Circulation*, 37: 1 (Supp. 1), 1968.

Shorey, R., Sewell, B., and O'Brien, M. Efficacy of diet and exercise in the reduction of serum cholesterol and triglyceride in free-living adult males. *Am. J. Clin. Nutr.*, 29: 512–520, 1976.

Thompson, R., Lazarus, B., Cullinane, E., et al. Exercise, diet, or physical characteristics as determinants of HDL levels in endurance athletes. *Atherosclerosis*, 46: 333–339, 1983.

13

················FAT, FIBER AND THE················
CARDIOVASCULAR CONNECTION

FAT AND CVD

TOTAL fat in the diet has been correlated with elevated cholesterol,[1] and even moderate lowering of dietary fat reduces serum cholesterol by 10 percent, with a subsequent reduction of 20 percent in CVD risk.[2-3] A recent study divided twenty-four patients with femoral atherosclerosis into a control group and a lipid-lowering group. The results showed a 60 percent reduction in atherosclerosis progression in those consuming the low-fat diet. The lipid-lowering treatment group showed twice as many cases of improvement as the control group. This study confirmed the effectiveness of a low-fat diet on reducing and perhaps reversing atherosclerosis.[4]

Even in vegetarian populations, a higher fat diet promotes elevated serum lipid levels. Mean fasting plasma total cholesterol, LDL-cholesterol and total triglycerides were 6 percent, 7 percent, and 19 percent lower in vegetarian males than in a non-vegetarian matched control group. This is to be expected, since vegetarian diets are high in fiber, polyunsaturated fats and essential fatty acids. No correlation was found, however, between the subjects' widely varying egg (and therefore cholesterol) consumption and plasma lipid levels. The amount of total dietary fat did affect serum cholesterol levels. Total mean serum cholesterol was 11 percent lower and serum triglycerides were 21 percent lower in the low-fat vegetarian group, which consumed 23 percent to 33 percent of its total calories from fat, when compared to the high-fat vegetarian group, which consumed a diet of 35 percent to 48 percent calories from fat. HDL-cholesterol was 14 percent higher in the low-fat vegetarian group.[5]

POLYUNSATURATED FATS

Fat-modified diets can lower serum cholesterol 30 percent or more depending on the amount and type of fat.[6] In addition to reducing the total number of calories derived from fat, the ratio of polyunsaturated to saturated fat must be increased. Reducing dietary cholesterol or increasing the polyunsaturated-saturated fat ratio lowers serum cholesterol.[7,8] In one study, polyunsaturated fats lowered serum cholesterol and reduced the incidence of myocardial infarction and sudden death by 47 percent.[9]

One cholesterol-lowering action of PUFA is a result of their strong antilipogenic ability. They lower liver lipoprotein synthesis and increase lipoprotein catabolism (breakdown) and removal.[10] A second cholesterol-lowering function of PUFA is a result of their essential fatty acid content (see p. 30). The essential fatty acid, linoleic acid, cannot be manufactured in the body and must be supplied through the diet. An essential fatty acid deficiency relative to the saturated fatty acid intake is associated with CVD.[10] Increased intake of safflower oil (high in linoleic acid), increases platelet linoleic acid, decreases platelet aggregation and decreases serum cholesterol. Some dietary lipids, particularly essential fatty acids, influence prostaglandin synthesis which in turn reduces blood platelet aggregation and thrombosis (see p. 151). Essential fatty acids may also influence other activities of prostaglandins, including smooth muscle contraction, renal functions and numerous cardiopulmonary functions.

As precursors to the prostaglandins, dietary essential fatty acids have the potential to affect the type and amount of prostaglandin synthesis. Dietary linoleic acid is converted to arachidonic acid, a precursor of prostaglandins. Arachidonic acid in the cardiovascular system is included in platelet membrane phospholipids where, in the presence of the enzyme thromboxane synthetase, it is converted to endoperoxide intermediates and the platelet aggregator thromboxane (TXA-2). In the arterial intima, thromboxane synthetase levels are low. Here arachidonic acid is acted upon by the enzyme protacyclin synthetase and is converted to prostacyclin (PGI-2), a platelet aggregation inhibitor. These two prostaglandins may maintain the delicate balance between abnormal blood clotting and prolonged bleeding time.

Dietary polyunsaturated fats have been associated with reduced platelet aggregation.[11] When subjects were fed 23 grams/day of high linoleic and oleic acid safflower oils for four weeks, platelet aggregation was reduced, as were blood pressure, platelet thromboxane release and the LDL/HDL ratio.[12] Thus, dietary linoleic acid, by influencing tissue concentrations of arachidonic acid and therefore TXA-2 and PGI-2, is of greatest interest in the manipulation of prostaglandin synthesis. Dietary linoleic acid does increase tissue arachidonic acid, although this elevation may vary from tissue to tissue. The amount of this essential fatty acid necessary to maintain prostaglandin synthesis is unknown.[13]

Essential fatty acids may also affect intravascular coagulation and myocardial metabolism. In studies where diets were enriched with linoleic or arachidonic acids, serum cholesterol was reduced 10 to 15 percent, incidence of CVD declined, and if heart attacks occurred, fewer deaths resulted.[10] The typical American diet contains high amounts of saturated fats, lesser amounts of polyunsaturated fats, and low vitamin E. The essential fatty acid needs may not be met by such a diet.

Despite the beneficial effects of polyunsaturated fats on the development and treatment of CVD, increased PUFA intakes have been correlated with increased risk of cancer (see p. 133). Although PUFA are not carcinogenic, they supply the essential fatty acid needs of rapidly growing cancer cells. It is the ratio of these fats to saturated fats that is important, not an increased intake of PUFA. To reduce the risk of heart disease without increasing the risk of cancer, saturated fat intake should be reduced and PUFA intake should be held constant or raised slightly. The goal is to reduce dietary fat in general with an emphasis on reducing saturated fats. (See p. 196.)

THE OMEGA-3 FATTY ACIDS

Eicosapentaenoic acid is a polyunsaturated fatty acid that belongs to the omega-3 fatty acid series. The omega-3 fatty acid series is derived from alpha-linolenic acid. Eicosapentaenoic acid might be a factor in reducing platelet aggregation and thrombosis.

The fatty acid omega-3-eicosapentaenoic acid (EPA) is found in cold-water fish and is believed to explain the low levels of serum cholesterol and high levels of HDL-cholesterol in Greenland Eskimos and fish-eating inhabitants of a village in Japan.[14-15] Eskimos have prolonged bleeding times, reduced serum triglycerides and total cholesterol and an increased ratio of HDL-cholesterol to total cholesterol when compared to groups consuming less of the omega-3 fatty acid.[16] These symptoms are associated with reduced thrombosis and impaired atherosclerotic progression. Given in supplementary form as MaxEPA (containing EPA and another omega-3 fatty acid, DHA), this oil has produced changes in blood platelets that are associated with a reduced risk of heart disease.[17-18] EPA inhibits the formation of the prostaglandin thromboxane A-2, a vasoconstrictor that enhances the aggregation of platelets. This omega-3 fatty acid also inhibits prostaglandin production in platelets and arteries and thus reduces platelet reactivity (see p. 150). Omega-3 fatty acid is the fatty acid required for the production of prostaglandin E-3 or PGE-3.[19] The PGE-3 series of prostaglandins has been found to affect the HDL and LDL-cholesterol ratio by lowering the latter. PGE-3 also reduces the blood's tendency to clot.[20-21]

Diets containing mackerel, salmon and sardines have been shown to lower the risk of atherosclerosis. Dietary patterns in the United States show a reduction in seafood intake over the years and thus a reduction in the omega-3 fatty acids.[22] At the same time, the American diet contains increased amounts of animal and hydrogenated fats and therefore, not surprisingly, the incidence of cardiovascular disease has increased. It appears that EPA is not efficiently manufactured by the body and must be obtained from the diet. Clinical studies have demonstrated that consumption of EPA supplements or fatty fish was paramount to the diet if sufficient amounts of EPA were to enter the body and perform its role as producer of PGE-3.[23]

EPA is not found in appreciable amounts in foods

other than fish. Therefore, until other foods containing significant amounts of the omega-3 fatty acid are identified, there will be restricted availability of naturally occurring EPA in the food supply. To reverse the shift away from the current Western food consumption pattern to a diet providing adequate amounts of EPA, individuals may need to include more fish or an EPA supplement in their diets.

A word of caution regarding EPA supplementation. Some evidence does imply that supplementation may cause adverse effects, including thrombocytopenia and hepatotoxicity.

MONOUNSATURATED FATS

In the Mediterranean countries, where olive oil, a vegetable oil high in monounsaturated fatty acids, is a daily addition to the diet, coronary artery disease is low in comparison to the American diet, which derives 16 percent of its calories from saturated fats. Fred Mattson, Ph.D., director of the Lipid Research Clinic at the University of California, San Diego, reported at the American Heart Association's fifty-sixth scientific session that monounsaturated fat and olive oil are effective in lowering serum cholesterol and LDL-cholesterol while maintaining HDL-cholesterol levels. Polyunsaturated fats were more effective in lowering total cholesterol but this may be due to a greater depression of HDL-cholesterol, an undesired side effect. Polyunsaturated fats have also been shown to cause cancer in laboratory animals, whereas monounsaturated fats have not.

SATURATED FATS

In a recent review of epidemiologic studies on cardiovascular disease, it was concluded that a positive association exists between dietary fat and ischemic heart disease and that, for the prevention of cardiovascular disease (CVD), dietary fat and cholesterol should be restricted.[24] As much as 80 percent of the serum cholesterol variability can be explained by the level of saturated fat in the diet.[25] Teaspoon for teaspoon, saturated fats are twice as effective in raising serum cholesterol as polyunsaturated fats are in lowering it.[8]

Saturated fat is the predominant fat in most animal foods. These foods are also the only source of cholesterol. The role of saturated fat in elevating serum cholesterol goes beyond its association with cholesterol in the diet. Its intake stimulates cholesterol biosynthesis in the liver and increases bile production,

the only means of cholesterol elimination. Saturated fats alter homeostasis of lipoprotein metabolism, which results in elevation of LDL-cholesterol and improper accumulation and clearance of cholesterol and its esters from arterial walls.[10]

HYDROGENATED VEGETABLE OILS

Animal fats have taken the blame for their high saturated fat and low polyunsaturated fat contribution to the diet, but hydrogenated vegetable fats (see p. 30), supply less PUFA than meats and dairy products. Americans consume 600 million pounds of these frying fats each year, more than all the corn oil manufactured in the 50 states. Although vegetable fat consumption has increased from 24.0 to 43.1 pounds per person per year between 1950 and 1975, two-thirds of that fat was hydrogenated to make margarines and shortening.[26] These fats contain more saturated fats than butter, whole milk and meat, and few—if any—vitamins and minerals.

Unsaturated fatty acids contain one or more double bonds in the cis configuration. When unsaturated vegetable oils are hydrogenated, various amounts of the cis form are converted to a more stable trans configuration. The amount of this trans form varies between 8 percent and 70 percent depending on the brand.[29] The majority of dietary trans fatty acid intake comes from hydrogenated oils, and with the increases in consumption of these processed fats, their intake escalates as well. Dietary need for essential fatty acids such as linoleic acid increases with increased consumption of trans fatty acids; however, hydrogenated fats contain little linoleic acid.[27] Trans fatty acids also reduce prostaglandin production and interfere with the conversion of linoleic acid to arachidonic acid in the formation of prostaglandins (see p. 33).[28] Trans fatty acids have been found to elevate serum cholesterol and liver glycerides in rabbits.[28]

Trans fatty acids are absorbed, but do not appear to be used as readily in cellular energy metabolism. When they are used they appear to act more like saturated than unsaturated fats. In addition, metabolism of these abnormal fatty acids may impair cellular function and their presence in heart and smooth muscle may be a factor in the development of CVD.[30] Normal mitochondria in heart muscle contain a high concentration of polyunsaturated fatty acids; however, since mitochondria fatty acid composition appears to mirror dietary intake,[28] a diet high in trans fatty acids may alter this lipid composition. In one study, rats fed hydrogenated fats had heart mitochondria which oxidized fatty acids at a slower rate than rats fed corn oil, high in PUFA.[31] The corn oil-fed rats' mitochondria were more efficient in oxygen uptake and energy (ATP) synthesis than the mitochondria from the hydrogenated fat-fed rats. Since mitochondria are the cellular components responsible for energy production, their impairment could have far-reaching effects on heart function.

THE PHOSPHOLIPIDS

Lecithin is a generic term for a phospholipid. It is composed of glycerol, two fatty acids and a phosphatidic acid. The major phosphatides in lecithin are phosphatydlcholine (PC) and phosphatylethanolamine (PE).

The phosphatidylcholine (PC) in lecithin may be useful in reducing serum cholesterol. Clinical studies have shown that lecithin can reduce serum lipid levels and thus favorably affect the risk of CVD.[32] PE is more effective at lowering serum cholesterol and increasing bile acid excretion than PC, which implies a varying potency for lecithin, depending on its composition.[33] In one study, no decrease in serum lipoproteins and liver lipids was found when rats were fed only soybean phosphatidylcholine. But when they were fed egg yolks which contain phosphatidylethanolamine and phosphatidylcholine, serum cholesterol and apoprotein A-I declined and serum apoprotein B and liver cholesterol increased.[34] All phospholipids increase fecal excretion of neutral sterols and therefore help to reduce the entry of dietary cholesterol and the reentry of endogenous cholesterol into the body. The ability of phosphatidylcholine to emulsify cholesterol may make the fat more soluble and less likely to form gallstones.[35]

FIBER AND CVD

Dietary fiber can be defined as nondigestible plant materials that are cellulosic and free of calories (see p. 16). In groups in which fiber constitutes a major portion of the diet, diseases such as constipation, diarrhea, hemorrhoids. gallstones, hiatus hernia, varicose veins, appendicitis and heart disease are unknown. The well-known ability of fiber to normalize bowel activity, reduce transit time of food through the intestines, influence the intestinal microbial flora, and possibly reduce the formation of intestinal carcinogens,

has made it a prime protector against cancer of the bowel and other intestinal disorders. Some types of fiber, wheat bran excluded, have been implicated in lowering blood cholesterol, and people consuming a high-fiber diet have a relatively low mortality rate from heart disease.[36]

Pectin, a form of dietary fiber found in apples and other fruits, selectively lowers LDL-cholesterol,[37] lowers serum cholesterol levels and aortic cholesterol levels in humans, and reduces cholesterol synthesis in ilial and jejunal cells of the small intestine in hamsters.[38–39]

The fiber in oats also affects serum cholesterol. When men were fed either a control or an oat-fiber diet (100 grams of oat fiber), serum cholesterol levels remained stable on the control diet but declined 13 percent on the test diet. Plasma LDL-cholesterol declined 14 percent and fecal excretion of bile acids increased 54 percent in the oat-fiber test group.[40] Another study reported a 21 percent reduction in serum cholesterol following the addition of oat bran to the diet.[41]

Several of the dietary gums are classified as fibers and have a cholesterol-lowering effect. Guar gum and konjac mannan fed to chicks reduces plasma and hepatic cholesterol while elevating hepatic triglycerides. Pectin and guar gum suppress the synthesis of liver fat. Locust bean gum lowers cholesterol and LDL-cholesterol while increasing the HDL/LDL ratio.[42]

The cholesterol-lowering effect of beans may be due to their saponin content. Saponins are steroids or triterpene glycosides found in soybeans, chickpeas and peanuts. When saponins are ingested in isolated or food-borne forms, they form large mixed micelles with bile salts and significantly reduce serum cholesterol by increasing fecal excretion of bile salts, thus inhibiting cholesterol reabsorption. Saponins have been reported to reduce cholesterol significantly without altering the level of HDL.[43] It is proposed that their mode of action includes increasing fecal excretion of endogenous and exogenous neutral steroids and bile acids.

Alfalfa contains a high number of saponins and has been shown to reduce elevated serum lipids. Monkeys were fed a diet containing 1.2 g of cholesterol for six months, at which time eighteen were investigated for atherosclerosis. The remaining monkeys were divided into three groups of eighteen monkeys each and fed semipurified diets containing 0.34 g of cholesterol with or without alfalfa meal. With the addition of alfalfa, cholesterolemia and plasma phospholipid levels declined, plasma lipoprotein levels normalized and aortic and coronary atherosclerosis regressed. Saponins were found to bind with cholesterol in the intestines and facilitate its removal via the feces.[44] Studies on primates indicate that an alfalfa-enriched diet not only reduced blood cholesterol levels but also reversed atherosclerotic plaque.

Although some fiber in the diet is beneficial for prevention and treatment of cardiovascular disease, excessive fiber intake can bind trace minerals and interfere with their absorption. Excessive fiber intake also can irritate intestinal lining. A diet containing about 37 grams of dietary fiber daily provides the protective effect without contributing to malnutrition or intestinal disorders (see p. 190).

REFERENCES

1. Ershow, A., Nocolosi, R., and Hayes, K. Separation of the dietary fat and cholesterol influences on plasma lipoproteins of rhesus monkeys. *Am. J. Clin. Nutr.*, 34: 830–840, 1981.

2. Connor, W. and Connor S. The dietary treatment of hyperlipidemia. *Med. Clin. North. Am.*, 66: 485–518, 1982.

3. Miettinen, M., Turpeinen, O., Karvonen, M, et al. Effects of cholesterol-lowering diet on mortality from CHD and other causes: A 12-year trial in men and women. *Lancet*, 2:835, 1972.

4. Duffield, R. Treatment of hyperlipidemia retards progression of symptomatic femoral atherosclerosis. *Lancet*, II:639–641, 1983.

5. Liebman, M. and Bazzarre, T. Plasma lipids of vegetarian and non-vegetarian males: Effects of egg consumption. *Am. J. Clin. Nutr.*, 38: 612–619, 1983.

6. Anderson, J., Grande, F., and Keys, A. Cholesterol-lowering diets. *JAMA*, 62: 133–142, 1973.

7. Anderson, J., Grande, F., and Keys, A. Independence of the effects of cholesterol and degree of saturation of the fat in the diet on serum cholesterol in man. *Am. J. Clin. Nutr.*, 29: 1184–1189, 1976.

8. Keys, A., Anderson, J., and Grande, F. Serum cholesterol response to changes in the diet. IV. Particular saturated fatty acids in the diet. *Metabolism*, 14: 776, 1965.

9. Hjermann, I., Velve Bure, K., Holme, I., et al. Effect of diet and smoking intervention on the incidence of coronary heart disease. *Lancet*, II: 1303-1309, 1981.

10. Oliver, M. Diet and coronary heart disease. *Hum. Nutr. Clin. Nutr.*, 36: 413–427, 1982.

11. Bazan, N., Paoletti, R., and Iacono, J. (eds) *New Trends in Nutrition, Lipid Research, and Cardiovascular Disease.* New York: Alan R. Liss, Inc., 1981.

12. Sacks, F., Stampfer, M., Schafer, A., et al. Dietary unsaturated fats affect blood pressure, platelet thromboxane production, and HDL subfractions in normal subjects. *Arterioscl. Council Abstracts*, 3: 483A–484A, 1983.

13. Galli, C. Dietary influences on prostaglandin synthesis. *Advances in Nutritional Research*, vol. 3, H.H. Draper, ed. New York: Plenum Press, 1980, pp. 95–126.

14. Fish oil for prevention of atherosclerosis. *The Medical Letter*, 24: 622: 99–100, 1982.

15. Connor, W. *Medical World News*, January, 1982.

16. Bang, H. and Dyerberg, J. Lipid metabolism and ischaemic heart disease in Greenland Eskimos, in *Advances in Nutritional Research*, H.H. Draper, ed. New York: Plenum Press, 1980, pp. 1–22.

17. Fish oil for prevention of atherosclerosis. *The Medical Letter*, 24: 622: 99–100, 1982.

18. *Ibid.*

19. Bennet, A. Recent advances in clinical pharmacology. *Prostaglandins*, 1978, 17–30.

20. Von Lossonczy, T., Ruiter, A., et al. Effect of a fish diet on serum lipids in healthy human subjects. *Am. J. Clin. Nutr.*, 31: 1340–1346, 1978.

21. Siess, W., Roth, P. et al. Platelet membrane fatty acids, platelet aggregation and thromboxane formation during mackerel diet. *Lancet I*, 441-443, 1980.

22. Korsan-Bengsten, K., et al. Thrombosis diathesis. *Haemorrh.*, 1972.

23. Williams, R., Bailey, A., and Robinson, D. High-density lipoprotein and coronary risk factors in normal men. *Lancet*, 1: 72–75, 1979.

24. Sidney, S. and Farquhar, J. Cholesterol, cancer, and public health policy. *J. Med.*, 75: 494–508, 1983.

25. Keys, A. *Seven Counties—Death and Coronary Heart Disease in 10 Years.* Cambridge, Mass.: Harvard University Press, 1970.

26. Brewster, L. and Jacobson, M. *The Changing American Diet: A Chronicle of American Eating Habits from 1910–1980*, Washington, D.C.: Center for Science in the Public Interest, 1983.

27. Beare-Rogers, J., Gray, L., and Hollywood, R. The linoleic acid and trans fatty acids of margarines. *Am. J. Clin. Nutr.*, 32: 1805–1809, 1979.

28. Ruttenberg, H., Davidson, L., Little, N., et al. Influence of trans unsaturated fats on experimental atherosclerosis in rabbits. *J. Nutr.*, 113: 835–844, 1983.

29. Beare-Rogers, J., Gray, L. and Hollywood, R. *Op. cit.*

30. McGill, H., Geer, J., and Strong, J. The natural history of atherosclerosis, in *Metabolism of Lipids as Related to Atherosclerosis*, F. A. Kummerow, ed. Springfield, Ill.: Charles C. Thomas, 1965, 36.

31. Hsu, C. and Kummerow, F. Influence of elaidate and erucate on heart mitochondria. *Lipids*, 12: 486, 1977.

32. Vroulis, G., Smith, R., Schoolar, J., et al. Reduction of cholesterol risk factors by lecithin in patients with Alzheimer's disease. *Am. J. Psychiatry*, 139: 1633–1634, 1982.

33. Imdizumi, K. The contrasting effect of dietary phosphatidylethanolamine and phosphatidylcholine on serum lipoproteins and liver lipids in rats. *J. Nutr.*, 113: 2403–2411, 1983.

34. Murata, M., Imaizum, K. and Sugano, M. Effect of dietary phospholipids and their constituent bases on serum lipids and apolipoproteins in rats. *J. Nutr.*, 112: 1805–1808, 1982.

35. ter Well, H., van Gent, C. and Dekker, W. The effect of soya lecithin on serum lipid values in Type II hyperlipoproteinemia. *Acta. Med. Scan.*, 195: 267–271, 1974.

36. Albrink, M., Davidson, P., and Newman, T. Lipid-lowering effect of a very high carbohydrate, high fiber diet. *Diabetes*, 25: 324, 1976.

37. Baig, M. and Cerda, J. Pectin: Its interaction with serum proteins. *Am. J. Clin. Nutr.*, 34: 50–53, 1981.

38. Schwartz, S., Starr, C., Bachman, S., et al. Dietary fiber decreases cholesterol and phospholipid synthesis in rat intestine. *J. Lipid. Res.*, 24: 746–752, 1983.

39. Sable-Amplis, R., Sicart, R., and Buthe, E. Decreased cholesterol ester levels in tissues of hamsters fed with apple fiber enriched diet. *Nutr. Rep. In.* 27: 881–889, 1983.

40. Kirby, R., Anderson, J., and Sieling, B. Oat-bran intake selectively lowers serum low-density lipoprotein cholesterol concentrations of hypercholesterolemic men. *Am. J. Clin. Nutr.*, 34: 824–829, 1981.

41. Anderson, J., Chen, W., Story, L., and Sieling, B. Hypocholesterolemic effects of soluble fiber-rich foods for hypercholesterolemic men. *Am. J. Clin. Nutr.*, 37: 699, 1983.

42. Zavoral, J., Hannan, P., Fields, D., et al. The hypolipidemic effect of locust bean gum food products in familial hypercholesterolemic adults and children. *Am. J. Clin. Nutr.*, 38: 285–294, 1983.

43. Malinow, M., Connor, W., McLaughlin, P., et al. Cholesterol and bile balance in Macaca fascicularis. *J. Clin. Invest.*, 67: 156–162, 1981.

44. Malinow, M., McLaughlin, P., Naito, H., et al. Effect of alfalfa meal on shrinkage (regression) of atherosclerotic plaques during cholesterol feeding in monkeys. *Atherosclerosis*, 30: 27–43, 1978.

Additional Reading

Connor, W., Cerqueira, M., Connor, R., et al. The plasma lipids, lipoproteins, and the diet of the Tarahumara Indians of Mexico. *Am. J. Clin. Nutr.*, 31: 1131, 1978.

Hutchinson, K., Oberle, K., Crockford, P., et al. Effects of dietary manipulation on vascular status of patients with peripheral vascular disease. *JAMA*, 249: 3326–3330, 1983.

Stamler, J. Prima vegetarian and non-vegetarian males: Effects of egg consumption. *Am. J. Clin. Nutr.*, 38(4): 612–619, 1983.

14

················VITAMINS AND MINERALS: THEIR ················
RELATIONSHIP TO CARDIOVASCULAR DISEASE

THE HEART DISEASE ISSUE is complex, and focusing on one food factor may be a simplified approach to the prevention and treatment of this disease. It is now recognized that the types and amounts of several nutrients, including protein, fiber, carbohydrates, vitamins, and minerals, are important components of the CVD puzzle. Approximately 70 percent to 80 percent of blood cholesterol is manufactured by the liver and intestines. The building materials of cholesterol are protein, fat and carbohydrates. This biosynthesis and the body's mechanisms for excretion can be influenced by such dietary components as amino acids, the vitamins, inositol and general nutritional status.

PROTEIN

Protein and its building blocks, amino acids, may reduce or elevate serum cholesterol levels. Vegetable-based protein products reduce serum cholesterol levels[1-4] regardless of egg consumption.[5] Soybeans are relatively high in arginine and low in lysine, a combination that apparently lowers cholesterol. Other studies have reported that lysine and arginine are the two key amino acids that appear to influence the body's production of cholesterol.[6] Supplementation with lysine, however, may be a double-edged sword. Whereas studies are researching the possible effect lysine may have on the prognosis and incidence of herpes, cholesterol levels are increased when supplemental lysine is added to the diet, suggesting that lysine may stimulate cholesterol biosynthesis.[7]

VITAMINS

THE B VITAMINS

The B vitamins play a role in lipid metabolism. Pantothenic acid, vitamin B2 and niacin are converted to coenzymes involved in fatty acid synthesis and oxidation reactions. Niacin has been shown to lower cholesterol in hypercholesterolemic subjects,[8] and nicotinic acid and its derivatives increase HDL-cholesterol while reducing LDL-cholesterol, thus positively affecting the LDL/HDL ratio and reducing the risk of cardiovascular disease.[9] When colestipol, a cholesterol-lowering drug, is administered in conjunction with niacin to subjects with hypercholesterolemia, a significant reduction in LDL-cholesterol and elevation of HDL-cholesterol also is seen.[10]

Inadequate intakes of vitamin B6 may contribute to atherosclerotic lesions and place people at a greater risk of CVD.[11] Vitamin B6 deficiency results in an elevation of homocysteine similar to that seen in homocystenuric individuals prone to atherosclerosis. In one study, pigs were placed on a vitamin B6-deficient diet and the aorta and major organs were checked twelve weeks later by light microscopy. Spots of intimal degeneration and thickening were observed in renal arteries, resembling the initial stage of atherosclerosis.[12]

In the American diet, substantial amounts of vitamin B6 are lost in processing of grains and other foods, and this vitamin is not one of the four nutrients added back when refined foods are "enriched." In addition, since vitamin B6 needs depend on protein intake, the typical American diet, high in protein, could aggravate an already borderline deficiency and thus contribute to the development of CVD.

VITAMIN C

A mere ten milligrams a day, the amount of vitamin C found in 3½ tablespoons of orange juice or one banana, is adequate to prevent the bleeding gums and loose teeth characteristic of scurvy. Meeting the body's needs for this vitamin seems simple, and if only the overt deficiency signs are considered, then neglecting the fruit and vegetable section at the grocery store may be condoned. A lack of produce in the daily diet, however, may contribute to heart disease and hypertension.

The fragility of brain capillaries, arterioles and arteries in hypertension may be associated with a low vitamin C intake above the level necessary to eliminate scurvy. In one study, a low intake of fruits and vegetables was correlated with an increased incidence of CVD.[13] If the vitamin C content of fruits and vegetables is the determining factor, the effect may be due to the role of vitamin C in the synthesis of collagen, the ground substance of blood vessel walls responsible for strengthening and supporting the tissue.

Vitamin C deficiency may cause petechial hemorrhages (as are seen under the skin in scurvy) beneath the endothelium of the blood vessels, which could result in thrombosis on the damaged wall.[14] Vitamin C was administered in 500-mg doses to preoperative surgical patients to test the theory that the vitamin would reduce postoperative deep venous thrombosis (DVT). Although no difference was found in the incidence of DVT during or after surgery, on the sixth and ninth postoperative days leucocyte ascorbic acid was significantly lower in those with DVT versus those without it.[15] Researchers at the University of Kentucky have also found that leukocyte ascorbic acid levels are low in patients with coronary atherosclerosis,[16] suggesting an association between low vitamin C intake and the development of CVD.

Vitamin C plays a crucial role in cholesterol metabolism and serum cholesterol status. When vitamin C intake is inadequate, the body cannot effectively convert cholesterol to bile acids and with poor elimination of excess cholesterol, serum cholesterol remains high.[17] Studies have shown that 500 mg of supplemental vitamin C benefits patients who have elevated serum cholesterol levels, and a low vitamin C intake encourages maintenance of elevated serum levels.

Vitamin C not only affects the total cholesterol content of the blood but also positively influences lipoprotein ratios and triglyceride levels. A study of men and women with heart disease showed them to have elevated triglycerides and a reduced HDL-cholesterol/total cholesterol ratio. Vitamin C supplementation for six weeks resulted in increased HDL-cholesterol/total cholesterol, a reduction in total serum cholesterol, and, in men, a reduction in LDL-cholesterol.[18-19] The influence of vitamin C on lowering cholesterol and elevating HDL-cholesterol has been substantiated by some studies[20-21] and refuted by others.[22]

The lipoprotein-vitamin C connection is further affected by the vitamin's possible role in transporting cholesterol to the liver. When animals are fed a diet high in cholesterol, deposits of this fat are found in the aorta. If vitamin C is added to the diet, cholesterol is found in the liver and adrenals but not in aortic tissue.[23] In healthy persons, vitamin C is associated with a decline in serum cholesterol, whereas in persons with atherosclerosis, the levels rise.[24] If this rise is due to vitamin C mobilization of atherosclerotic cholesterol deposits, then the vitamin C-dependent mechanism for transportation of cholesterol may be verified. Aged persons with atherosclerosis, when treated with vitamin C, show marked improvement in symptomology in spite of insignificant changes in serum cholesterol.[25] Again, it would appear that arterial cholesterol was being mobilized, elevating cholesterol levels from arterial deposits but improving circulation. Other serum lipids are positively affected by vitamin C. Reductions in LDL-cholesterol[26] and increased lipoprotein lipase activity[25] have been reported.

An association also appears to exist between vitamin C and prostaglandin synthesis. Prostacyclin, a prostaglandin, dilates large coronary arteries and may encourage collateral circulation to ischemic areas of the heart. Prostacyclin is an antiaggregator and deaggregator of platelets, the cell fragments responsible for blood clotting and perhaps associated with the initiation and progression of atherosclerosis. If prostacyclin levels decline, cholesterol and another prostaglandin responsible for enhanced platelet aggregation, TXA-2, increase, platelet aggregation escalates, vasoconstriction occurs and smooth muscle proliferates, all symptoms of atherosclerosis. If prostacyclin is elevated the symptoms are reversed. Nutrients which encourage prostacyclin synthesis are vitamin C,[29] pyridoxine (vitamin B6), essential fatty acids (linoleic and arachidonic acids), zinc and possibly niacin.

Prostaglandin synthesis in rabbit cornea epithelial cells is highly responsive to vitamin C intake.[27] Vitamin C has been shown to cause significant increases in the conversion of 14C-dihomogamma-linolenic acid to prostaglandin E1, a vasodilator and antiaggregator similar to prostacyclin.[28]

Studies at the University of Birmingham in England demonstrated a direct correlation between vitamin C intake and reduced cardiovascular death rates. The findings showed that the higher the ascorbic acid intake, the lower the cardiovascular death rate.[30] The effectiveness of the vitamin may be the result of its various functions: maintaining capillary wall strength, reducing total cholesterol, improving cholesterol transportation, increasing the HDL-cholesterol/total cholesterol ratio, indirectly influencing blood coagulation and thrombosis, mobilizing arterial deposits of cholesterol and maintaining elevated vitamin C in leukocytes.

Vitamin C is found predominantly in fruits and vegetables. It is easily destroyed when these foods are exposed to air, stored for long periods, overcooked or reheated, or when cooking water and juices are discarded. Daily tensions and frustrations tend to deplete the small body stores, as do cigarette smoke,[31] the birth control pill,[32] and alcohol. In addition, increased consumption of fast foods may contribute to low intakes, since these menus feature foods high in fat, salt and sugar to the detriment of vitamin C-rich selections. Although the potato is a reasonable source of the vitamin, once it has been sliced, stored, fried in hot oil and held under warming lights, little, if any, of the original vitamin C remains. If potatoes are julienned, shredded, dehydrated, canned, frozen or turned into potato chips, the vitamin C has been cut by half, if not more.

Vitamin C intake can be increased by choosing fresh vegetables and fruits, refrigerating foods, cooking in a minimal amount of water and time, preparing enough food for one meal (reheating destroys more of the vitamin content), including several vitamin C-rich foods in the diet daily and taking vitamin C supplements. (See pp. 53–56.)

THE FAT-SOLUBLE VITAMINS: A, E AND D

The fat-soluble vitamins may both encourage and help prevent CVD. Vitamin A and E protect endothelium, function as antiperoxidants, are antiaggregants,

affect O_2 transport and utilization, increase HDL-cholesterol and enhance the hypolipidemic action of niacin. They may therefore play a protective role in CVD. Vitamin D in excess has been shown to promote atherosclerotic lesions in the aorta and coronary arteries, especially when fed in conjunction with cholesterol.[33–35]

The role of vitamin E in cardiovascular disease has been a topic of interest for over 40 years. Vitamin E has not been shown to reduce angina; however, the ingestion of three daily doses (100 mg each) has been shown to relieve intermittent claudication and lameness associated with peripheral occlusive heart disease.[36] In a sixteen-year study in Sweden, patients were reported to show improved arterial flow as a result of vitamin E administration. Half the group reported improvement in gait and endurance when walking.[37]

Since the 1940s, researchers have studied the possible importance of vitamin E in dissolving and preventing blood clots. In 1964, alpha tocopherol (vitamin E) was identified as a thrombin inhibitor which did not induce excessive bleeding. It was therefore recommended as a safe therapy against thrombosis.[38]

Vitamin E may also reduce platelet aggregation. Platelet aggregation was induced in a group of volunteers by collagen ADP and the hormone epinephrine. One group was given daily vitamin E doses of 400 IU to 1200 IU, a second group received 300 mg of aspirin and a third group was given a combination of vitamin E and aspirin. Weekly measurements showed aspirin to be ineffective in altering platelet adhesiveness. A significant reduction was seen in the vitamin E and the vitamin-E-plus-aspirin groups. The conclusion was drawn that vitamin E was a mild antiaggregatory agent when taken in doses up to 1200 IU, especially in women.[39–40]

This antiaggregatory function may not be due directly to vitamin E but rather to one of its derivatives. An oxidative product of tocopherol, vitamin E quinone, is a structural analog to vitamin K and may compete for the vitamin K-dependent enzyme in carboxylation reactions during blood coagulation. If vitamin E quinone is a vitamin K antagonist, it would inhibit the role of vitamin K as a cofactor for the enzyme carboxylase, which converts glutamyl residues to omega carboxyglutamyl residues found on coagulation proteins. This would interfere with the cascade of reactions in blood clotting. Another theory suggests that vitamin E quinone may function directly as an antiaggregatory agent.

Destruction of the body's cell membranes by metabolic byproducts such as superoxide, peroxides and free radicals may encourage arterial wall damage, thus initiating platelet aggregation and the beginnings of atherosclerosis. Vitamin E is a powerful antioxidant that can reduce the blood's burden of fat peroxides, and thus possibly prevent the deteriorating action of these highly reactive substances.[41–42]

This research suggests a possible advantage to vitamin E supplementation for the prevention of blood clotting and other complications of atherosclerosis. Questions still remain to be answered which evoke a word of caution on this practice. People with vitamin K deficiencies could worsen a poor blood-clotting mechanism by the ingestion of large amounts of vitamin E. Vitamin E supplementation in the presence of oxidants such as cigarette smoke and other pro-oxidant substances which would encourage the formation of vitamin E quinone, could explain the varied effects in platelet adhesion observed in different individuals.[43]

MINERALS

Studies in humans and animals have shown optimal intakes of minerals such as sodium, magnesium, chromium, zinc, calcium and iodine to be important in reducing the risk of CVD. The cholesterol-lowering effect of pectin may be due to its silicon content, although this has not been confirmed in some studies.[44] Inadequate dietary intake and foods grown on trace element-depleted soil can contribute to these deficiencies.[45]

CADMIUM

Cadmium may accelerate the development of cardiovascular disease. Geographical differences in CVD incidence have been correlated with environmental cadmium concentrations,[46] and cadmium concentrations similar to those consumed by the average American have been found to cause cardiovascular lesions and alterations in systolic blood pressure in rats.[47] Calcium protects against cadmium- and lead-induced aortic atherosclerosis and hypertension, whereas magnesium may accelerate their effects.[48]

CHROMIUM

Chromium intake has declined with the popularization of refined and processed foods. This decline could have implications for heart disease since sub-clinical chromium deficiency has been reported to elevate blood

cholesterol levels.[49] In a study of hypercholesterolemic elderly patients, chromium supplementation led to improvements in serum cholesterol.[50] In another study, a daily dose of 200 micrograms of chromium chloride reduced total cholesterol and increased HDL-cholesterol.[51] Patients consuming chromium-rich brewer's yeast for eight weeks showed a slight reduction in cholesterol and elevation in HDL-cholesterol. The amount of chromium consumed was far less than in the above-mentioned group supplemented with chromium chloride. The brewer's yeast used was specially produced; normal torula and other yeasts do not have sufficient amounts of chromium in the biologically active form (glucose tolerance factor [GTF]) to affect serum lipids substantially.

COPPER

Copper and cholesterol metabolism have been linked in animals and man because of certain similarities in copper deficient animals and ischemic heart disease patients. Low hepatic copper is associated with hypercholesterolemia. When male rats are given clofibrate, a drug used for this condition, a copper deficiency develops. This suggests that the drug's cholesterol-lowering effect lies in the alteration of copper metabolism.[52] How copper effects cholesterol synthesis and management is still not understood.

Copper deficiency may affect heart disease by altering tissue metabolism. Copper-induced deficiency in rats results in depressed Purkinje system conductivity and S and T segment depression in the heart. Significant metabolic changes are observed in cardiac, renal and hepatic tissue, including decreased ATP and phosphocreatine levels and increased inorganic orthophosphate and ADP levels. Microscopic examination of heart tissue shows severe abnormalities of mitochondrial fine structure, with fragmentation of the cristae and the inner and outer mitochondrial membranes.[53] These changes mirror myocardial changes in heart disease and suggest a link between CVD and copper deficiency.

MAGNESIUM

Magnesium is the second most abundant cation and is involved in over 300 enzymatic reactions, of which many are associated with normal cardiovascular function. Magnesium influences the configuration and stability of phospholipids, cell membranes and nucleic acids and is therefore important for the maintenance of myocardial function and structure. In addition, a deficiency can cause cardiac vulnerability to cardiotoxic agents.

Drugs such as diltiazem and nifedipine, which are calcium channel blockers, enhance collateral blood flow. Magnesium, a calcium antagonist, has been shown to do the same.[54] This mineral may therefore play a role in maintaining normal blood pressure and reducing irregular heartbeat. Magnesium also dilates large coronary arteries and encourages collateral circulation, further promoting normal blood pressure and protection from heart disease.

Magnesium is an anti-arrhythmic. This mineral participates in the regulation of the heart's electrical activity, and abnormalities of this function can lead to coronary vasospasms, the cause of spontaneous resting angina[55-56] and arrhythmia—often the ultimate cause of death from heart failure. A magnesium deficiency combined with digitalis poisoning encourages arrhythmias. Hypomagnesiaemia is common in digitalis poisoning and administration of the mineral has been used for arrhythemias characteristic of digitalis overdose.[57]

The potassium retention capabilities of magnesium may explain the way it functions in digitalis toxicity. If magnesium also retains potassium in hypoxic tissue, then it would play a role in maintenance of the heart's normal resting potential and in the reduction of cardiac arrhythmias. This has been suggested in several studies. Magnesium injections elevate the threshold for premature ventricular contractions and fibrillation in dog heart.[58] Successful defibrillation has been achieved with administration of magnesium to open heart surgery patients.[59] When dog heart is ligated, administration of the mineral reduces tachycardia (abnormally fast heart rate),[60] suggesting that pretreatment may have a possible protective effect from coronary occlusion. Large daily doses of the mineral in rats limit destruction of cardiac tissue resulting from coronary ligation,[61] and rats fed a magnesium-deficient diet show multiple necrosis of the cardiac muscle.[62]

Magnesium is significantly reduced in cardiac tissue following a myocardial infarction (heart attack).[63-66] The normal magnesium content of 200 mg/kg wet weight is reduced by as much as 50 percent in diseased tissue and between 12 percent and 33 percent in unaffected but coronary-prone tissue. It is not yet recognized whether magnesium deficiency precedes or is a result of the myocardial infarction.

Serum levels of magnesium are usually lower preceding and following a heart attack. Results are contradictory, however, perhaps as a result of differences in research design and protocol. It has been theorized that the reduced serum levels are due to increased adipose tissue uptake and urinary excretion of the mineral.[67] In animal studies, catecholamines (hormones and neurotransmitters such as epinephrine [adrenalin] and norepinephrine [noradrenalin]) reduce magnesium content in cardiac tissue and elevate calcium. Magnesium deficiency stimulates catecholamine release, which further perpetuates magnesium deficiency through increased excretion of urinary magnesium, increased adipose tissue uptake or both.[68] The stress-induced elevation of plasma-free fatty acids, in conjunction with the stress hormones epinephrine and norepinephrine, reduces free ionized levels of magnesium in the blood and thus creates a possible association between chronic stress, coronary vasospasms, ischemia (reduced blood supply to the heart) and destruction of heart tissue.

The typical American diet discourages adequate magnesium intake, absorption and utilization. Diets high in refined and processed carbohydrates are low in magnesium as well as vitamin B6, vitamin E, pantothenic acid, biotin, folic acid, vitamin C, potassium, copper, zinc and iron.[69] In addition, excessive intake of calcium, phosphorus or vitamin D can cause a serious magnesium loss.[70-72] Poor magnesium absorption is amplified by the high fat content of American diets. A life of chronic stress and strains can also antagonize magnesium metabolism.

This chronically low intake, nutrient interference, malabsorption, or metabolic interference may be counteracted by the magnesium content in hard water. Those living in soft water areas would obviously not benefit from this additional source. Although the issue is still being debated, the reduced risk of CVD in areas with hard water has been attributed to the water's magnesium content.[73] When cardiac tissue is analyzed, soft water regions have 7 percent less magnesium then cardiac tissue from hard water areas.[74-75]

OTHER FOOD FACTORS

There is more to food than the six classes of nutrients—protein, carbohydrates, fats, vitamins, minerals and water. Other substances in foods can enhance, interfere with or independently contribute to the effect these nutrients have on health.

Daily intake of garlic oil (15 mg or the equivalent of eight to nine cloves of garlic) lowers total cholesterol levels, increases HDL-cholesterol, and lowers LDL-cholesterol.[76]

Inositol, an accessory food factor manufactured in the body and supplied by the diet, may contribute to lipid metabolism. As a member of the lipotrophic family of nutrients, inositol functions to prevent fatty liver infiltration. In conjunction with folic acid, vitamin B6, choline, vitamin B12, betaine and the amino acid methionine, inositol stimulates normal liver management of fats.[77] Good sources of dietary inositol include grapefruit juice, cantaloupe, oranges, stoneground wholewheat bread, cooked beans, grapefruit, limes and green beans.

Age and fasting affect serum cholesterol levels. Cholesterol synthesis is regulated by the amount of hydroxymethylglutaryl CoA (HMG-CoA) reductase. This enzyme fluctuates with age and nutritional status and can decline by 50 percent to 90 percent during the aging process. Cholesterol concentrations increase with age, however, in spite of this reduction in enzymatic activity, implying an accompanying decline in cholesterol degradation. Fasting lowers HMG-CoA reductase activity and may have a temporary effect on lowering serum cholesterol levels.

CONTROLLING OR REVERSING CARDIOVASCULAR DISEASE

The decline in mortality from atherosclerosis and cardiovascular disease implies that Americans are doing something right. Efforts to control blood pressure, lower LDL-cholesterol, raise HDL-cholesterol, eliminate or reduce smoking and increase aerobic exercise have undoubtedly contributed to this trend. But for the 33 million dying of heart disease each year, the millions suffering from related disorders, and the children who may eventually die or be severely handicapped by CVD, more needs to be done.

Generalized atherosclerosis may be prevented, its progress may be stopped and, in some cases, it may be reversed if the individual takes responsibility for changing life-threatening dietary and sedentary habits. Three of the four primary risk factors—hypertension, elevated serum cholesterol and elevated LDL-cholesterol—can be partially or totally controlled with a diet high in complex carbohydrates, fiber and nutrient-dense foods, and low in fats, cholesterol, salt and sugar. It has been proposed that essential hypertension may be controlled or eliminated in as many as 85 percent of subjects who restrict fats and salt and maintain ideal weight.[78] In addition, several of the secondary risk factors, including diabetes, obesity and high serum triglycerides, are also affected by dietary practices. Some preliminary research estimates that 90 percent of atherosclerotic plaques will regress when an individual follows a diet which places him in negative cholesterol balance.[79] LDL receptors on cell surfaces are saturated when daily dietary cholesterol intakes are 100 mg or more. A diet which limits cholesterol to this level or less may in future research studies show a negative dietary cholesterol balance that will result in the regression of existing atherosclerotic lesions.[80] Although this severe reduction in dietary fats is recommended by some, a more moderate reduction is proposed by several leading nutrition organizations and governmental agencies.

The dietary recommendations in the next section are designed to optimize a person's chances of living a long and healthy life. No essential nutrients have been eliminated, and the potentially damaging ones, such as cholesterol, fats and salt, have been minimized. Cholesterol deficiency diseases have not been identified in man since, even on cholesterol-free diets, the human body produces all the cholesterol needed for intracellular metabolism. A reduction in salt carries no known health risks. And, in spite of a need for dietary fat to supply the essential fatty acids and provide a route for absorption of the fat-soluble vitamins, Americans could cut their fat consumption in half and still ingest more than enough oils. Dietary changes can be made successfully and with little discomfort; they even can be fun. With a few tools and techniques, eating healthful meals can be an adventure and a delight.

REFERENCES

1. Van Vaaij, J., Katan, J. and Hautvast, J. Effects of casein versus soy protein diets on serum cholesterol and lipoproteins in young healthy volunteers. *Am. J. Clin. Nutr.*, 34: 1261–1271, 1981.

2. Carroll, K. Dietary protein in relation to plasma cholesterol levels and atherosclerosis. *Nutr. Rev.*, 36: 1–5, 1978.

3. Sirtori, C., Gatti, E., and Manter, O. Clinical experience with the soybean protein diet in the treatment of hypercholesterolemia. *Am. J. Clin. Nutr.*, 32: 1645–1658, 1979.

4. Kritichevsky, D., Tepper, S., Czarnecki, S., et al. Atherogenicity of animal and vegetable protein. *Atherosclerosis*, 41: 429–431, 1982.

5. Check, W. Switch to soy protein for boring but healthful diet. *JAMA*, 247: 3045–3046, 1982.

6. Hermes, R., and Dallinga-Thie, G. Soya, saponins, and plasma cholesterol. *Lancet* II: 48, 1979.

7. Schmeisser, D., et al. Effect of excess dietary lysine on plasma lipids of the chick. *J. Nutr.*, 113, 1777–1783, 1983.

8. Saudek, C. Hyperlipidemia—A diabetic emergency. *Geriatrics*, 37: 81–89, 1982.

9. Fidanza, A., and Audisio, M. Vitamins and lipid metabolism. *Acta Vitaminol. Enzymol.*, 4: 105–114, 1982.

10. Brown, B. G., Albers, J. J. and Brunzell, J. D. Normalization of elevated apolipoprotein-B with niacin plus colestipol in subjects with familiar combined hyperlipidemia. *Atherosclerosis*, 3:A477, 1983.

11. McCully, K. and Wilson, R. Homocysteine theory of atherosclerosis. *Atherosclerosis*, 22: 215–227, 1975.

12. Smolin, L., Crenshaw, T., Kurtycz, D., et al. Homocysteine accumulation in pigs fed diets deficient in vitamin B-6: Relationship to atherosclerosis. *J. Nutr.*, 113: 2022–2033, 1930.

13. Acheson, R. and Williams, D. Does consumption of fruit and vegetables protect against stroke? *Lancet*, I: 1191–1193, 1983.

14. Clemetson, C. Some thoughts on the epidemiology of cardiovascular disease (with special reference to women "on the Pill"). Role of ascorbic acid. *Med. Hypotheses*, 5: 25–34, 1979.

15. Taylor, T., Raferty, A., Elder, J., et al. Leucocyte ascorbate levels and post-operative deep venous thrombosis. *Br. J. Surg.*, 66: 583–585, 1979.

16. Ramirez, J. and Flowers, C. Leukocyte ascorbic acid and its relationship to coronary artery disease in man. *Am. J. Clin. Nutr.*, 33: 2079–2087, 1980.

17. Ginter, E. Ascorbic acid in cholesterol and bile metabolism. *Ann. NY. Acad. Sci.*, 258: 410–421, 1975.

18. Horsey, J., Livesley, B., and Dickerson, J. Ischemic heart disease and aged patients : Effects of ascorbic acid on lipoproteins. *J. Hum. Nutr.*, 35: 53–58, 1981.

19. Ginter, E. Pretreatment serum-cholesterol and response to ascorbic acid. *Lancet*, II: 958–959, 1979.

20. Bates, C., Burr, M., and Leger, A. Vitamin C high density lipoproteins and heart disease in elderly subjects. *Age and Aging*, 8: 177–182, 1979.

21. Burr, M., Bates, C., Milbank, J., et al. The relationship between plasma ascorbate and lipid concentrations in fasting men. *Hum. Nutr. Clin. Nutr.* (England), 36: 135–139, 1982.

22. Joshi, V., Joshi, L., and Gokhale, L. Effect of ascorbic acid on total and high density lipoprotein cholesterol of plasma in normal human subjects. *Indian. J. Physiol. Pharmacol.*, 25: 348–350, 1981.

23. Zaitsev, N. Myasnokov, L., and Sheikman, M. Effect of ascorbic acid on distribution of cholesterol-4-C-14 in tissues of animals with experimental atherosclerosis. *Kardiologyia*, 4: 30, 1964.

24. Spittle, C. Atherosclerosis and vitamin C. *Lancet*, II: 1280, 1971.

25. Sokoloff, B., Michiteru, H., and Sailhof, C. Aging, atherosclerosis, and ascorbic acid metabolism. *J. Am. Geriat. Soc.*, 14: 1239, 1966.

26. Zaitsev, N., Myasnikov, L., and Sheikman, M. *Op. cit.*

27. Taylor, L., Menconi, M., Leibaowitz, M., and Polgar, P. The effect of ascorbate, hydroperoxides, and bradykinin on prostaglandin production by corneal and lens cells. *Invest. Ophthalmol. Vis. Sci.*, 23: 378–382, 1982.

28. Manku, M., Oka, M., and Horrobin, D. Differential regulation of the formation of prostaglandins and related substances from arachidonic acid and from dihomogammalinolenic acid. II. Effects of vitamin C. *Prostaglandins Med.*, 3: 129–137, 1979.

29. Polgar, P. and Taylor, L. Alterations in prostaglandin synthesis during senescence of human lung fibroblasts. *Mech. Ageing. Dev.*, 12: 305–310, 1980.

30. Knox, E. Ischemic heart disease, mortality and dietary intake of vitamin C. *Lancet* 1: 1465–1467, 1973.

31. Brook, M. and Grimshaw, J. Vitamin C concentration of plasma and leukocytes related to smoking habit, age, and sex of humans. *Am. J. Clin. Nutr.*, 21: 1254, 1968.

32. Briggs, M. and Briggs, M. Vitamin C requirements and oral contraceptives. *Nature*, 238: 277, 1972.

33. Kunitomi, M., Kinoshita, K., and Bando, Y. Experimental atherosclerosis in rats fed a vitamin D, cholesterol-rich diet. *J. Pharmacobiodyn.*, 4: 718–723, 1981.

34. Seelig, M. Vitamin D: Risks vs. benefit. *J. Am. Col. N.*, 2: 109–110, 1983.

35. Huang, W., Kamio, A., Yeh, S., et al. The influence of vitamin D on plasma and tissue lipids and atherosclerosis in swine. *Artery*, 3: 439, 1977.

36. Haeger, A. Long-term study of alpha-tocopherol in intermittent claudication. *NY. Acad. Sci.*, 392:369–375, 1982.

37. Meerson, F. and Ustinova, E. Prevention of stress injury to the heart and its hypoxic contracture by using natural antioxidant alpha-tocopherol. *Kardiologiia (USSR)*, 22: 89–94, 1982.

38. Ochsner, A. Preventing and treating venous thrombosis. *Postgrad. Med.*, 44: 91, 1968.

39. Steiner, M. Effect of alpha-tocopherol administration on platelet function in man. *Thrombosis and Hemeostasis*, 49: 73–77, 1983.

40. Challen, A., Branch, W., and Cummings, J. The effect of aspirin and linoleic acid on platelet aggregation, platelet fatty

acid composition and haemostasis in man. *Hum. Nutr. Cl.*, 37: 197–208, 1983.

41. Wilson, C., Middleton, C. and Sun, G. Vitamin E, antioxidants, and lipid peroxidation in experimental atherosclerosis of rabbits. *J. Nutr.*, 108: 1858–1867, 1978.

42. Chan, A., Pritchard, T. and Choy, P. Differential effects of dietary vitamin E and antioxidants on eicosanoid synthesis in young rabbits. *J. Nutr.*, 113: 813–819, 1983.

43. Megavitamin E supplementation and vitamin K dependent carboxylation. *Nutr. Rev.*, 41: 268–270, 1983.

44. Truswell, A. Diet and plasma lipids—a reappraisal. *Am. J. Clin. Nutr.*, 31: 977–985, 1978.

45. Mertz, W. Trace minerals and atherosclerosis. *Fed. Proc. United States*, 41: 2807–2812, 1982.

46. Lener, J. and Bibr, B. Calcium and hypertension. *Lancet*, I: 970, 1971.

47. Kopp, S., Glonek, T., Perry, H., et al. Cardiovascular actions of cadmium at environmental exposure levels. *Science*, 217: 837–839, 1982.

48. Revis, N. and Zinsmeister, A. Atherosclerosis and hypertension induction by lead and cadmium ions: An effect prevented by calcium ion. *Proc. Natl. Acad. Sci.*, 78: 6494–6498, 1981.

49. Boyle, C. Chromium depletion in the pathogenesis of diabetes and atherosclerosis. *S. Med. J.*, 70: 1449–1453, 1977.

50. Offenbacher, E. and Sunyer, X. Beneficial effect of chromium-rich yeast on glucose tolerance and blood lipids in elderly subjects. *Diabetes*, 29: 919–925, 1980.

51. Riales, R. Effect of chromium chloride supplementation on glucose tolerance and serum lipids including high-density lipoprotein of adult men. *Am. J. Clin. Nutr.*, 34: 2670–2678, 1981.

52. Klevay, L. Clofibrate hypocholesterolemia associated with increased hepatic copper. *Am. J. Clin. Nutr.*, 26: 1060, 1973.

53. Kopp, S. Klevay, L., and Feliksik, J. Physiological and metabolic characterization of a cardiomyopathy induced by chronic copper deficiency. *Am. J. Physl.*, 245: H855–H866, 1983.

54. Turlapaty, P. and Altura, B. Magnesium deficiency produces spasms of coronary arteries: Relationship to etiology of sudden death ischemic heart disease. *Science*, 208: 198–200, 1980.

55. *Ibid*.

56. Altura, B. Sudden-death ischemic heart disease and dietary magnesium intake: Is the target site coronary vascular smooth muscle? *Med. Hypoth.*, 5: 843, 1979.

57. Ghani, M. and Smith, J. The effectiveness of magnesium chloride in the treatment of ventricular tachyarrhythmias due to digitalis intoxification. *Am. Heart. J.*, 88: 621, 1974.

58. Ghani, M., et al. Effect of magnesium chloride on electrical stability of the heart. *Am. Heart. J.*, 94: 609, 1977.

59. Scheiman, M., Sullivan, R. and Hyatt, K. Magnesium metabolism in patients undergoing cardiopulmonary bypass. *Circulation*, 39/40 (Supple.): 235–241, 1969.

60. Harris, A., Estandia, A., Smith, H., et al. Magnesium sulfate and chloride in suppression of extopic ventricular tachycardia accompanying acute myocardial infarction. *Am. J. Physiol.*, 172: 251, 1953.

61. Bajasz, E. and Selye, H. The chemical prevention of cardiac necroses following occlusion of coronary vessels. *Can. Med. Assoc. J.*, 82: 212, 1960.

62. Lehr, D., Tissue electrolyte alteration in disseminated myocardial necrosis. *Ann. NY. Acad. Sci.*, 156: 344–378, 1969.

63. Cummings, J. Electrolyte changes in heart tissue and coronary arterial and venous plasma following coronary occlusion. *Circ. Res.*, 8: 865–870, 1960.

64. Seelig, M. Magnesium interrelationships in ischemic heart disease: A review. *Am. J. Clin. Nutr.*, 27: 59–79, 1974.

65. Shakibi, J., Nazarian I. and Moezzi, B. Myocardial metal content in patients who expired from cyanotic congenital heart disease and acute rheumatic heart disease. *Jpn. Heart. J.*, 23: 717–723, 1982.

66. Manthey, J., Opherk, D., Stockins, B., et al. Magnesium in serum of patients with coronary heart disease. *Dtsch. Med. Wochenschr.*, 107: 732–735, 1982.

67. Ebel, H. and Gunther, T. Role of magnesium in cardiac disease. *J. Clin. Chem. Clin. Biochem.*, 21: 249–265, 1983.

68. Vormann, J., Gunther, T, and Ising, H. Magnesium deficiency and catecholamine release. *Magnesium Bul.*, 3:140–142, 1981.

69. Heaton, K., Emmett, P., Henry, C., et al. Not just fiber—the nutritional consequences of refined carbohydrate foods. *Clin. Nutr.*, 37C: 31–35, 1983.

70. Seelig, M. Excessive nutrient consumption and magnesium loss. *Magnesium Bul.*, 3: 26–47, 1981.

71. Seelig, M. *Magnesium Deficiency in the Pathogenesis of Disease*. New York: Plenum Books Co., 1980.

72. Irwin, M. and Feeley, R. Frequency and size of meals and serum lipids, nitrogen and mineral retention, fat digestibility, and urinary thiamin and riboflavin in young women. *Am. J. Clin. Nutr.*, 20: 816–824, 1967.

73. Altura, B. *Op. cit*.

74. Anderson, T., Neri, L., Schreiber, G., et al. Ischemic heart disease, water hardness and myocardial magnesium. *Can. Med. Assoc. J.*, 113: 199–203, 1975.

75. Crawford, T. and Crawford, M. Prevalence and pathological changes of ischemic heart disease in hard water and in soft water areas. *Lancet*, I: 229–232, 1967.

76. Bordia, A. Effect of garlic on blood lipids in patients with coronary heart disease. *Am. J. Clin. Nutr.*, 34: 2100–2103, 1981.

77. Gavin, G., and McHenry, E. Inositol: A lipotropic factor. *J. Bio. Chem.*, 139: 485, 1941.

78. Basta, L., et al. Regression of atherosclerotic stenosing lesions of the renal arteries and spontaneous cure of systemic hypertension through control of hyperlipidemia. *Am. J. Med.*, 61: 420–421, 1976.

79. Wissler, R. Conference on the health effects of blood lipids: Optimal distributions for populations. Workshop Report: Laboratory Experimental Section, American Health Foundation. *Prev. Med.*, 8: 715–732, 1979.

80. Inkeles, S. and Eisenber, D. Hyperlipidemia and coronary atherosclerosis: A review. *Medicine*, 60: 110–123, 1981.

Additional Reading

Bates, C., Mandal, A., and Cole, R. HDL-cholesterol and vitamin C status. *Lancet*, II: 611. 1977.

Lindeman, R., et al. *Magnesium in Health and Disease*. Jamaica, N.Y.: SP Medical and Science Books, 1980.

Seelig, M. Vitamin D: Risk vs. benefit. *J. Am. Col. N.*, 2: 109–110, 1983.

Serfontein, K., Urbink, J. and de Villiers, L. Further evidence on the effect of vitamin E on the cholesterol distribution in lipoproteins with special reference to HDL subfractions. *Am. J. Clin. Pathology*, 79: 604–606, 1983.

Part V
DIETARY
RECOMMENDATIONS

15

·············· ESTABLISHING THE DIETARY GOALS ···············
FOR THE UNITED STATES

THE DIETARY GOALS
FOR THE UNITED STATES

1. To avoid overweight, consume only as much energy (calories) as is expended; if overweight, decrease calories and increase calorie expenditure (through exercise).

2. Increase the consumption of complex carbohydrates and "naturally occurring" sugars from 28 percent of calorie intake to 48 percent of calorie intake (with a range of 45 percent to 51 percent).

3. Reduce the consumption of refined and processed sugars by 45 percent to account for 10 percent of total calorie intake (with a range of 4 percent to 16 percent).

4. Reduce overall fat consumption from 40 percent to 30 percent of calorie intake (with a range of 27 percent to 33 percent).

5. Reduce saturated fat consumption to account for 10 percent of total calorie intake and balance that with polyunsaturated and monounsaturated fats, which should account for about 10 percent of calorie intake each (with a range for saturated, polyunsaturated and monounsaturated fats of 8 percent to 12 percent each).

6. Reduce cholesterol consumption to 300 mg a day (with a range of 250 mg to 350 mg).

7. Limit the intake of sodium by reducing the intake of salt to about 5 g a day (with a range of 4 g to 6 g).

The Senate Select Committee on Nutrition and Human Needs was formed in 1968 to investigate and make recommendations regarding the nutritional status of the American people. Initially, the committee focused on hunger and undernutrition in various population sections and geographical locations. In time, it became apparent that the pressing nutritional concerns of the nation stemmed more from overnutrition and its relation to the high incidence of degenerative disease. As a result of the committee's investigation, the *Dietary Goals for the United States* were published in 1977. The *Goals* were a landmark in health and dietary policy and were the beginning of a movement in political, scientific and social areas to acknowledge lifestyle habits and their relationship to health and disease. (See Figure 16.) At the same time, the nation was turning its attention to the staggering and accelerating costs of medical care. Two years following the publication of the *Goals*, the Surgeon General released *Healthy People*, a national announcement of the need for health promotion and disease prevention in the treatment and avoidance of the nation's worst enemies—cardiovascular disease and cancer. The main target for modification was the American lifestyle. Both government bodies recognized that improved nutrition was a key component in developing a solution.

The redirection in health care, from a disease and treatment model to one of health and prevention, was not confined to the United States. Canada published a national health policy statement in 1974 entitled *A New Perspective on the Health of Canadians*. This report emphasized the need for preventive health care approaches, individual responsibility and economic conservation in health care.

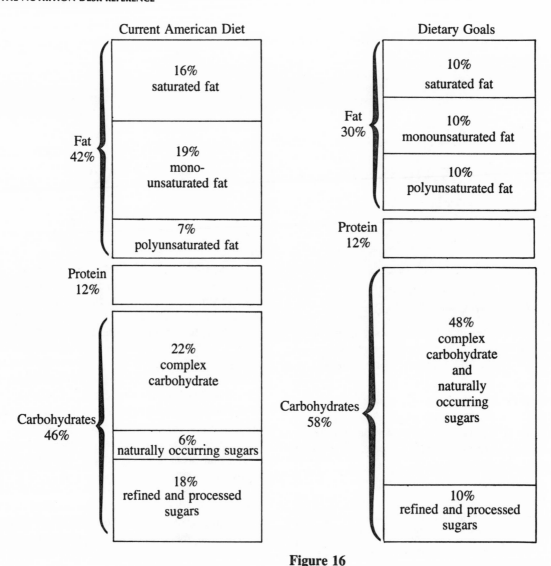

Figure 16

Comparison of current American diet pattern to the Dietary Goals

The Dietary Goals were not welcomed with open arms but were met with heated debate and controversy among the nation's health and nutrition professionals. In fact, the debate was so active that the popular journal *Nutrition Today* compared the diet controversy to the eruptions of Mount St. Helens. Some argued that the *Goals* were timely and provided needed guidelines for the American people; others claimed that they were premature and inadequately supported by research. The primary concern was the appropriateness of generalized and restrictive guidelines for the general public when only a segment of that population seemed to be

at risk. Middle-aged men are the population at greatest risk (elevated cholesterol creates a similar risk to women but to a reduced degree) and some researchers felt that recommendations for this group should not be forced on all segments of the population. Some people are more susceptible to dietary cholesterol and fat, and it was argued that a beneficial dietary change for one should not be generalized to all.

The retaliation to this argument stated that atherosclerosis is developing from childhood in the average artery at a rate of 1 percent to 2 percent per year. Its development goes unnoticed until clinical manifestations develop in later life or the person has a stroke or heart attack. For many heart disease victims their first symptom is their last. Secondary prevention (treatment after the diagnosis of atherosclerosis) may not be as effective as primary prevention. In addition, a reduction in plasma cholesterol through dietary modification may further decrease the risk for cardiovascular disease even for those with serum cholesterol in the "normal" range.[1] In countries with low dietary fat and cholesterol intakes, incidence of cardiovascular disease is low or nonexistent, implying a protective effort for others besides the known high-risk population.[2] Without universal screening for cardiovascular disease, identifying at-risk people is impossible. Reducing fat, cholesterol, salt and sugar poses no nutritional or health risk for anyone and may benefit not only high-risk but perhaps low-risk individuals. The current American diet does raise serum cholesterol levels and high cholesterol is directly associated with the development of atherosclerosis and cardiovascular disease.

Others felt that the *Goals* were unrealistic and doomed to failure as a result of noncompliance. The rebuttal to this argument was that there is nothing sacred about the typical American diet. In the course of development over the past several million years, the human body's nutritional needs developed to support the complex biochemical processes of life. Adequate intake of over forty nutrients is needed for the optimal health of modern man. The current style of food selection is not based on optimal nutrient intake to meet these needs, nor has it been intentionally designed for even basic biological needs. The typical American diet has been strongly influenced by agricultural trends, industry advertising and marketing, convenience, the accelerating pace of life and the development of technology capable of providing a greater selection of easily stored and prepared foods. As a consequence, the modern diet of processed, synthesized and convenience foods is nutritionally depleted as compared to food in its original state and, with the addition of fats, salt and sugar, this diet actually may contribute to morbidity and mortality rates in America. Advocates of the *Dietary Goals* voiced their opinion that there was no reason not to make recommendations which could help people make informed and appropriate food choices.

As Americans become more nutrition conscious, dietary values and attitudes are shifting to reflect health values. Eating patterns are taking some of their cues from Mediterranean and Far Eastern practices, with increased consumption of grains, vegetables and fiber.

Studies show that dietary habits can change and that the biggest obstacle to that change is the first step. When asked to rate the "prudent diet"—consisting of 30 to 35 percent of calories from fat, less than 10 percent from saturated fat, less than 3 grams of sodium and high in fiber—only 26 percent of physicians considered it "very palatable." After trying the diet, 64 percent gave the diet the same rating.[3] People eat out of habit and social custom. Habits are developed and can be changed or modified and social custom can be influenced by education and social evolution.

OTHER DIETARY RECOMMENDATIONS

Since the *Dietary Goals* were published, several documents have been developed that in whole or in part support the same recommendations. In 1980, the U.S. Departments of Agriculture and Health, Education and Welfare (now Health and Human Services) jointly issued the *Dietary Guidelines for Americans*. This set of dietary recommendations mirrored the *Goals* without providing specific target figures. It also included a recommendation that if alcohol is consumed, it should be in moderation. The recommendation to "reduce fats" was less specific than the *Goal's* statement to "reduce fats to 30 percent of calories intake," yet the *Guidelines* added fuel to the fires of critics.

The National Academy of Science/National Research Council's (NAS/NRC) Food and Nutrition Board (the same agency responsible for developing the Recommended Dietary Allowances) published its own set of guidelines entitled *Toward Healthful Diets* in 1980. Many of the same diet and disease issues were addressed but this document ignored the fat and cholesterol issue, thus further fueling disagreements among nutrition and diet advocates. Because of the food industry ties, and possible vested interests of several of the members of the NAS/NRC Board, some of the report's credibility waned.

The American Heart Association's dietary guidelines have been gradually modified, so that the 1981 version is in agreement with the *Dietary Goals*. Maintenance of ideal weight and salt restriction, as well as goals for specific fat and cholesterol reductions and ratios, reflect the Goals set in 1977.[4] The AHA has recommended dietary changes for the healthy American as well as identification and treatment of high-risk individuals; these recommendations are in agreement with the *Dietary Goals*.

THE CHANGING AMERICAN DIET

While the heated debates regarding proper food patterns have persisted for decades, Americans have continued to pass the potatoes, bake pies, prepare turkey on holidays and socialize over a good meal. In the process, food patterns have changed. In fact, the American diet has changed more radically and quickly since the beginning of the twentieth century than at any other time in human history. In addition, the food supply of the 1980s mirrors the complex relationship between technology, economics and social changes.[5]

By replacing manual labor with machines, industrialization has reduced the body's need for a high-calorie diet. New technologies have revamped the food supply by extending "shelf-life," developing hundreds of new processed food products, and using flavor enhancers, colorings, preservatives, emulsifiers, stabilizers, surfactants, antioxidants and a host of other laboratory-derived additives. These substances alter the taste, texture, color, feel, flavor, smell and nutrient content of products lining supermarket shelves. The average grocery store of the 1920s stocked 800 items. Today, a store with fewer than 10,000 items is said to carry a limited selection.[6] This escalation in diversity has been bought at a high price. The nutritional quality of many convenience and preprepared meals and snack foods bears little resemblance to that of the basic foodstuffs. These "fabricated" foods are ones which are processed more than necessary—"doing more to it than we need to," according to George Briggs, professor of nutrition at the University of California, Berkeley.[7] Processed foods may be fortified with some nutrients but usually ignore several trace minerals and fiber. Many are high in fat, salt and sugar.

Only half the calories consumed by the average American are derived from wholesome foods in the basic four food groups—vegetables and fruits, whole grains, lean meats and legumes, and milk and milk products. The rest are derived from sugar, white flour and fat.[8] A University of California study showed that even well-balanced and nutritious meals may degenerate into a poor diet when diluted with sugar and other processed foods. In an experiment on laboratory animals, the researchers noted that when a diet resembling the "typical American diet" was given to the animals they demonstrated a strong craving for sugar and alcohol when compared to animals eating the same diet that was supplemented with 12 vitamins and 13 minerals. The satisfaction of this craving further undermines the quality of the diet.[9]

Life in the 1980s is more affluent than at the beginning of the century. People eat out more often,[10] snack frequently, and choose more "finished" convenience foods.[11] Some basic American customs have changed too. The composition of the American family is shifting, with more women in the work force, more single-parent families, and a larger proportion of single-person households.[12-13] No behavior, except perhaps religion, more closely reflects a society's character than its eating habits. It is no wonder, with these changes in the American lifestyle, that nutritional and dietary trends have undergone such profound changes in the past eighty years.

Americans today are eating less than their ancestors[5] and gaining more weight. The shift from physical labor to office jobs has resulted in a reduced calorie expenditure, which offsets the moderate decrease in energy intake. Protein intake has remained constant but the type of protein has changed. Earlier in the century, plant protein made a major contribution to total protein intake. Today, meals revolve around meat, poultry, fish or eggs. Meat is eaten once or twice a day by 83 percent of Americans.[14] The large proportion of high-fat animal proteins, accompanied by an increased use of margarine and oils, has contributed to a sharp increase in fat consumption.

Sugar consumption has followed the path of meat and fats, while starches have become the dietary black sheep. Refined carbohydrates such as sugars and white flour, white bread and white rice have replaced high-fiber selections. This dietary pattern is considered a major contributor to the degenerative diseases (obesity, heart disease, cancer, diabetes mellitus) and to gastrointestinal diseases.

The increased consumption of fat, the decreased intake of whole grains and the high percentage of sugar in today's diet have resulted in a shift away from nutrient-dense foods. The metabolism of protein, carbohydrate and fats for energy requires vitamins and minerals. A nutrient-dilute, calorie-rich diet may not supply ample amounts of these necessary components for proper energy metabolism, growth, repair and maintenance of normal body functions.

The results of the USDA Nationwide Food Consumption Survey (1977–1978) indicated that the national diet probably supplies adequate nutrient density for protein, phosphorus, vitamin A, vitamin C, thiamin, riboflavin, niacin and vitamin B12. It does not provide adequate iron, magnesium, calcium and vitamin B6. Trace minerals and folic acid were not tested so it can only be estimated that a diet of highly refined foods, with 60 percent of calories coming from fats and sugar, would predispose to deficiencies of these nutrients as well. Magnesium and vitamin B6 play crucial roles in the metabolism of all energy nutrients. These nutrient deficiencies in the American diet have been linked to heart disease. Obviously, this survey is based on the average diet; some diets are better and some are worse than this average.

Cardiovascular disease has dropped since 1968 and the evidence suggests that improvements in lifestyle are the cause.[15] The increased popularity of exercise, reduced smoking and control of hypertension have made significant contributions to this trend. Since publication of the *Dietary Goals* in 1977, sugar consumption has dropped 1.3 percent and starch consumption has risen 1.5 percent. This is modest improvement,

considering that sugar still accounts for more than half of the carbohydrate content of the American diet. Fat intake, unfortunately, has continued to rise.[5]

Public opinion has modified with the growing awareness of health and nutrition. In response to the demands of health-conscious consumers, the food industry has introduced new lines of "light" and "wholesome" foods lower in calories, sugar, fats and additives or produced with less processing. Over the years the fat in pork has declined over 25 percent, fat in beef has diminished 6–7 percent and low-fat ham and some luncheon meats are available. The American Meat Institute is requesting changes in USDA fat requirements which would allow further fat reductions. The continuation of this trend would mean an increase in products which are economically profitable for industry and nutritionally profitable for consumers.

REFERENCES

1. Stamler, J. Public health aspects of optimal serum lipid-lipoprotein levels. *Prev. Med.*, 8: 733, 1979.

2. McGill, H. (ed). *The Geographic Pathology of Atherosclerosis*. Baltimore: Williams and Wilkins, 1968, p. 41.

3. Kottke, T. et al. Short report: Perceived palatability of the prudent diet: Results of a dietary demonstration for physicians. *Prev. Med.*, 12: 588–593, 1983.

4. AHA Nutrition Committee Report. Rationale of the diet-heart statement of the American Heart Association. Special Report. *Arteriosclerosis*, 4: 177–191, 1982.

5. Brewster, L. and Jacobson, M. *The Changing American Diet: A Chronical of American Eating Habits from 1910–1980*. Washington, D.C.: Center for Science in the Public Interest, 1983.

6. Gussow, J. Can industry afford a healthy America? *CNI Weekly Report* IX, No. 22: 5, June 7, 1979.

7. Puzo, D. Fabricated foods are not sufficient. *The San Diego Union*, June 8, 1978, D-14.

8. Bland, J. *Your Health Under Siege: Using Nutrition to Fight Back*. Brattleboro, Vt.: The Stephen Greene Press, 1981.

9. Jenks, R. Well-rounded diets may be nutritionally deficient. *University of California Clip Sheet*, 49: 35, April 16, 1974.

10. A new perspective on eating out. *Am. J. Diet. Assoc.*, 73: 171, 1978.

11. The revolution in American food intake. *J. Am. Diet. Assoc.*, 74: 369, 1979.

12. U.S. Department of Labor, Bureau of Labor Statistics, 1980.

13. U.S. Department of Commerce, Bureau of Census Current Population Reports, Series P-20, No. 345: Projections—Series P-25, No. 805.

14. A new perspective on eating out. *Am. J. Diet. Assoc.*, 73: 171, 1978.

15. Stamler, J. Diet and coronary heart disease. *Biometrics*, 38(Supple.): 95–118, 1982.

Additional Reading

Study finds U.S. diet means lots of meat. *The Nation's Health*, Sept. 2, 1978.

Dietary Goals for the United States, prepared by the Select Committee on Nutrition and Human Needs, United States Senate. December, 1977. U.S. Government Printing Office.

Food and Nutrition Board, Division of Biological Sciences, Assembly of Sciences—National Research Council. *Toward Healthful Diets*, Washington, D.C. National Association of Sciences, 1980.

The National Nutrition Consortium. Guidelines for a national nutrition policy. *Nutrition Reviews*, 38: 96–98, 1980.

Healthy People: The Surgeon General's Report on Health Promotion and Disease Prevention. U.S. Department of Health, Education, and Welfare. Publ. No. 79-55071. 1979.

Report of the AHA Nutrition Committee. Rationale of the Diet-Heart Statement of the American Heart Association. *Arteriosclerosis*, 4: 177–191, 1982.

Windham, C., Wyse, B. and Hanse, G. Nutrient density of diets in the USDA Nationwide Food Consumption Survey, 1977–1978: II: Adequacy of nutrient density consumption practices. *J. Am. Diet. Assoc.*, 82: 34–43, 1983.

16

APPLYING THE DIETARY GOALS: A RATIONALE FOR HEALTHFUL EATING

HOW TO USE THE DIETARY GOALS

THE DIETARY GOALS are intended to be used in conjunction with the Recommended Dietary Allowances (RDA) in menu planning. They extend the RDA individual vitamin and mineral recommendations to include necessary and healthful ranges of intake for carbohydrate, fat, cholesterol and salt. The Dietary Goals should be used as ranges of intake, with the specific recommendation as the average amount. As the name implies, these recommendations are goals for which the people of the United States are to aim. They do not demand instant dietary restructuring but recognize that dietary changes occur in steps; they provide direction and magnitude for this change.

To apply the Dietary Goals the following food selection and preparation habits should be practiced:

1. Increase the intake of wholegrain cereals and breads, and fruits and vegetables.
2. Reduce the intake of refined and processed sugars and foods high in sugars.
3. Reduce the intake of animal and plant foods high in fats, especially saturated fats. Reduce the intake of animal fats.
4. Except for young children, chose low- and nonfat dairy foods.
5. Reduce the intake of high-cholesterol foods such as butter, eggs, fatty meats and organ meats.
6. Reduce the intake of salt and salty foods.

THE DIETARY GOALS AND WEIGHT CONTROL

GOAL 1: To avoid overweight, consume only as much energy (calories) as is expended. If overweight, decrease energy intake and increase energy expenditure.

One in three Americans is overweight. The alarming prevalence of obesity is partially the result of marked changes in lifestyle which include increased affluence and reduced physical exercise, but no proportionate reduction in food consumption. Obesity is a major risk factor in the development of cardiovascular disease, cancer, gout, congestive heart failure, diabetes mellitus, hypertension and numerous other degenerative diseases. It is associated with elevated blood lipids and glucose intolerance,[1] and is a risk factor for heart disease independent of its association with other complications.[2] Data from the Framingham study indicated that a 10 percent reduction in weight by men ages thirty-five to fifty-five would reduce the rate of heart disease by 20 percent. The evidence that obesity reduces life expectancy and can diminish the quality of life has been verified repeatedly by studies.

Cholesterol synthesis is elevated in overweight subjects. The reduction of fat tissue results in mobilization of cholesterol stores which are picked up in the blood by HDL-cholesterol and transported to the liver for removal. With sustained weight loss, fasting blood sugar levels decline, serum cholesterol drops, and glucose tolerance is improved.[3]

The *Dietary Goals* recommend reducing nutrient-dilute foods high in fats, refined and processed foods and sugars, and increasing high-fiber foods such as fruits, vegetables, whole grains and legumes. This recommendation, combined with the guidelines set down in the Four Food groups and the RDAs, forms the foundation of any eating plan, whether for weight loss, maintenance or gain.

The calorie contribution of alcohol should be acknowledged in the maintenance of ideal weight. Alcohol provides 7 calories/gram compared to the 4 calories/gram of protein and carbohydrate, and the 9 calories/gram of fat. Since alcohol contributes minimal or no nutrients to the diet other than calories, it is considered nutrient dilute. In spite of its low nutrient density, alcohol comprises 10 percent of the average American woman's daily calorie intake and 7½ percent of the average man's intake. The 3½ ounce glass of wine before dinner is not calorie-free; it supplies 85 calories. If it is dessert wine, it contributes 140 calories to the day's total.

The *Dietary Goals* do not recommend simply restricting calorie intake for those in need of weight loss. Exercise should play an equally important role. Exercise increases energy expenditure and protects against the restriction of calories to sub-optimal levels in order to loss weight. Weight-loss programs that rely only on calorie restriction provide fertile ground for malnutrition because of food intake that is inadequate in nutrients for daily needs.

THE DIETARY GOALS AND CARBOHYDRATES

GOAL 2: Increase carbohydrate consumption to account for 55–60 percent of the energy (calorie) intake.

Studies of food patterns since the turn of the century show a gradual reduction in carbohydrate consumption and an increasing consumption of fat. Sugar outranks starch as a carbohydrate contributor in the diet. As of the mid-1970s, starches represented only 22 percent of the total calorie intake; sugars accounted for 24 percent. Less than half the flour and cereal are consumed today as were consumed in 1910.[4] Americans are not as imaginative as their forefathers in the variety of grains selected; rye, barley, buckwheat and corn flour

and meal do not grace the American table with the frequency seen in 1910.

This reduction in starch consumption may be due to the rise in income and the relative lack of prestige of starchy foods. Advertising has encouraged the decline by promoting highly refined and processed foods containing increasing amounts of sugars, fats and salt. Fruits, vegetables, whole grains and legumes combined do not get the equivalent air time of processed cereals. The popularization and credence given to fad diets also has had an effect.

Many diet claims falsely represent carbohydrates as "fattening" and this myth has influenced the food choices of the weight-conscious millions. Complex carbohydrates are not "fattening" unless, as with any food, they are consumed in excess of calorie needs. Since they supply less than half the calories of fats, a greater quantity of carbohydrate-rich foods can be consumed than fatty foods, thus satisfying appetite without adding poundage. For example, a tablespoon of salad dressing contains many more calories than the two cups of lettuce and vegetables beneath it. A baked potato contains 100 calories plus trace minerals, protein, vitamins and fiber; the added tablespoon of sour cream or butter doubles the calories with no nutrient benefits.

Carbohydrates need to be increased to provide the calories lost when fats are reduced in the diet. Besides making up the calorie deficit, complex carbohydrates found in legumes, fruits, vegetables and wholegrain breads and cereals contribute trace minerals, vitamins, fiber, inositol and other food factors found to reduce the incidence of cardiovascular disease. (See pp. 169–177.)

These carbohydrate-rich foods are also low in saturated fats and are devoid of cholesterol. Populations consuming a high carbohydrate diet have a lower incidence of cardiovascular disease.[5] Increasing dietary fiber from such sources as oats, apples and other fruits, legumes and grains has been effective in lowering serum cholesterol and reducing the risk of cardiovascular disease. (See p. 169.)

The fact that some fiber in the diet is beneficial does not mean more is better. Excessive dietary fiber can reduce the absorption of trace minerals and irritate the intestinal lining. A diet containing 37 grams of fiber will provide enough protective roughage without negatively affecting trace mineral status or damaging the intestinal mucosa. This amount can be obtained daily from:

6 servings of wholegrain breads and cereals
(1 serving = 1 slice of bread, ½ cup
cooked pasta, rice or cereal, or 1 cup
high-fiber cold cereal) .... 13 grams

4 servings of fresh fruits and vegetables
(1 serving = 1 piece of fruit, 1 cup raw
vegetables, or ½ cup cooked vegetable). 15–23 grams

1 serving dried beans (1 serving = ½ cup) .. 9 grams.
Total 37–45 grams

TABLE 15
Dietary Fiber in Foods

Food	Amount	Dietary Fiber (grams)
Milk and Milk products		0

Vegetables

Food	Amount	Dietary Fiber (grams)
Asparagus	4 med. spears	0.9
Avocado	½ whole	2.2
Beets, boiled	½ cup	2.1
Broccoli	½ cup	3.2
Brussels sprouts	½ cup	2.3
Cabbage, boiled	½ cup	2.0
Carrots, boiled	½ cup	2.3
raw	1	2.3
Celery, raw	1 stalk	0.7
Corn, off the cob	⅓ cup	3.1
on the cob	1 ear	5.9
Eggplant, peeled, cooked	½ cup	2.5
Lettuce	⅙ head	1.4
	6 med. leaves	0.7
Mushrooms, raw	½ cup	0.9
Peas, boiled	½ cup	4.2
Potato, baked with skin	1 med	3.0
boiled, peeled	1 med	2.7
french fried	10	1.6
mashed, with milk	½ cup	0.9
Spinach, cooked	½ cup	5.7
Sweet potato, cooked	1 5"×2"	3.5
Tomato, raw	1 med	2.0
juice		0
sauce	½ cup	2.6

Fruits

Food	Amount	Dietary Fiber (grams)
Apple, with peel	1 med	3.3
juice		0
sauce	½ cup	2.6
Apricots	2 med	1.6

Food	Amount	Dietary Fiber (grams)
Banana	½ med	1.6
Cantaloupe	¼	1.6
Dates, dried	5	3.1
Fig, dried	1 med	2.4
Grapefruit, fresh	½ whole	0.6
Grapes, seedless	12	0.3
Nectarine	1 med	3.0
Orange	1 small	2.4
Peach, fresh	1 med	1.4
Pear, fresh	1 med	2.6
Pineapple, fresh	½ cup	0.9
Prunes, uncooked	2 med	2.0
Raisins	2 Tbs	1.2
Raspberries	½ cup	4.6
Strawberries	½ cup	1.7

Bread and Cereals

Bread:

Food	Amount	Dietary Fiber (grams)
Cracked wheat	1 slice	2.1
Frankfurter bun	1	1.2
Hamburger bun	1	1.2
Pumpernickel	1 slice	1.2
Raisin	1 slice	0.4
Rye	1 slice	1.2
White	1 slice	0.8
Wholewheat	1 slice	2.1

Cereals

Food	Amount	Dietary Fiber (grams)
All-Bran	⅓ cup	9.0
Bran Buds	⅓ cup	8.0
Cracklin' Bran	⅓ cup	4.0
Raisin Bran	⅓ cup	4.0

Crackers

Food	Amount	Dietary Fiber (grams)
Rye	3 3½"	2.3
Saltines	4 squares	0
Popcorn	1 cup	0.4
Beans, baked	½ cup	11.0
Chili with beans	½ cup	8.6
Meats		0
Eggs		0
Fats: dressings, margarine, mayonnaise, etc.		0

Nuts

Food	Amount	Dietary Fiber (grams)
Peanut butter	2 Tbs	2.4
Peanuts, roasted	¼ cup	2.9
Spanish	10	0.7
Walnuts, chopped	¼ cup	1.6

To consume 55–60 percent of the total calories as carbohydrate, meals should feature complex carbohydrates, not the traditional eight-ounce steak, eggs and bacon, or corned beef sandwich. Meat becomes a condiment, as in Oriental cooking, and noodles, rice, pasta or other starches form the main dish.

The following are suggestions for increasing complex carbohydrates and fiber in the diet.

1. Select a good balance of fresh, frozen and canned fruits and vegetables. The nutrient contribution from fruits and vegetables has declined as canned and processed produce has replaced fresh. Vegetables and fruits gathered fresh from the garden are superior to frozen, canned or processed selections. Frozen produce is processed within hours of harvesting and may be nutritionally superior to fresh produce that has been stored or damaged in shipping. Canned produce is generally inferior to both frozen and fresh.

2. Choose whole and fresh foods over processed and refined, since the latter are typically of inferior nutrient quality and often have added fats, salt and sugars. If fresh produce or whole foods are not available, choose foods that have undergone minimal processing. For example, if fresh broccoli is not available or is inconvenient, choose fresh-frozen broccoli, rather than broccoli in sauces, pies, freeze-dried in soups or processed into vegetable patties. When white flour is refined from whole wheat, the milling removes varying amounts of the bran and wheat germ. The average white flour used in the United States is 76 percent extraction, meaning that 76 percent of the original wheat grain is retained. Wholewheat flour would be 100 percent extraction. Figure 17 shows a portion of the nutrient loss from processing whole wheat into white flour; the degree of milling apparently affects the degree of nutrient loss.

   Wholegrain flour, when processed into white flour, loses 10 percent to 100 percent of its trace mineral, vitamin and fiber content. Flour nutrients—niacin, riboflavin, thiamin and iron—are added back in the "enrichment" process; the other nutrients are not. In general, the more any food is processed, the fewer the nutrients and the greater the cost.

3. Select grain products for breakfast. Choices include wholewheat toast, hot or cold cereal, pancakes, waffles, muffins, biscuits or breads. Leftovers from the night before of brown rice, bulgar, kasha, or noodles can be used as a breakfast cereal. Hot cereals tend to undergo less processing than cold ready-to-eat cereals and, if whole grain, will be more nutritious. In spite of extensive enrichment campaigns, cold cereals are made from refined grain products with a few or several nutrients added back in varying proportions. Many trace minerals and fiber are neglected in the "fortification" process, thus making wholegrain cereals and breads the preferred choice.

4. Lunches and dinners can include chili without beef, salads, soups, sandwich spreads made from beans and vegetables, fresh fruit desserts, wholegrain spaghetti, lasagna, brown rice and vegetable dishes, East Indian curries, pocket bread sandwiches, vegetable and pasta casseroles. The list is endless.

5. Snacks can be chosen from a similar listing of foods—fruits, grains, vegetables and legumes.

GOAL 3: Reduce the consumption of refined and other processed sugars by about 45 percent to account for about 10 percent of total energy intake.

Each year, Americans eat their weight in sugar (sucrose) and sweeteners (130 pounds or more). This equals 40 teaspoons of sugar a day—almost one cup or 640 calories—a large contribution for a food for which the body has no need. At the same time, tooth decay and obesity are rampant. Sugar consumption has increased since the turn of the century, and the type of sugar consumed today is different. While our grandmothers added sugar in homemade baked goods and jams, 75 percent of the sugar consumed today is added by industry. Sugar is the leading ingredient added to commercial foods.[6]

Sugar is obtained from several sources, some obvious and many not. The most obvious source is the spoonful added to coffee or cereal or the cupfuls that are an ingredient in desserts. The hidden sugars are found in processed and refined foods. Read labels. Sugar can be found in commercial frozen pizzas, salad dressing, chili mix, meat extenders, soup, fruit drinks, chicken pie, spaghetti sauce, frozen entrees, fruited yogurt, catsup, luncheon meats and hundreds of unsuspected foods. See Table 16.

Ready-to-eat cereals are a major sugar contributor. The addition of this sweetener to cold cereals, beginning in 1948, is held responsible for saving the cereal

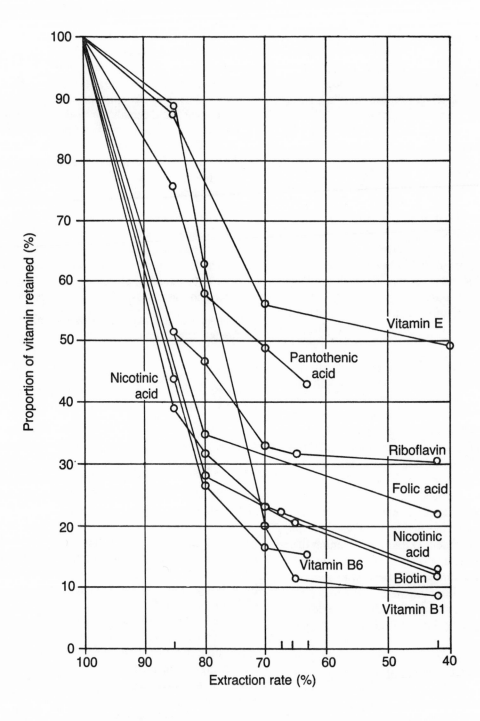

Figure 17

*Relation between extraction rate and proportion of
total vitamins of the grain retained in flour*

Source: Dietary Goals for the United States, 2nd ed. Select Committee
on Nutrition and Human Needs, United States Senate. Washington,
D.C.: U.S. Government Printing Office, 1977.

market. Since then, the variety of sugar-laden, and candy-coated cereals has sky-rocketed. These foods comprise a large portion of supermarket stock and sometimes claim one full aisle for their territory. Often they are no more than sugar-coated vitamin substitutes, and some contain more sugar than a candy bar. See Table 17.

TABLE 16
Added Sugar in Selected Foods

Food	Portion	Sugar content (tsp)
Applesauce (unsweetened)	½ cup	2
Apricots, canned	4 halves/1 Tbs. syrup	3½
Beets, pickled	½ cup	2.1
Beverages		
Kool-aid	1 cup	6
Tang	4 oz.	3
Whiskey Sour	3 oz.	1½
Brownies	2″ × 2″ × ¾″	3
Catsup	2 Tbs.	1 ½
Chewing Gum	1 stick	½
Cake		
Chocolate	1/12 of 2 layer	15
Angel food	1/12 of large	6
Banana	4 oz.	4
Pound	4 oz.	5
Sponge	1/10 of average	6
Cookies, chocolate chip	1	2–3
Gingersnaps	1	1 ½
Macaroons	1 lg.	3–6
Oatmeal	1	2
Oreo	1	1½
Vanilla Wafer	1	1
Cool Whip	1 Tbs.	0.23
Cranberry sauce	½ cup	12
Doughnut, plain	3″ diameter	4
glazed	1	6
Fruit cocktail	½ cup	5
Graham cracker	2	0.9
Grape juice, frozen conc	6 oz. serving	1
Grape juice drink	6 oz.	3.9
Honey	1 Tbs.	3
Ice cream	½ cup	5–6
Jam, strawberry	1 Tbs.	4
Jello	1/3 cup	4.5
Jelly	1 Tbs.	4–6
Marmalade, orange	1 Tbs.	4–6

Food	Portion	Sugar content (tsp)
Meats, processed		
Bacon	2 slices	.05
Bologna	2 slices	0.35
Cured ham	3 oz.	.1
Luncheon meat	2 slices	0.35
Pork sausage	3 links	.3
Salami	6 slices	0.15
Spam	3 oz.	.8
Milk drinks, chocolate	1 cup	6
Eggnog	1 cup	4.5
Orange juice, imitation	6 oz.	5.4
Peas, sweet, canned	1/3 cup	0.95
Peaches, canned in syrup	2 halves	3.5
Peanut butter	2 Tbs.	0.325
Pie, apple	1/6 med. pie	12
Boston cream	1/6 of 8″	11
Cherry	1/6 med. pie	14
Lemon	1/6 med. pie	13–14
Raisin	1/6 med. pie	13
Pumpkin	1/6 med. pie	10
Pop Tarts	1	3.8
Salad dressing		
blue cheese	1 Tbs.	0.25
French	1 Tbs.	0.75
Italian	1 Tbs.	0.25
Sherbet	½ cup	6–8
Soft drinks		
Cola drinks	12 oz.	9
Ginger ale	12 oz.	7
Seven-Up	12 oz.	9
Sweet roll, plain	1	4
iced	1	7
Syrup, maple	1 Tbs.	2.5
Yogurt, fruited	1 cup	7.5
Frozen	1 cup	5.3

One quarter of America's sugar is consumed in soft drinks, over 490 eight-ounce servings per person each year. Promotional campaigns have been successful; soft drink sales doubled between 1960 and 1975 and are still on the rise. A beverage which supplies six to nine teaspoons of sugar per twelve-ounce serving and is often high in phosphates, caffeine and additives has become the national drink, second only to coffee. As a result, the marketing, sales and consumption of soft drinks has overtaken and bypassed that of more nutritious beverages, such as non-fat milk.

TABLE 17
Sugar (Sucrose) Content of Ready-to-eat Cereals

The dentists who published this information suggested, tentatively, that to avoid promoting the development of dental decay the consumer should choose cereals containing less than 20 percent refined sugar.

CEREAL	Sucrose (percent)	CEREAL	Sucrose (percent)
LESS THAN 10 PERCENT SUCROSE		**20 TO 29 PERCENT SUCROSE**	
Shredded Wheat, large biscuit	1.0	All Bran	20.0
Shredded Wheat, spoon-sized biscuit	1.3	Granola, with almonds and filberts	21.4
Cheerios	2.2	Fortified Oat Flakes	22.2
Puffed Rice	2.4	Heartland	23.1
Uncle Sam Cereal	2.4	Super Sugar Chex	29.0
Wheat Chex	2.6	**30 TO 39 PERCENT SUCROSE**	
Grape Nut Flakes	3.3	Bran Buds	30.2
Puffed Wheat	3.6	Sugar Sparkled Corn Flakes	32.2
Alpen	3.8	Frosted Mini Wheats	33.6
Post Toasties	4.1	Sugar Pops	37.8
Product 19	4.1	**40 TO 49.5 PERCENT SUCROSE**	
Corn Total	4.4	Alpha Bits	40.3
Special K	4.4	Sir Grapefellow	40.7
Wheaties	4.7	Super Sugar Crisp	40.7
Corn Flakes, Kroger	5.1	Cocoa Puffs	40.7
Peanut Butter	6.2	Cap'n Crunch	43.3
Grape Nuts	6.6	Crunch Berries	43.4
Corn Flakes, Food Club	7.0	Kaboom	43.8
Crispy Rice	7.3	Frankenberry	44.0
Corn Chex	7.5	Frosted Flakes	44.0
Corn Flakes, Kellogg	7.8	Count Chocula	44.2
Total	8.1	Orange Quangarooa	44.7
Rice Chex	8.5	Quisp	44.9
Crisp Rice	8.8	Boo Berry	45.7
Raisin Bran, Skinner	9.6	Vanilly Crunch	45.8
Concentrate	9.9	Baron Von Redberry	45.8
10 TO 19 PERCENT SUCROSE		Cocoa Krispies	45.9
Rice Crispies, Kellogg	10.0	Trix	45.9
Raisin Bran, Kellogg	10.6	Froot Loops	46.6
Heartland, with raisins	13.5	Honeycomb	47.4
Buck Wheat	13.6	Pink Panther	49.2
Life	14.5	**50 TO 59 PERCENT SUCROSE**	
Granola, with dates	14.5	Cinnamon Crunch	50.3
Granola, with raisins	14.5	Lucky Charms	50.4
Sugar-Frosted Corn Flakes	15.6	Cocoa Pebbles	53.5
40% Bran Flakes, Post	15.8	Apple Jacks	55.0
Team	15.9	Fruity Pebbles	55.1
Brown Sugar-Cinnamon Frosted Mini Wheats	16.0	King Vitamin	58.5
40% Bran Flakes, Kellogg	16.2	**MORE THAN 60 PERCENT SUCROSE**	
Granola	16.6	Sugar Smacks	61.3
100% Bran	18.4	Super Orange Crisp	68.0

Sugar indirectly contributes to malnutrition. Besides this century's increase in sugar consumption and the dramatic shifts in the source of that sugar, the proportion of daily calories supplied by this sweetener has increased. Sugar accounts for 24 percent of the total calories; refined sugar accounts for 82 percent of that, or 18 percent of calorie intake. People today consume fewer calories than their counterparts in 1910, but sugar consumption has increased. More calories are being supplied by a food which provides no nutritional benefits other than calories. These calories still require vitamins and minerals to be metabolized for energy in the body, but must rob the body's stores to get them. In addition, a person either eats sugared foods over and above the other foods that supply the daily needs for nutrients, thus predisposing him- or herself to weight gain, or the sugared foods replace nutritious foods and the daily needs are not met. Either choice is a step away from optimal nutrition and health.

If a person is very active, burning extra calories each day in sports or vigorous manual work, then a few "empty" calories can be tolerated. The proportion of sugar to nutritious foods should remain constant no matter what the allowed calorie intake; increased activity allows for greater food intake and sugar would still be only 10 percent of that. To consume more than 15 to 20 percent of calories as sugar reduces the nutrient density of the entire diet.

Sugar has been linked with numerous diseases including heart disease, cancer, and diabetes. Although the research is not conclusive, excessive intake of sugar (more than 30 percent of total calories) may disturb hormonal balance and produce a wide range of biochemical abnormalities similar to those seen in cardiovascular disease.[7,8]

Sugars, especially those which are sticky, eaten frequently or retained in the mouth, are associated with tooth decay, dental cavities in all ages, gum disease and eventual loss of teeth. In the United States, over 90 percent of school-aged children have some form of tooth decay. Half of adults over fifty-five years have no teeth. In cultures where sugar consumption is nonexistent or minimal, tooth decay is considerably less common.

The *Dietary Goals* recommend reducing sugar to 10 percent of the diet. If the daily calorie intake is 2000, then a day's allotment of sugar would be $.10 \times 2000$ calories $= 200$. These calories add up quickly. A cup of commercial fruited yogurt and a fruit drink for lunch supply the day's allotment for sugar.

TABLE 18
Recommended Sugar Calories Per Day

Age		Average Calorie intake	Maximum Calories From sugar
Children	4–6 years	1300–2300	130–230
	7–10	1650–3300	165–330
Males	11–14	2000–3700	200–370
	15–18	2100–3900	210–390
	19–22	2500–3300	250–330
	23–50	2300–3100	230–310
	51–75	2000–2800	200–280
	76+	1650–2450	165–245
Females	11–14	1500–3000	150–300
	15–18	1200–3000	120–300
	19–22	1700–2500	170–250
	23–50	1600–2400	160–240
	51–75	1400–2200	140–220
	76+	1200–2000	120–200

To reduce sugar in the diet:

1. Read labels. Sugar has many aliases, including sucrose, raw sugar, glucose, brown sugar, turbinado, honey, dextrose, fructose, corn syrup, corn sweetener and natural sweetener. Industry is required to list the sugar content of most foods, but it does not have to identify the amount of sugar. The consumer can make a guess at the amount of sugar by reading labels. Since labels list ingredients in descending order of amounts, the closer sugar is to the top of the listing, the greater is its caloric contribution.

2. Substitute fruit juices, non-fat milk, unsweetened tea, mineral water with a slice of lemon, vegetable juice and water for sugared fruit-flavored drinks and soft drinks. A mixture of carbonated water and undiluted frozen fruit juice makes a low-sugar "natural" soft drink. Although commercial diet soft drinks are low in sugar, they are high in phosphates, additives and often caffeine. Use them in moderation.

3. Reduce desserts, candies, baked products, doughnuts, pies, cakes, soft drinks, ice cream, cookies, jams and jellies.

4. Choose fresh fruits or fruits canned in their own juices, in unsweetened juices or in water.

TABLE 19
Nutrient and Percentage of U.S. R.D.A. Composition of Various Sweeteners
(One Tablespoon)

	White Sugar	Strained Honey	Dark Brown Sugar	Corn Syrup	Light Molasses	Medium Molasses	Blackstrap Molasses
CALORIES	46	64	52	57	50	46	43
%CALORIES** Female, 15–22	2.1	3.0	2.4	2.7	2.3	2.1	2.0
%CALORIES*** Male, 15–22	1.5*	2.1	1.7*	1.9*	1.6*	1.5*	1.4*
PROTEIN	—	—	—	—	—	—	—
VITAMIN A	—	—	—	—	—	—	—
VITAMIN C	—	trace*	—	—	—	—	—
THIAMIN	—	trace*	—	—	0.9*	—	3
RIBOFLAVIN	—	0.5*	—	0.1*	0.7*	—	3
NIACIN	—	trace*	—	—	trace*	—	2
CALCIUM	trace*	0.1*	1*	—	3	6	13
IRON	—	0.1*	2	4	4	7	16
VITAMIN E				Figures not available			
VITAMIN B6	—	—	—	—	2	2	2
VITAMIN B12	—	—	—	—	—	—	—
PHOSPHORUS		0.3*	0.5*	0.3*	0.9*	1.4*	1.7*
MAGNESIUM				Figures not available			
ZINC				Figures not available			
COPPER		0.4*	2	3	14	14	14

*Less than 2%—not a significant source
**2100 calories
***2850 calories

5. Choose ready-to-eat cereals without sugar or with sugar lower than the third or fourth item on the ingredients list. Hot cereals are less likely to contain sugar, but read the labels before buying. Sweeten cereal with fruit, not sugar.

6. Reduce sugar in recipes. Prepare favorite recipes with three quarters of the required sugar. As the sweet tooth adjusts, reduce the sugar to one-half, one-quarter or one-eighth of the original amount. Use apple juice concentrate in place of sugar in recipes.

7. Reduce the frequency of sugar intake as well as the amount.

8. Brown sugar, raw sugar, turbinado and honey are sugar. The minuscule amount of vitamins or minerals is insignificant in terms of meeting daily needs and these sweeteners should not be relied upon as a source of anything but calories. For example, almost 300 tablespoons of honey must be consumed to provide the calcium in one cup of non-fat milk or collard greens. The exception is blackstrap molasses, which supplies some nutrients in appreciable amounts.

THE DIETARY GOALS AND FAT

GOAL 4: Reduce overall fat consumption from approximately 40 percent to 30 percent of energy intake.

GOAL 5: Reduce saturated fat consumption to account for about 10 percent of total energy intake, and balance that with polyunsaturated and monounsaturated fats, each of which should account for about 10 percent of energy intake.

GOAL 6: Reduce cholesterol consumption to about 300 milligrams a day.

Dietary fat, especially saturated fats and cholesterol, is strongly associated with increased risk of atherosclerosis, cardiovascular disease, hypertension, obesity and other degenerative diseases. (For a detailed account of fat and cardiovascular disease refer to pages 166–169.) Polyunsaturated fats are associated with an increased risk of cancer as well.

Many of today's popular foods were not in use nationwide at the turn of the century. For example,

TABLE 20
Fatty Acid Composition of Oils and Fats

source	polyunsat. (%)	monounsat. (%)	saturated (%)	P/S ratio
Beef fat	2	44	54	<0.1
Butter	4	37	59	<0.1
Chicken fat	27	29	44	0.6
Coconut oil	2	6	92	<0.1
Corn oil	60	26	14	4.3
Egg yolk	14	51	35	0.4
Lard	14	46	40	0.4
Olive oil	15	69	16	0.9
Palm oil	10	37	53	0.2
Peanut oil	35	45	20	1.8
Safflower oil	78	11	11	7.1
Soybean oil	58	27	15	3.9
Sunflower oil	70	18	12	5.8

french fries are the common accompaniment to most fast-food meals. These processed potatoes are 40 percent fat calories; the original potato had only a trace of fat. The rapid increase in doughnut, fried chicken and pizza shops will attest to the popularity of high-fat foods. Coconut oil and hydrogenated vegetable oils are found in hundreds of commercially packaged convenience foods, including non-dairy creamers, whipped cream substitutes, granola, and numerous frozen foods. The Center for Science in the Public Interest has investigated these preprepared frozen selections and found several dinners, entrees, frozen vegetables in pastry and side dishes to be high in fat. One manufacturer's frozen croissant contained 200 calories, 118 of which came from butter.

Fat is the most concentrated source of food energy. One gram of this oily substance provides nine calories in comparison to the four provided by proteins and carbohydrates. Fat comprises over 40 percent of the calories in the typical American diet. Many of the foods promoted as high-protein sources are actually far higher in fat content. The ubiquitous hamburger, whether fried, grilled or barbequed, derives as much as 75 percent of its calories from fat; whole milk is 3.5 percent fat by weight but 50 percent fat calories; sixty-three of an egg's eighty calories come from fat; two strips of crispy bacon may leave some grease in the pan but retain enough to provide 80 percent of the calories as fat. A common meal at a roadside restaurant might contain steak, baked potato with sour cream and butter, salad with dressing, roll and butter, and coffee with cream. The fat calories total 75 percent of the meal.

Fat and sugar are high in calories, low in nutrients. These two dietary components, however, comprise over 60 percent of the calories in the American diet. Fat consumption, therefore, should be viewed in terms of what it crowds out. When fat comprises a large portion of the diet, other, more nutrient-dense foods, such as whole grains and fruits and vegetables, are cut back or eliminated. Not only do these foods provide trace minerals, vitamins, fiber and other nutrients in a high nutrient-to-calorie ratio, but they are not linked with the disease-promoting qualities that are attributed to dietary fats. Reducing dietary fat would promote the consumption of more nutritious foods and would reduce the intake of concentrated calories, both positive factors in the treatment of obesity and degenerative disease.

Some fat in the diet is necessary to provide the essential fatty acids. These fats are polyunsaturates and are found abundantly in vegetable oils. About 2 percent of calories provided as essential fatty acids is enough to prevent obvious signs of deficiency. All fats contain a mixture of polyunsaturated, monounsaturated and saturated triglycerides. Oils tend to be high in polyunsaturates and low in saturates; they have a high P/S ratio. The hidden fat in nuts, whole grains and fish is also high in polyunsaturates. Olive oil is a good source of monounsaturated fat. Most animal fats are higher in saturated fats and have a low P/S ratio. Reducing fat intake to 30 percent of calories with 10

TABLE 21
Cholesterol Content of Foods

Food	Weight	Cholesterol (mg)
Liver	3 oz.	372
Egg	1	252
Ladyfingers	4	157
Custard	½ cup	139
Sardines	3-¼ oz.	129
Apple or custard pie	⅛ of 9″ pie	120
Waffles, mix, egg, milk	1 (9 × 9″)	112
Lemon meringue pie	⅛ of 9″ pie	98
Veal	3 oz.	86
Turkey, dark meat, no skin	3 oz.	86
Lamb	3 oz.	83
Beef	3 oz.	80
Pork	3 oz.	76
Spaghetti, meatballs	1 cup	75
Lobster	3 oz.	72
Turkey, light meat, no skin	3 oz.	65
Chicken breast	½ breast	63
Noodles, whole egg	1 cup, cooked	50
Clams	½ cup	50
Macaroni and cheese	1 cup	42
Chicken drumstick	1	39
Oysters	3 oz.	38
Fish fillet	3 oz.	34–75
Whole milk	8 oz.	34
Salmon, canned	3 oz.	30
Hot dog	1	27
Cheddar or Swiss cheese	1 oz.	28
Rice pudding with raisins	1 cup	29
Ice cream	½ cup	27–49
American processed cheese	1 oz.	25
Low-fat milk (2%)	8 oz.	22
Heavy whipping cream	1 tbs.	20
Mozzarella, part skim	1 oz.	18
Brownies	1 (1¾″ × 1¾″ × 1⅛″)	17
Yogurt, plain	8 oz.	17
Cream cheese	1 tbs.	16
Cottage cheese	½ cup	12–24
Butter	1 pat/tsp.	12
Mayonnaise	1 tbs.	10
Sour cream	1 tbs.	8
Half and half	1 tbs.	6
Cottage cheese, dry curd	½ cup	6
Non-fat milk/buttermilk	8 oz.	5
Margarine		0
Beans, grains, nuts, fruits, vegetables		0

on safflower oil announcing that the product contains no cholesterol is a marketing gimmick; no vegetable oil contains cholesterol. Foods which are especially high in this fat are eggs, liver and organ meats, red meats, fish and shellfish, animal fats such as lard and chicken fat, and high-fat dairy products. Cholesterol is found in the lean and the fatty portions of all meats. The cholesterol content of marbled meat is not much greater than that of lean cuts of meat. It occurs in greater concentrations in the organ and glandular meats—heart, kidney, sweetbreads, and liver—than in regular cuts with or without fat. Discarding the fatty portion of meat will reduce the cholesterol and saturated fat, but if a larger portion of lean meat is served, there will be little reduction in cholesterol intake. Egg yolk is one of the most concentrated sources of dietary cholesterol, while egg white contains no cholesterol.

RECOMMENDED DAILY FAT CALORIES
(30 percent of total calorie intake)

Age	Average Daily Calorie Needs	Maximum Fat Calories
Children		
4–6	1300–2300	390–690
7–10	1650–3300	495–990
Males		
11–14	2000–3700	600–1100
15–18	2100–3900	630–1170
19–22	2500–3300	750–990
23–50	2300–3100	810–930
51–75	2000–2800	600–840
76+	1650–2450	495–735
Females		
11–14	1500–3000	450–900
15–18	1200–3000	360–900
19–22	1700–2500	510–750
23–50	1600–2400	480–720
51–75	1400–2200	420–600
76+	1200–2000	360–600
Pregnant	+300	+90
Lactating	+500	+150

percent from each of the three fats—saturated, monounsaturated and polyunsaturated—would meet the daily essential fatty acid needs and positively alter the P/S ratio.

Cholesterol is found only in animal foods. The label

SUGGESTIONS FOR MODIFYING THE DIET TO REDUCE FAT AND CHOLESTEROL

• Eat dried beans and peas as the main source of

protein. Be careful of nuts and seeds—as much as 90 percent of their calories comes from fat.

- Limit meat portions to no more than three or four ounces of lean, well-trimmed meats a day.
- Avoid fried and sautéed foods. If a dish must be fried, use non-stick vegetable sprays or a non-stick pan, or brush the pan lightly with oil. Never reuse frying oils.
- Fish, chicken and turkey: Remove the skin before preparing. Limit consumption of fish canned in oil.
- Goose and duck: High in fat and cholesterol and should be avoided or used sparingly.
- Meats: Beef—choose lean cuts (less than 15 percent fat), such as rump, round and tenderloin. Trim all extra fat before cooking. Ground beef—do not buy preground unless it is extra lean. Have it ground to order from lean round. Lamb—the leg and loin sections are the leanest; trim visible fat. Eliminate organ meats, luncheon meats, bacon, hot dogs and sausages—all are processed meats high in saturated fats and cholesterol.
- Dairy: Choose skim milk and skim-milk cottage cheese or yogurt. Whole milk and hard cheeses are high in saturated fats and cholesterol. (An ounce of cheddar contains 70 percent fat calories and about 30 mg of cholesterol.) Choose low-fat and non-fat cheeses. Dietary emphasis on cultured milk products, such as buttermilk, kefir and yogurt, has been demonstrated to yield significant reductions in blood cholesterol.[9]
- Eggs: Egg yolks supply more cholesterol per serving than any other typically eaten American food. In recipes, use the whites and throw the yolks away. This can be done in pancakes, cakes, cookies, etc.; it does not work in recipes requiring many eggs, such as sponge cake or soufflé. Eat no more than three to four whole eggs a week.
- Fruits and vegetables: Except for avocados and olives, fruits and vegetables are low in fat and all are cholesterol-free. They can be eaten in abundance.
- Breads and cereals: Grains tend to be low in fats; all are devoid of cholesterol unless eggs are used in the recipe. Egg noodles can be used in moderation, but if noodles are eaten in quantity, choose an eggless brand. Avoid baked goods high in saturated fat and cholesterol. This includes doughnuts, pastries, desserts, breakfast rolls, croissants, pie crusts, and waffles and pancakes made with eggs and fat.
- Desserts: Choose desserts low in fats. Gelatin desserts, sherbet, ice milk, corn-starch puddings made with skim milk, fruit, angel food cake, and skim milk yogurt with fruit are excellent choices.
- Salad dressing: Make your own from non-fat yogurt, puréed vegetables, non-fat cottage cheese, garlic, onion, spices, vinegar and other seasonings.

WHEN EATING OUT:

- Appetizers may include fresh fruits and vegetables, juices, seafood cocktail. No sour cream, seasoned butter or seasoned cream.
- Ask for baked potatoes without butter, margarine or sour cream. Use pepper, chives or cottage cheese as a garnish.
- Choose soups such as consommé, barley, vegetable, rice, and split pea. Avoid cheese, egg, onion or cream soups.
- Vegetables are desirable as long as they are not seasoned with butter or oil, cooked in egg yolk batter or served with cheese or other fatty sauces.
- Salads and salad bars offer a wide selection of low-fat items. These may include all vegetables and fruits, turkey, chicken, seafood, lean roast beef, lean ham or low-fat cheese. Potato salad, cole slaw and Waldorf salad should be prepared with little mayonnaise. Use the salad dressing sparingly or use lemon or vinegar.
- All varieties of fish, chicken, Cornish hen, and lean hind-quarter cuts of beef, lamb, pork, and veal may be chosen. Avoid goose, duck and prime cuts, and preparation methods such as fried or batter-dipped, breaded or sautéed. Select broiled, poached, steamed or baked foods.
- Breads are acceptable, especially wholegrain, sourdough or enriched rolls, bagels, muffins and tortillas, or matzos and rye crisp. Be careful of commercial crackers, which are high in fat and salt, and avoid biscuits, croissants, corn muffins, blueberry muffins and butter rolls.
- Cereals and legumes are good selections if prepared without fat. Check the menu or ask the waiter for the style of preparation.
- Desserts can include gelatins, fruit ices, fresh fruit or angel food cake.
- Terms like refried, creamed, cream sauce, au gratin, Parmesan, in cheese sauce, escalloped, au lait, à la mode, marinated, prime, pot pie, au fromage, stewed, basted, casserole, hollandaise, or crispy may imply that fat is used in preparation.

- Foods described as steamed, in broth, in its own juice, poached, garden-fresh, roasted, in tomato sauce or marinara sauce, in broth or in cocktail sauce suggests a low-fat selection.
- Any restaurant that prepares each meal from scratch can accommodate low-fat alterations in the menu.
- Beverages which are common in restaurants and which are low in fat include: fruit and vegetable juices, skim buttermilk or milk tea or coffee.

WHEN SHOPPING:

- Read labels to identify amounts and types of fat. If a fat or fat-rich ingredient is listed first, the product is high in fat calories. If these ingredients appear last on the ingredients list, the product is low in fat. If the package includes a nutrition information panel, this will provide information about the grams and thus the percentage of fat per serving. It also may include the percentage of polyunsaturated to saturated fat and the milligrams of cholesterol.

The following is an example of a vegetable oil label:

Portion size	1 Tablespoon
	(14 grams)
Portions per container (1 Pint)	32
Calories	120
Protein	0 grams
Carbohydrate	0 grams
Fat	14 grams
Percentage of calories from fat**	100%
Polyunsaturated**	8 grams
Saturated**	2 grams
Cholesterol** (0 mg/100 gr)	0 mg
Sodium (0 mg/100 gr)	0 mg

Percentage of the U.S. Recommended Daily Allowances (U.S. RDA)

Contains less than 2 percent of the U.S. RDA of protein, vitamin A, vitamin C, thiamin, riboflavin, niacin, calcium and iron.

**Information on fat and cholesterol content is provided for individuals who, on the advice of a physician, are modifying their total dietary intake of fat and/or cholesterol.

INGREDIENTS: Corn oil with isopropylcitrate and methyl silicone added to preserve freshness.

- Read labels for fat-containing additives. Avoid the following:

Animal fat	Egg and egg	Palm oil
Bacon fat	yolk solids	Shortening
Butter	Lard	Vegetable fat

Coconut	Hydrogenated	Whole-milk solids
Coconut oil	vegetable oil	
Cream and	Milk chocolate	
cream sauce		

Use the following in moderation:

Cocoa butter	Peanut oil
Mustard seed oil	
Olive oil	

WHEN COOKING:

- Trim visible fat from all meats, fish and poultry. This is especially important if the meat is to be roasted or broiled.
- When roasting, elevate the meat off the rack so that it does not sit in the drippings. Do not baste the meat with these drippings; instead, use wine, fruit juices or broth.
- Low temperature roasting (325-350°F) enhances flavor and fat removal. High temperatures tend to seal fats into the meat. High-temperature deep fat fryers produce foods that may contain heart-toxic materials.[10] Steaming, baking, broiling and braising foods are recommended.
- Do not bread or flour meat before roasting; the flour will absorb more fat.
- Remove fat from drippings before making gravies or sauces. Chill the drippings to harden the fat for easy removal.
- Roast chicken and turkey with carrots or onions rather than breaded stuffing, which absorbs and retains fat.
- Use non-stick pans rather than fats in cooking; eliminate or reduce fat intake at the table (for example, reduce 1 tablespooon of butter to 1 teaspoon).
- If fat is used in cooking, use polyunsaturated vegetable oils such as safflower or corn.
- Experiment with herbs and spices to compensate for the loss of excess fat.
- Poach fish for a mild, low-fat method of preparation. Use a small amount of water, white wine or herbs and onion. Simmer—do not boil—the poaching liquid.
- Cook fish only until it is flaky. Overcooking causes fish to be dry and tough.
- Fillets can be wrapped in foil with wine and herbs and baked at 375° until tender.
- Sauté vegetables in defatted chicken stock.
- Mash potatoes with skim milk.
- Use defatted beef or chicken stock for soup base.

TABLE 22
Percentage of Fat Calories in Selected Foods

Food	Amount	Fat Calories	Total Calories	Percent Fat
Beverages				
Beer, wine	1 serving	0	85–150	0
Coffee, tea	1 serving	0	0	0
Fruit, juice	6 oz.	0	75-110	0
Dairy Products				
Milk chocolate				
Cocoa mix	1 cup	108	245	44
Milk, whole	1 cup	81	160	50
2 percent	1 cup	45	145	31
non-fat	1 cup	trace	90	<1
buttermilk	1 cup	trace	90	<1
Cheese,				
Cheddar	1 oz.	81	115	70
Cottage, creamed	1 cup	90	260	35
Cottage, uncreamed	1 cup	9	170	5.3
cream	1 cu. in.	54	60	90
Parmesan	1 oz.	81	130	2
Swiss	1 oz.	72	105	69
processed	1 oz.	81	105	77
Cheese food	1 Tbs.	27	45	60
Cream, half & half	1 cup	252	325	78
sour	1 cup	423	485	87
Whipping, light	1 cup	675	715	94
Whipping, heavy	1 cup	810	840	96
Imitation creamers				
Powdered	1 tsp	9	10	90
Liquid	1 Tbs.	18	20	90
Custard	1 cup	135	305	44
Ice cream	1 cup	126	255	49
Ice milk	1 cup	63	200	31
Yogurt, low fat	1 cup	36	125	29
whole	1 cup	72	150	49
Meat, Poultry, Fish, Shellfish; Related Products				
Bacon	2 slices	72	90	80
Beef				
Hamburger, regular	3 oz.	153	245	63
lean	3 oz.	90	185	49

Food	Amount	Fat Calories	Total Calories	Percent Fat
Steak, broiled				
(lean only)	2.0 oz.	36	115	31
(lean and fat)	3 oz.	243	330	74
Roast, oven-cooked				
rib (lean only)	1.8 oz.	63	125	50
(lean and fat)	3 oz.	306	375	81
Roast, oven-cooked heel of round				
(lean only)	2.7 oz.	27	125	22
(lean and fat)	3 oz.	63	165	38
Canned, corned	3 oz.	90	185	49
Chicken, flesh only				
(broiled)	3 oz.	27	115	23
Drumstick (fried)	2.1	36	90	40
Chili con carne				
with beans	1 cup	135	335	40
without beans	1 cup	342	510	67
Pork				
Ham, light cured	3 oz.	171	245	70
Luncheon, ham	2 oz.	90	135	67
Roast pork	3 oz.	216	310	70
Sausage	1 oz.	63	90	70
Bologna	2 slices	63	80	79
Fish				
Clams	3 oz.	9	45	20
Crab meat	3 oz.	18	85	21
Oysters	1 cup	36	160	23
Salmon	3 oz.	45	120	38
Shrimp	3 oz.	9	100	9
Tuna, canned in oil	3 oz.	63	170	37

Mature Beans, Peas, Nuts; Related Products

Almonds	1 cup	693	850	82
Beans				
Great Northern	1 cup	9	210	4
Navy	1 cup	9	225	4
Cashews	1 cup	576	785	73
Peanuts	1 cup	648	840	77
Peas, split	1 cup	9	290	3

Vegetables

Asparagus through Zucchini		trace		<1
exceptions:				
Candied sweet potatoes	1	63	295	21
All fried, sauteed, or buttered vegetables				

Food	Amount	Fat Calories	Total Calories	Percent Fat

Fruits

Apples through Watermelon ... trace ....<1
exceptions:
    Avocados ....1 ....333 ....370 90

Grain Products·

Breads and cereals...<12
exceptions:
    Biscuits ....1 ....45 ....105 43
    Cupcake ....1 ....27 ....90 30
    Devil's food cake .1 piece ......81 ....235 35
    Gingerbread .....⅛ of 8".......36 ....175 20
    Fruitcake.......1 slice........18 ....55 33
    Cookies.........1 ....27 ....50 54
    Brownies........1 ....54 ....95 57
    Corn muffins ....1 ....36 ....125 29
    Crackers (saltines) .4 ....9 ....50 18
    Danish pastry ....1 ....135 ....275 49
    Pancakes........1 ....18 ....60 30
    Waffles ....1 ....63 ....210 30

All fats: butter, lard, vegetable oils, shortening, margarine, salad dressing, mayonnaise and chicken fat 100

Of the above foods, those which are less than 20 percent fat should provide the bulk of the diet. Those foods containing 20 percent to 35 percent fat should be eaten in moderation. Foods containing more than 35 percent fat should comprise a small portion of the diet; selections from this group should total fewer than two or three a day.

TABLE 23
Sodium Content of Foods

Food	Amount	Sodium (mg)
A-1 Sauce	1 Tbs.	278
Accent	1 tsp.	518
Anchovy paste	1 Tbs.	1540
Bacon	1 slice	209
Baking soda	1 tsp.	1200
Baking powder	1 tsp.	400
Barbeque sauce	½ cup	1019
Beans, dried, no salt	1 cup	13
Beef bouillon	1 cube	960
Bisquick	1 cup	1475
Broccoli, frozen in cheese sauce	½ cup	331
Bouillon cube	1	900
Catsup	1 Tbs.	177
Cabbage, fresh, shredded	½ cup	7
Celery	1 stalk	50
Celery seasoning	1 tsp.	1430
Cereal, corn flakes	1 cup	251
oatmeal, regular, no salt	¾ cup	trace
instant	¾ cup	255
shredded wheat	1 cup	2
Cheese, cheddar	½ cup	350
cottage (2% fat)	½ cup	459
processed	½ cup	812
Cheese soufflé, homemade	1 cup	346
Cherries, raw	1 cup	2
Cherry pie	⅙ of 9"	480
Chicken, no skin	2 pieces	32
Chili, canned	1 cup	1354

Food	Amount	Sodium (mg)
Chili sauce	1 Tbs.	200
Chocolate, baking	100 grams	3
Chocolate fudge topping (Hershey)	100 grams	115
Cocoa mix (Hershey)	100 grams	505
Dill pickle	1	928
Fast foods		
McDonald's*		
Egg McMuffin	1	885
Big Mac	1	1010
Hamburger	1	520
Quarter Pounder	1	735
Quarter Pounder with cheese	1	1236
Strawberry Sundae	1	96
Arby's**		
Roast Beef	1	880
Super Roast Beef	1	1420
Turkey Deluxe	1	1220
Club Sandwich	1	1610
Dairy Queen***		
Brazier Chili Dog	1	939
Super Brazier Dog	1	1552
Frozen dinners (approximate values)		
Beef chop suey with rice	12 oz.	2040
Beef pie	10 oz.	1600
Broccoli au gratin	10 oz.	470
Chicken crepes with mushroom sauce	8 oz.	1040
Chicken pie	10 oz.	1530
Corn soufflé	12 oz.	510
Green bean mushroom casserole	9.5 oz.	1350
Green pepper steak with rice	10 oz.	1500
Ham and asparagus crepes	6 oz.	840
Pizza, cheese	10.5 oz.	850
sausage	12 oz.	1320
Pot pie	1	1807
Spaghetti with meat sauce	14 oz.	1970
Tuna noodle casserole	11.5 oz.	670
Fruit, fresh	½ cup	0
Fruit Pie, Hostess	1	605
Garlic salt	1 tsp.	1850
Lemon juice	1 Tbs.	trace
Macaroni and cheese, packaged	1 cup	574–1086
Margarine, Nucoa	1 Tbs.	160
Margarine, Mazola	1 Tbs.	115
Margarine, Diet Mazola	1 Tbs.	135
Mayonnaise	1 Tbs.	84
Meats, processed		
Bologna	1 oz.	369
Chipped beef	½ cup	3526
Corned beef	3 oz.	802
Cured ham	3 oz.	863
Frankfurters	2 oz.	627
Pepperoni	1 oz.	425
Sausage	1 link	290
Turkey ham	3 oz.	865
Meat tenderizer	1 tsp.	1700
Milk, whole	1 cup	227

Food	Amount	Sodium (mg)
2 percent	1 cup	276
non-fat	1 cup	233
Monosodium glutamate (MSG)	1 tsp.	750
Mr. Goodbar	100 grams	45
Mustard	1 tbs.	150
Olives	10	686
Onion salt	1 tsp.	1620
Orange juice	1 cup	0.2
Pancake: mix, egg, milk	1	412
Peanut Butter, Skippy brand	2 tbs.	150
Peanut Butter Cups, Reese's brand	100 grams	320
Pickle, dill	1 small	800
Pizza, cheese	1 piece	768
Potato, baked, plain	1	6
Potato chips, Ruffles brand	1 oz.	364
Pudding, instant vanilla	½ cup	406
Ravioli, canned	1 cup	1349
Salad dressing, bottled	1 tbs.	200
Salt	1 tsp.	2132
Salt, lite	1 tsp.	1188
Sardines, drained	1 oz.	2093
Sauerkraut, canned	½ cup	878
Soups, commercial		
Bean and pork	1 cup	2136
Chicken gumbo	1 cup	1940
Chicken noodle	1 cup	979
Chicken and rice	1 cup	1872
Clam chowder	1 cup	1915
Cream of asparagus	1 cup	984
Cream of celery	1 cup	1950
Cream of chicken	1 cup	1982
Cup of soup	1 pkg.	900
Split pea	1 cup	1956
Turkey noodle	1 cup	2038
Vegetable beef	1 cup	2135
Vegetable with beef broth	1 cup	1725
Soy sauce	1 tsp.	440
Taco chips, Dorito brand	1 oz.	193
Tomato, raw	1 cup	40
canned	1 cup	313
juice	1 cup	486
sauce	1 cup	1662
Tuna, canned	½ cup	679
TV Dinner	1	1400
V-8 Juice	1 cup	700
Worcestershire sauce	1 Tbs.	315

(Source: Nutritive Value of American Foods in Common Units. Agricultural Handbook 456, USDA, 1975.)

(*Source: McDonald's Corporation, Oak Brook, Illinois: Nutritional Analysis by Raltech Services, Inc. Madison, Wisconsin.)

(**Source: Consumer Affairs, Arby's Inc., Atlanta, Georgia: Nutritional Analysis by Technological Resources, Camden, New Jersey.)

(***Source: International Dairy Queen Inc., Minneapolis, Minn. Nutritional Analysis by Raltech Services Inc. Madison, Wisconsin.)

Use skim milk and flour instead of cream or whole milk when preparing creamed soups.

GOAL 7: Limit the intake of sodium by reducing the intake of salt (sodium chloride) to about 5 grams/day.

In the body, salt (sodium) is found in tears, blood, sweat and every tissue and cell. The saltiness of the human body is akin to sea water. Under normal circumstances, the human body requires about .2 grams of sodium a day to maintain this saltiness, yet the daily consumption in the United States is as high as 20 grams. In spite of sodium's essential role in numerous metabolic functions (see p. 75) an excess of this mineral is associated with the development of hypertension (see p. 76 and pp. 156–157).

Commercially prepared foods are high in salt. Salt is used as a flavoring agent, and in some cases, such as canned and instant soups, it is the primary flavoring agent. It may be used to mask less pleasant tastes in packaged foods.

The *Dietary Goals* recommend limiting salt intake to 5 grams or one teaspoon a day. Since salt is 40 percent sodium, this amount is equivalent to 2 grams of sodium.

To reduce salt:

- Avoid the heavy-handed salt shaker. Reduce or eliminate salt in cooking, at the table or both.
- Reduce consumption of foods processed in brine (olives, sauerkraut, pickles).
- Avoid commercial snack items (potato and corn chips, salted peanuts or popcorn, pretzels, crackers)
- Reduce consumption of salted or smoked meats, sandwich meats, bacon, hot dogs, corned or chipped beef, sausage and salt pork.
- Reduce consumption of salted or smoked fish, pickled herring, caviar, salted and dried fish, sardines and smoked salmon.
- Be aware that prepared catsup, mustard, Worcestershire sauce, horseradish, bouillon cubes, barbeque and soy sauce contain salt and contribute to the total sodium intake.
- Limit cheeses, especially processed selections. These are high in salt.
- Eliminate canned and instant soups, packaged meat extenders, seasoning mixes and packaged gravies and sauces.
- Read the labels on foods and medications to identify sodium additives and unsuspected sodium-containing items, such as baking soda, monosodium glutamate (MSG), cough medicines, laxatives, aspirin, sedatives and the food additives sodium phosphate, sodium alginate, sodium nitrate and many more.

REFERENCES

1. Angel, A. and Roncarl, D. Medical complications of obesity. *Can. Med. Assoc. J.*, 119: 1408, 1978.

2. Hubert, H., Feinleib, M., McNamara, P. et al. Obesity as an independent risk factor for cardiovascular disease—a 26-year follow-up of participants in the Framingham Heart Study. *Circulation*, 67: 968–977, 1983.

3. Farinaro, E., Stamler, J. and Upton, M. Plasma glucose levels: Long term effect of diet in the Chicago coronary prevention evaluation program. *Ann. Int. Med.*, 86: 147, 1977.

4. Brewster, L. and Jacobson, M. *The Changing American Diet: A Chronicle of American Eating Habits from 1910–1980.* Washington, DC: Center for Science in the Public Interest, 1983.

5. Connor, W. and Connor, S. in *Present Knowledge in Nutrition*, Washington DC.: The Nutrition Foundation, 1976.

6. Lecos, C. Sugar: How sweet it is—and isn't. *Consumer*, Feb. 1980, 21–23.

7. Yudkin, J. Dietary factors in arteriosclerosis: Sucrose. *Lipids*, 13: 370–372, 1980.

8. Reiser, S., Hallfrisch, J., Michaelis, O., et al. Isocaloric exchange of dietary starch and sucrose in humans: I. Effects on levels of fasting blood lipids. *Am. J. Clin. Nutr.*, 32: 1659–1669, 1979.

9. Hepner, G., Fried, R., Fusetti, L., et al., Hypocholesterolemic effect of yogurt and milk. *Am. J. Clin. Nutr.*, January 1979: 19–24.

10. Kummerow, F. Nutrition imbalance and angiotoxins as dietary risk factors in coronary heart disease. *Am. J. Clin. Nutr.*, January 1979: 58–83.

Part VI
NUTRITION AND DRUGS

17

·················DRUG-NUTRIENT INTERACTIONS·····················

INTRODUCTION

NUTRIENTS AND DRUGS have a great deal in common. They can share common routes of absorption and compete for transport mechanisms, binding sites and excretion. The molecular structure of certain drugs may actually be very similar to all or part of a vitamin's structure. Because of these similarities and shared metabolic pathways, nutrients can affect drug activity and drugs can affect the nutritional status of individuals.

Although nutrients can affect drug activity and alter the expected therapeutic outcome, this type of nutrient-drug interaction is generally addressed by the pharmacist through the use of warning labels at the time the drug is dispensed. But the effects of prescription and over-the-counter drugs on the patient's nutritional status are rarely considered, outside of the potassium recommendation with certain diuretics. Current research now suggests that the nutrient losses induced by many popular prescription and OTC drugs may impair the patient's health to the extent that the disease for which the medication was originally prescribed is actually encouraged!

The greatest impact of drug-induced nutritional deficiencies is on the elderly, the group that consumes the majority of prescription and OTC drugs. It has been estimated that in the next few years, 70 percent of all prescriptions will be written for individuals over the age of fifty. This group of 25 million individuals is at risk for nutritional inadequacy even before they are placed on medications or elect to self-medicate.[1] Drugs that can further impair the nutritional status of these individuals will have a significant effect on their overall health status.

Another area of concern with regard to drug-nutrient interactions is substance abuse. The nutrient losses induced by alcohol and the opiates have been studied for many years. But only recently has it been suggested that the nutritional impairment induced by drug abuse may actually perpetuate the craving for continual drug usage. Models using nutrition and exercise as neurochemical modulators for improving compliance with alcohol and drug treatment programs are currently being explored.

This section is divided into two chapters. Chapter 17 deals with prescription and OTC drugs and their nutritional interrelationships. Chapter 18 reviews the basis for a nutritional approach to improve the recovery process for alcoholics and drug addicts.

DRUG EFFECTS ON NUTRIENT INTAKE

The side effects of some drugs can increase appetite, while the side effects of others can decrease it. And certain drugs can have a dual effect, depending upon age and situational factors. Although drugs that can increase appetite may be of concern, it is the drug-induced appetite suppression that presents the more serious problem. Populations that may already be at risk for nutritional adequacy, such as the elderly, those with chronic disease, dieters, alcoholics, cigarette smokers, new mothers, adolescents and certain ethnic minorities, could have their health severely compromised by drugs that suppress appetite.

DRUGS THAT INCREASE APPETITE

Certain tricyclic antidepressants, e.g., amitriptyline (Elavil), can produce a significant increase in appetite, food intake and a craving for sweets, resulting in considerable weight gain. Sometimes these drugs produce agitation in the elderly, which in turn affects appetite.

Chlordiazepoxide (Librium) and diazepam (Valium) at low dosages may increase appetite and food intake in the elderly. But at higher dosages these drugs may create lethargy and disinterest. The antihistamine cyproheptadine (Periactin) can also stimulate appetite in the elderly.

DRUGS THAT DECREASE APPETITE

Cancer drugs can produce significant anorexia and weight loss.[2] A recent study suggests that the anorexia associated with chemotherapeutic agents may be due to alterations in serotonin metabolism rather than solely to the nausea that is produced.[3] Methotrexate, mithramycin (Mithracin), carmustine (BICNU), doxorubicin (Adriamycin), cyclophosphamide (Cytoxan), asparaginase (Elspar) and daunorbucin (Cerubidine) commonly cause anorexia, thereby further compromising the patient's immune system.

Alcohol abuse can cause anorexia, especially in the elderly.[4] Anorexia in alcoholics may be due to thiamin, zinc or protein deficiencies. It may also be caused by gastritis, pancreatitis, hepatitis, lactose intolerance, ketoacidosis, cirrhosis and other related disorders.

High doses of digitalis can cause anorexia, as can the antiarthritic drug d-penicillamine (Cuprimine). D-pencillamine produces anorexia by impairing taste acuity due to drug-induced deificiencies of zinc and copper.

Conditions that might cause anorexia, as opposed to anorexia resulting from the drugs used to treat these conditions, include: acute bronchitis, acute cholecystitis, acute confusional psychoses, burns, fractures, generalized dermatitis or other dermatoses with severe itching, intestinal obstruction, oral candidiasis (yeast infections of the mouth), other viral and bacterial infections and pneumonia (viral or bacterial).

DRUG EFFECTS ON NUTRIENT ABSORPTION

There are a number of mechanisms whereby a drug can impair the absorption of a nutrient. A drug can absorb a nutrient, change the characteristics of the nutrient so that it is rendered insoluble, alter pH, produce maldigestion or impair mucosal function, which results in nutrient malabsorption.

Laxatives such as phenolphthalein (Alophen, Ex-Lax, Feen-a-Mint), senna (Senokot) and bisacodyl (Dulcolax) may cause calcium and vitamin D losses because of an increase in gut motility coupled with mucosal change.[5] Another laxative, mineral oil, impairs the absorption of beta-carotene and vitamins A, D and K.[6-9] Beta-carotene becomes solubilized in mineral oil and therefore unavailable for absorption.[10]

The cholesterol-lowering agent cholestyramine (Questran) may induce steatorrhea and malabsorption of fat-soluble vitamins.[11] It can also reduce absorption of folic acid by absorbing this nutrient onto the anion-exchange resin.[12]

The magnesium and aluminum hydroxide antacids (Maalox, WinGel, Kolantyl, Aludrox, Creamalin, Mylanta, Gelusil, DiGel, etc.) are another category of drugs that can impair nutrient absorption. These antacids can precipitate dietary phosphate and lead to secondary osteomalacia.[13,14] Other drugs that can lead to bone disorders by impairing calcium absorption are listed in Table 24. The elderly, who frequently have a decreased capacity for calcium absorption, are particularly at risk for drug-induced bone disorders.

Antacids can also decrease the absorption of folacin by altering the pH of the small intestine.[15] Drug-induced alterations of intestinal pH can have a serious impact on the availability of another nutrient, vitamin B12. Cimetidine (Tagamet) and the slow-release potassium drugs (Slow-K, Micro-K, Kaon-Cl, K-Tab, Klotrix) can reduce B12 absorption.

Alcohol is particularly damaging to the intestinal mucosa, which contributes to alcohol-induced nutrient deficiencies. Thiamin and folacin are two of the many nutrients at risk in the alcoholic which have impaired absorption due to decreased intestinal function.[19,20] The range of nutrients that may be at risk in the alcoholic is summarized below. Table 25 summarizes some of the major drug-induced nutrient malabsorption mechanisms.

NUTRIENT DEPLETION IN ALCOHOLISM	
1) Vitamin Depletion	2) Mineral Depletion
Folic Acid	Magnesium
Thiamin	Zinc
Riboflavin	
Niacin	3) Electrolyte Depletion
Ascorbic Acid	
Vitamin B6	4) Amino Acid Depletion
Vitamin B12	
	5) Fatty Acid Depletion

TABLE 24
Major Drug-Induced Calcium Malabsorption Mechanisms

Drugs	Malabsorption	Usage	Mechanism
Prednisone (other gluco-corticoids)	Calcium	Allergic and collagen disease	Calcium transportation
Diphosphonates	Calcium	Paget's disease	1,25-DHCC formation
Glutethimide	Calcium	Sedative	Accelerated catabolism of vitamin D and active metabolites
Phenobarbital	Calcium	Anticonvulsants	
Diphenylhydantoin	Calcium	Anticonvulsants	
Primidone	Calcium	Anticonvulsants	" "

TABLE 25
Major Drug-Induced Nutrient Malabsorption Mechanisms

Drugs	Malabsorption	Usage	Mechanism
Biguanides: Metformin Phenformin	Vitamin B12	Hypoglycemic agents (in diabetes)	Competitive inhibition of B12 absorption
Cholestyramine	Fat, Vit. A, K, B12, D, Fe	Hypocholesterolemic agent	Binding of bile acids (salts) and nutrients, e.g. Fe
Colchicine	Fat, carotene, Na, K, Vit B12, lactose	Anti-inflammatory agent in gout	Mitotic arrest Structural defect Enzyme damage
Mineral Oil	Carotene, Vit. A, D, K	Laxative	Physical barrier Nutrients dissolve in mineral oil & are lost micelle formation
Neomycin	Fat, nitrogen, Na, K, Ca, Fe, lactose, sucrose, Vit. B12	Antibiotic to "sterilize" gut	Structural defect Pancreatic lipase Binding of bile acids (salts)
Para-amino salicylic acid	Fat, folate, Vitamin B12	Anti-tuberculosis agent	Mucosal block in B12 uptake
Phenolphthalein	Vitamin D, CA	Laxative	Intestinal hurry K depletion, loss of structural integrity
Potassium Chloride	Vitamin B12	Potassium repletion	Ileal pH altered
Salicylazo-sulfpyridine (Azulfidine)	Folate	Anti-inflammatory agent in ulcerative colitis, and regional enteritis	Mucosal block in folate uptake

DRUG EFFECTS ON NUTRIENT UTILIZATION

Drug effects on nutrient bioavailability are considerably more complex and diverse than drug-induced nutrient malabsorption. Drugs that are structurally similar to vitamins can actually block metabolic processes. Certain drugs have chemical groupings that can block metabolic processes by binding to active sites on enzymes. Whether a drug interferes with a nutrient component or components of a single biological system or impairs nutrient-dependent and enzymatic function, the consequences can lead to both acute and chronic toxic effects.

When all drug-induced vitamin deficiencies are considered, the absorption and utilization of three nutrients in particular appear to be affected more frequently than others. These nutrients are vitamin B6, folate and vitamin B12.

VITAMIN B6

Five major categories of drugs are known to act as vitamin B6 antagonists or to increase the turnover of B6. These are: alcohol; hydrazine drugs (INH; hydralazine); anti-Parkinson drugs (levodopa); anti-Wilson drugs (D-pencillamine); and oral contraceptives.

Vitamin B6 is converted in the body to a key coenzyme, pyridoxal-5-phosphate (PLP), which plays a crucial role in at least nine different pathways for amino acid metabolism. Drugs that have an amino group are those that are most likely to form complexes with PLP, resulting in decreased drug activity and inactivation of the coenzyme.

Generally, the vitamin B6 deficiencies induced by drugs do not produce clinical symptoms. This is not to say that drug-induced marginal deficiencies are insignificant, especially in individuals who have an increased B6 requirement that may be many times that of the RDAs. Brin and others have demonstrated that significant physiological and behavioral changes take place in marginal deficiency states prior to the appearance of clinical symptoms (Table 26).[21] Table 27 lists the personality changes recorded on the Minnesota Multiphasic Personality Inventory in individuals with certain marginal nutrient deficiencies.[22-24]

The alterations in behavior that can occur in subclinical malnutrition prior to the appearance of a specific deficiency syndrome can worsen life habits that have been associated with some of the major degenerative diseases. Lack of sleep, irritability, lack of energy and decreased ability to adapt to stress may not appear to

TABLE 26
The Progressive Development of Vitamin B1 Deficiency

Deficiency Stage	Symptoms
1. Preliminary	Depletion of tissue stores (due to diet, malabsorption, abnormal metabolism, etc.). Urinary excretion depressed.
2. Biochemical	Enzyme activity reduced due to coenzyme insufficiency. Urinary excretion negligible.
3. Physiological and behavioral	Loss of appetite with reduced body weight, insomnia or somnolence, irritableness, adverse changes of MMPI scores.
4. Clinical	Exacerbated nonspecific symptoms plus appearance of specific deficiency syndrome.
5. Anatomical	Clear specific syndromes with tissue pathology. Death ensues unless treatment initiated.

TABLE 27
Minnesota Multiphasic Personality Inventory in Human Subjects with Marginal Deficiencies for Thiamine (B1), Ascorbic Acid (C) and Riboflavin (B2)

Personality Change Scales	Deficiency B1	Deficiency B2	C
Hypochondriasis	X	X	X
Depression	X	X	X
Hysteria	X	X	X
Psychopathic deviation		X	
Hypomania		X	

be life-threatening conditions. But these symptoms of sub-clinical micronutrient deficiences, often drug-induced, are not conducive to exercise and dietary programs that can reduce the risk of heart disease and cancer. Therefore, drug-induced vitamin or mineral deficiencies, no matter how minor they might appear, need to be addressed by all health care practitioners.

Alcohol

Alcohol-induced malnutrition is complex and is now known to affect neurotransmission and opiate receptor sites. The resulting behavioral effects may actually play a role in perpetuating the drive for alcohol. This subject is discussed in chapter 18 of this section but is mentioned here as it relates to vitamin B6 status.

The impaired neurological function seen in alcoholism is due in part to an alcohol-induced B6 deficiency. Alcohol interferes with B6 function, as demonstrated by decreased PLP values. Animal studies suggest that alcohol may actually impair the synthesis of PLP.[25] Other studies have demonstrated that there is increased catabolism of PLP in chronic alcoholism. Either way, B6 function is altered and PLP-dependent systems are impaired.

Hydrazine-Derived Drugs

There are a number of drugs that are hydrazine derivatives. The antituberculous drugs (such as INH), antihypertensive agents (such as hydralazine [Apresoline]), antidepressants, MAO inhibitors, and some anticarcinogenic agents all have antivitamin B6 activity. Hydrazine-derived drugs can readily form a hydrazone with PLP, thereby inactivating this essential coenzyme.

The antituberculous drug INH is well known for the behavioral and neurological effects it causes as a result of decreased B6 function. INH-induced irritability, sleep problems, psychosis, peripheral neuropathy and convulsions are all readily corrected with adequate doses of B6.

The inhibitory neurotransmitter GABA is dependent upon the enzyme glutamate decarboxylase. This enzyme requires the coenzymatic function of the B6 derivative PLP. In some individuals, INH competitively inhibits glutamate decarboxylase to such an extent that seizures occur. Other INH-inducted symptoms are due to hydrazone formation with PLP.

Another drug used extensively in the treatment of tuberculosis, cycloserine, induces B6 deficiencies by acting as an antagonist. The drug forms a Schiff base with PLP, resulting in inactivation of the B6 coenzyme.

The metal chelator drug penicillamine can interfere with vitamin B6 metabolism. This drug, commonly used for the treatment of Wilson's disease, can combine with PLP to form a thiazolidine derivative, thereby inactivating PLP and producing neurological disorders.[26]

Generally, vitamin B6 administered along with the drugs mentioned so far will prevent the drug-induced nutrient deficiency. But in the case of the anti-Parkinson's drug L-DOPA, B6 supplementation can decrease the efficacy of the drug. The dopamine neurotransmitter system, which is impaired in Parkinson's disease, can be modulated by the administration of the dopamine precursor L-DOPA. L-DOPA can increase dopamine synthesis only if adequate B6 is available for decarboxylation of L-DOPA. But PLP can form a Schiff base with L-DOPA which in turn exerts an inhibitory action on L-DOPA decarboxylase, thereby decreasing the effectiveness of L-DOPA. The current approach of administering a decarboxylase inhibitor such as carbidopa along with the vitamin B6 can prevent this conflict.

One way in which drug-induced B6 deficiencies can cause behavioral problems is by decreasing the availability of the neurotransmitter serotonin. As indicated in Figure 18, the amino acid L-tryptophan is the precursor for serotonin. But if L-tryptophan is encouraged to enter the kynurenine pathway, serotonin synthesis will be discouraged. Steroid hormones can compete with the B6 coenzyme PLP for binding with apoenzymes and encourage L-tryptophan to enter the kynurenine pathway, thereby decreasing the synthesis of serotonin. The depression or mood swings observed in women using oral contraceptives may be due to this mechanism.

Commonly prescribed drugs that may induce a vitamin B6 deficiency are listed in the box below. Although many drugs can induce vitamin B6 deficiencies, supplements of the vitamin with certain drugs may decrease the drug's activity. (Vitamin B6 is not contraindicated with the drugs listed in the box.) High doses of either vitamin B6 or folic acid given to patients maintained on phenytoin and/or phenobarbital for seizure disorders can significantly lower drug blood levels and therapeutic efficacy.[27–29] (See Table 27 for suggested supplement dosages of these nutrients with phenytoin and phenobarbital.)

COMMONLY PRESCRIBED DRUGS THAT MAY INDUCE A B6 DEFICIENCY

APRESOLINE®	ORAL CONTRA-
DONNATAL®	CEPTIVES
DELTASONE®	PREMARIN®
MEDROL®	SERAPES®

VITAMIN B12 AND FOLATE

Vitamin B12 and folate are so closely associated that a drug-induced deficiency of either nutrient can result in megaloblastic anemia, thrombocytopenia, leukopenia, atrophic glossitis, and megaloblastic changes in any organ that has rapid cell turnover, such as the gastrointestinal tract or the uterine cervix. Drug-induced folic acid deficiencies appear to be more prevalent than drug-induced cobalamin deficiencies.

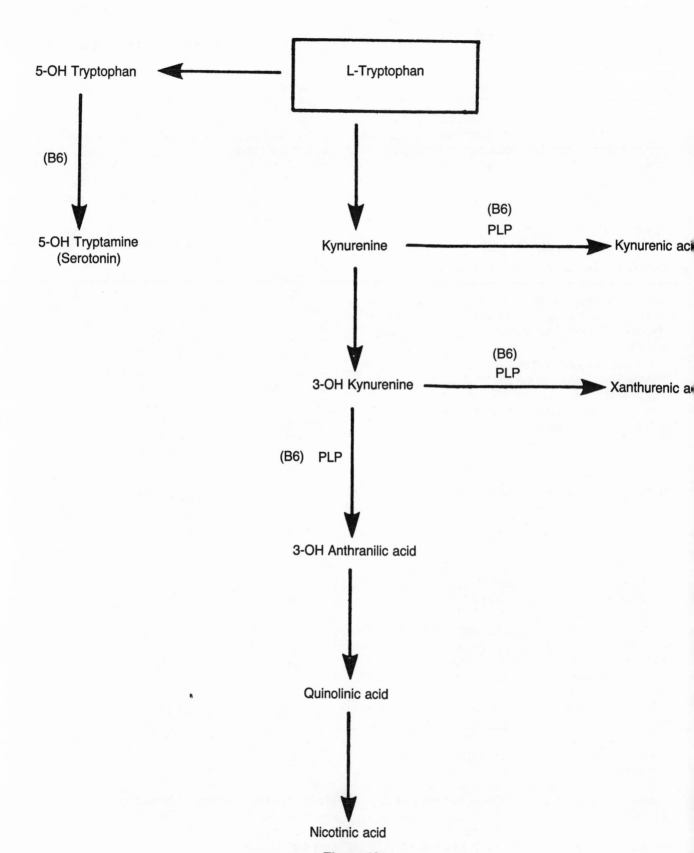

Figure 18

*The role of vitamin B6 and tryptophan in the forma-
tion of the neurotransmitter serotonin*

Oral contraceptives can induce low serum cobalamin levels, although the significance of this appears to be uncertain.[30–32] But a number of cases of megaloblastic anemia due to folate deficiency have been observed in women taking oral contraceptives. These drugs may cause an increased demand for folate, especially in the reproductive system. [30]

A significant number of patients taking anticonvulsants have subnormal serum, red cell and cerebrospinal fluid folate levels.[33] Although megaloblastic anemia is rare in these patients, macrocytosis is very common. There are a number of conflicting reports suggesting mechanisms for the interaction of these drugs with folate.

Folic acid therapy, as mentioned earlier, can interfere with the efficacy of certain anticonvulsant drugs, particularly phenytoin.[34,35] But many studies have shown no effect of supplemental folic acid therapy on the frequency of seizures.[36] Daphne Roe, M.D. suggests that patients maintained on phenytoin (Dilantin) supplement their diet with folic acid at levels up to 2 mg/day (see Table 28).

The incidence of megaloblastic anemia in alcoholics is anywhere from 1 percent to 40 percent depending on patient selection. Alcohol-induced folic acid deficiencies have long been recognized. The mechanism for this drug-induced nutrient deficiency is primarily through poor dietary intake, although alcohol also acts as a folate antagonist.[37,39,40] Alcohol-induced malabsorption may also contribute to folate deficiency.[38,41]

Methotrexate, a drug used extensively in the treatment of cancer and severe psoriasis, exerts its therapeutic effect by interfering with folate metabolism. This drug inhibits the enzyme dihydrofolate reductase, which is necessary for the conversion of folic acid to dihydrofolate, and dihydrofolate to tetrahydrofolate. The result of this drug-nutrient interaction is impaired DNA synthesis and cessation of cellular growth. Since this is the desired therapeutic outcome, folic acid supplementation is contraindicated with methotrexate.

There are other drugs that have as one of their side effects the inhibition of dihydrofolate reductase. Two commonly prescribed drugs with this side effect are trimethoprim (Bactrim, Septra) and triamterene (Dyazide, Dyrenium). These drugs can cause megaloblastic anemia, but generally only in individuals already at risk for nutrient adequacy, such as alcoholics, dieters and the elderly.[42] The brand names of frequently prescribed drugs that can induce a folate or vitamin B12 deficiency are listed in the box.

COMMONLY PRESCRIBED DRUGS THAT MIGHT INDUCE A B12 OR FOLATE DEFICIENCY

ACHROMYCIN	MICRO-K
ALDORIL	MACRODANTIN
ALDOMET	MEDROL
BACTRIM	ORAL CONTRACEPTIVES
BUTAZOLIDIN	PREMARIN
DYAZIDE	PERCODAN
DONNATAL	SEPTRA
DELTASONE	SLOW K
KLOTRIX	SUMYCIN
K-LYTE	STELAZINE
K-TAB	TAGAMET

DRUG-INDUCED MINERAL DEFICIENCIES

Many drugs, especially the cardiovascular drugs, can cause mineral deficiencies. Because of the delicate interrelationships among minerals, drug-induced mineral depletion may cause greater imbalances than the drug-induced vitamin deficiencies. It is not uncommon for patients, especially the elderly, to be taking several drugs at the same time that can cause serious mineral imbalances.

Hypokalemia with potassium depletion is a well-recognized side effect of diuretics. The thiazides, furosemide and ethacrynic acid can all cause potassium depletion. Other drugs that may cause hypokalemia and/or potassium depletion include levodopa, amphotericin B, phenolphthalein, senna, bisacodyl, corticosteroids, gentamicin, and salicylates at excessive dosages.

Recently it has become increasingly apparent that the diuretics mentioned above can cause serious magnesium imbalances. Most practitioners and pharmacists are aware of diuretic-induced potassium deficiencies and frequently prescribe potassium supplements. Since diuretic-induced magnesium deficiencies are less well known, this consequence of diuretic therapy may be more serious.

The thiazide diuretics are a major class of drugs that can induce a magnesium deficiency. This popular drug is used to treat hypertension, but it may increase the risk for cardiac disorders by inducing a magnesium deficiency.

Magnesium is an activator of numerous enzyme systems that control carbohydrate, fat and electrolyte metabolism; protein synthesis; nucleic acid synthesis and membrane transport and integrity. Magnesium deficiencies can lead to convulsions and cardiac arrhythmias. Mildred Seelig, M.D., suggests that Americans are at risk for magnesium adequacy, not necessarily because of inadequate intake, but because of excessive phosphate, fat, sugar and alcohol consumption.[43] Drugs such as the thiazide diuretics increase the risk for magnesium adequacy.

The thiazide diuretics, in addition to inducing magnesium deficiencies, can increase the risk for heart disorders through another mechanism. Thiazides can cause abnormalities in glucose and lipid metabolism.[44,45] Both short- and long-term treatment with the thiazide diuretics can increase LDL cholesterol and decrease HDL cholesterol. Plasma triglyceride levels may also be elevated by the thiazides. This effect may result from drug-induced insulin resistance that causes a secondary disturbance in carbohydrate and lipid metabolism. Now that cholesterol levels have been positively associated with an increased risk for heart disease, medical practitioners should become even more aware of the alterations in fat metabolism that occur with the thiazides. Magnesium supplementation in patients taking thiazide can play a significant role in decreasing some of the untoward effects of these popular diuretics.

Additional medications that can induce a magnesium deficiency include: furosemide, ethacrynic acid, gentamicin, cisplatin, neomycin and colchicine. Magnesium supplements should be recommended with these drugs.

The other mineral most frequently involved in drug-nutrient interactions is calcium. Drugs that impair calcium absorption have been discussed earlier and are listed in Table 24. There are additional drugs that increase the risk of osteomalacia or osteoporosis by inducing calcium imbalances through mechanisms other than malabsorption. The drugs that can lead to these conditions, either by decreasing absorption, increasing excretion or through other mechanisms, include furosemide, ethacrynic acid, phenolphthalein, phenobarbital, phenytoin, corticosteroids, aluminum and magnesium hydroxide, neomycin and colchicine.

Iron depletion may occur in individuals taking analgesics and NSAI agents. Aspirin and indomethacin (Indocin) are two examples of drugs that can cause iron deficiency.[46,47]

In selecting appropriate nutrients for supplementation during drug therapy, it is suggested that a balanced formula rather than single-entity nutrients be recommended. This is particularly true with mineral supplementation, where an excess of one mineral can impair the absorption and availability of another mineral. For a list of companies providing balanced formulas specifically designed to prevent drug-induced nutritional deficiencies, write: Health Media of America, P.O. Box 2173, Del Mar, CA 92014.

OTC DRUGS

Chien et al. reported in 1978 that 83 percent of all individuals over sixty years old take two or more drugs.[48] Of the total medications used by this population, 40 percent are over-the-counter drugs. In a similar study conducted the same year, Guttman reported that 61 percent of the elderly take OTC drugs, 31.7 percent take analgesics and 7.1 percent take laxatives. Analgesics and laxatives, along with antacids, are the major classes of OTC drugs that can cause nutritional deficiencies.[50] The significance of these nutrient losses depends upon the overall nutritional status of the patient. OTC drug-induced nutrient losses can cause serious disorders in the elderly individual who is marginally nourished or suffering from subclinical malnutrition. The nutritional effects of antacids, laxatives and non-narcotic analgesics are listed in the box.

NUTRITIONAL EFFECTS OF NON-NARCOTIC ANALGESICS

Iron deficiency
(Aspirin)
Folate depletion
(Aspirin)
Sodium depletion
(Acetaminophen)

NUTRITIONAL EFFECTS OF LAXATIVE USE AND ABUSE

Hypokalemia and potassium deficiency
(Bisacodyl, phenolphthalein, senna)
Malabsorption syndromes
(Bisacodyl, phenolphthalein, senna, mineral oil)
Protein-losing enteropathy (phenolphthalein)

NUTRITIONAL EFFECTS OF ANTACID USE AND ABUSE

Aluminum toxicity (aluminum hydroxide)
Folate malabsorption (sodium bicarb)
Magnesium overload (magnesium hydroxide)
Milk-alkali syndrome (sodium bicarb)
Phosphate depletion (aluminum/magnesium)
Sodium overload (sodium bicarb)

VITAMINS, MINERALS AND DRUG METABOLISM

All drugs must be detoxified or undergo biotransformation in order to be excreted. The biochemical reactions involved in this process are mainly enzymatic, and, as such, require certain vitamins and minerals as co-factors. Individuals at risk for vitamin and mineral adequacy, especially the elderly on poly drug therapy, may have an impaired ability to metabolize certain drugs.

Most drugs are metabolized in two phases. First, if they are not water-soluble, they are converted into water-soluble products to enable transport and excretion. Next, they may be conjugated to facilitate removal from the body. Ascorbic acid, calcium, copper, glycine, iron, magnesium, nicotinic acid, pantothenic acid, protein, riboflavin and iron play key roles in the first step of drug detoxification or biotransformation. If any

of these nutrients are deficient, incomplete drug metabolism is possible, leading to prolonged drug action or side effects from incomplete drug metabolites.

In the second step of drug biotransformation, the following nutrients, along with carbohydrates, amino acids and fats, play a key role: vitamin B12, nicotinic acid, folic acid, lipoic acid and pantothenic acid. It is important for the practitioner to note how essential vitamins and minerals are involved in drug metabolism.

It should be noted that there has been some discussion recently regarding the effects of large doses of single nutrients on drug metabolism. Additional research in this area is needed before any recommendations are made beyond those already mentioned in this chapter. Table 28, prepared by Daphne Roe, M.D., Professor of Nutrition at Cornell University, may be helpful in determining appropriate nutrient dosages for protecting against drug-induced nutritional deficiencies.

TABLE 28
Drug-Nutrient Interactions

Therapeutic Class	DRUG NAME Proprietary Examples	Generic/ Active Compound	Recommended Daily Vitamin/Mineral Supplement or Restriction During Drug Therapy*
Dermatological preparation	Accutane®	isotretinoin	Avoid vitamin A supplement
Antibiotics	Panmycin® Achromycin® Other Aureomycin®	tetracycline chlortetracycline	Riboflavin (B2), 5 mg Ascorbic acid, 100–200 mg Calcium, 0.8–1.5 gm**
Anticonvulsants	Dilantin® Mysoline®	phenytoin primidone	Vitamin D 400–800 IU† Vitamin K, 1–5 mg Folic acid, 0.4–1.0 mg (not > 2.0 mg/day) Vitamin K, 1–5 mg†
Anti-inflammatory	Azulfidine® Bayer aspirin® Bufferin® Other aspirin Indocin®	sulfasalazine aspirin indomethacin	Folic acid, 0.4–1.0 mg Ascorbic acid 50–100 mg Folic acid, 0.4–1.0 mg Iron, 20–50 mg Iron, 20–50 mg
Antilipemic	Questran® Colestid®	cholestyramine colestipol	Vitamin A, 2000–5000 IU Vitamin D, 200–800 IU Vitamin K, 2–25 mg‡ Folic acid, 0.4–1.0 mg
Antituberculous	INH Rifamate®	isoniazid rifampin-isoniazid	Vitamin B6, 25–50 mg Niacin, 15–25 mg Vitamin D, 400–800 IU

Therapeutic Class	DRUG NAME Proprietary Examples	Generic/ Active Compound	Recommended Daily Vitamin/Mineral Supplement or Restriction During Drug Therapy*
Anticoagulant	Coumadin®	coumarin anticoagulants	Avoid vitamin K
Diuretic	Dyrenium® Dyazide®	triamterene	Folic acid, 0.4–1.0 mg
Gastrointestinal	Agoral®	mineral oil	Vitamin A, 5000–10,000[11] IU Vitamin D, 400–800 IU
	Soda mint	antacids	Folic acid, 0.4–0.8 mg
Hypotensive	Apresoline®	hydralazine	Vitamin B6, 25–100 mg
Oral contraceptives	Norinyl® Demulen® Ovral® Ortho-Novum® Modicon® and others	estrogen/progestin	Vitamin B6, 1.5–5 mg Folic acid, 0.4–1.0 mg Avoid high doses of vitamin C (i.e. ≥ 1000 mg)
Tranquilizer	Thorazine® Mellaril®	chlorpromazine thioridazine other phenothiazines	Riboflavin, 2–5 mg
Other	Lardoopa®	levodopa	Vitamin B6, restrict supplement < 5 mg
	Depen®	penicillamine	Vitamin B6 24–100 mg

Pregnant or lactating women should consult their physicians for specific micronutrient recommendations.

*Short-term drug therapy may or may not necessitate specific vitamin/mineral supplementation.

**Calcium-containing foods and supplements should be given ≥ 2 hours away from drug dose.

†If Dilantin (phenytoin)-induced demineralization is identified, give vitamin D 2000 IU/day. Pregnant women or Dilantin or Mysoline should receive vitamin K, 5 mg/day for 3 days prior to delivery and neonate should receive 1 mg.

‡Routine use of vitamin K1 not required with Questran (cholestyramine) or Colestid (colestipol). Give vitamin K1 I.M. in stated dosage range if hypoprothrombinemia exists.

[11]When daily dose of mineral oil preparation equals or exceeds 30 ml/day, a vitamin supplement is required. Recommended supplement, vitamin A, 5000–10,000 IU/day plus vitamin D, 400–800 IU/day. Mineral oil should be taken at bedtime and never within 2 hours of a meal. Toxic signs of hypervitaminosis A may occur with chronic intake of vitamin A (retinol), ≥ 50,000 IU/day in the adult and ≥ 20,000 IU/day in the infant or child. Hypervitaminosis D may occur with chronic intake of vitamin D ≥ 4000 IU/day or ≥ 1000 IU/day in the infant or child.

Prepared by Daphne Roe, M.D., Professor of Nutrition, Cornell University, Ithaca, New York, as a service to the health profession by Hoffman-La Roche Inc.

REFERENCES

1. *Statistical Abstracts of the United States*, U.S. Dept. of Commerce, Bureau of the Census, Washington, D.C., 1980.

2. Johns, M.P. *Drug Therapy and Nursing Care*, New York: Macmillan, 1979, 263.

3. Chance, W.T., von Meyenfeld, M. and Fischer, J. Changes in brain amines associated with cancer. *Neuroscience and Biobehavioral Reviews*, 7: 471, 1983.

4. Roe, D.A. *Alcohol and the Diet*. Westport, Conn.: AVI 1979, 27.

5. Roe, D.A. *Drug-Induced Nutritional Deficiencies*. Westport, Conn.: AVI, 1983, 130.

6. Burrows, M.J. and Farr, W.K. The action of mineral oil per os on the organism. *Proc. Soc. Exp. Biol. Med.*, 24: 719, 1927.

7. Smith, M.C. and Spector, H. Calcium and phosphorus metabolism in rats and dogs as influenced by the ingestion of mineral oil. *J. Nutr.*, 20: 19, 1940.

8. Smith, M.C. and Spector, H. Some effects on animal nutrition of the ingestion of mineral oil. *Univ. Ariz. Coll. Agric. Exper. Sta. Bull.*, 84: 373, 1940.

9. Javert, C.T. and Macri, C. Prothrombin concentration and mineral oil. *Am. J. Obstet. Gynecol.* 42: 409, 1941.

10. Curtis, A.C. and Baliner, R.S. The prevention of carotene absorption by liquid petrolatum. *J.A.M.A.* 113: 1785, 1939.

11. Roe, D.A., *Drug-Induced Nutritional Deficiencies*. Westport, Conn.: AVI, 1983, 143.

12. West, R.J. and Lloyd, J.K. The effect of cholestyramine on intestinal absorption. *Gut*, 16: 95, 1975.

13. Lotz, M., Zisman, E. and Bartter, F.C. The effect of cholestyramine on intestinal absorption. *N.E.J. Med.*, 278; 409, 1868.

14. Bloom, W.L. and Flinchum D. Osteomalacia with pseudofractures caused by the ingestion of aluminum hydroxide. *J.A.M.A.*, 174: 1327, 1960.

15. Benn, A., Swan, C.H.J., Cooke, W.T., et al. Effect of intraluminal pH on the absorption of pteroylmonoglutamic acid. *Br. Med. J.*, 1: 148, 1971.

16. McGuigan, J.E. A consideration of the adverse effects of cimetidine. *Gastroenterology*, 80: 181, 1980.

17. Carmel, R., et al. Vitamin B12 uptake by human small bowel homogenate and its enhancement by intrinsic factor. *Gastroenterology*, 56: 548, 1969.

18. Palva, I.P., Salokannel, S.J., Timonen, T., et al. Drug induced malabsorption of vitamin B12. *Acta Med. Scand.*, 191: 355, 1972.

19. Tomasulo, P.A., Keter, R.M.H. and Iber, F.L. Impairment of thiamine absorption in alcoholism. *Am. J. Clin. Nutr.*, 21: 1340, 1968.

20. Halsted, C.H., Robles, E.A. and Mezey, E. Intestinal malabsorption in folate deficient alcoholics. *Gastroenterology*, 64: 526, 1973.

21. Bren, M. Erythrocyte as a biopsy tissue in the functional evaluation of thiamine status. *J.A.M.A.*, 187: 762, 1964.

22. Brozek, J. Psychologic effects of thiamine restriction and deprivation in normal young men. *Am. J. Clin. Nutr.*, 5: 109, 1957.

23. Hodges, R.E., Baker, E.M., Hood, J., et al. Experimental scurvy in man. *Am. J. Clin. Nutr.*, 22: 535, 1969.

24. Sterner, R.T. and Price, W.R. Restricted riboflavin: Within-subject behavioral effects in humans. *Am. J. Clin. Nutr.*, 26: 150, 1973.

25. Parker, T.H., Marshall, J.P., Roberts, R.K., et al. Effect of acute alcohol ingestion on plasma pyridoxal 5'-phosphate. *Am. J. Clin. Nutr.*, 32: 1246, 1979.

26. Rose, D.P. and Braidman, I.P. Excretion of tryptophan metabolites as affected by pregnancy, contraceptive steroids, and steroid hormones. *Am. J. Clin. Nutr.*, 24: 673, 1971.

27. Baylis, E.M., Crowley, J.M., Preece, J.M., et al. Influence of folic acid on blood phenytoin levels. *Lancet*, 1: 62–64, 1971.

28. Mattson, R.A., Gallagher, B.B., Reynolds, G.H., et al. Folate therapy in epilepsy: A controlled study. *Arch Neurol*, 29: 78–81, 1971.

29. Roe, D.A. Drug-nutrient interactions. *Med. Clin. N. Am.* 63: 985–1007, 1979.

30. Lindenbaum, J., Whitehead, N., and Reyner, F. Oral contraceptive hormones, folate metabolism and the cervical epithelium. *Am. J. Clin. Nutr.*, 28: 346, 1975.

31. Constanzi, J.J., Young, B.K., and Carmel, R. Serum vitamin B12-binding protein levels associated with oral contraceptives. *Texas Rep. Biol. Med.*, 36: 69, 1978.

32. Shojania, A.M. and Wylie B. The effect of oral contraceptives on vitamin B12 metabolism. *Am. J. Obs. Gyn.*, 135: 129, 1979.

33. Chanarin, I. *The Megaloblastic Anaemias*. Philadelphia: Blackwell, 1969.

34. Baum, C.L., Selhub, J. and Rosenberg, I.H. Antifolate actions of sulfasalazine on intact lymphocytes. *J. Lab. Clin. Med.* 97: 779, 1981.

35. Furlanut, M., Benetello, P., Avogaro, A., et al. Effects of folic acid on phenytoin kinetics in healthy subjects. *Clin. Pharmacol. Ther.*, 24: 294, 1978.

36. Norris, J.W. and Pratt, R.F. Folic acid deficiency and epilepsy. *Drugs*, 8: 366, 1974.

37. Lindenbaum, J. Folate and vitamin B12 deficiencies in alcoholism. *Semin. Hematol.* 17: 119, 1980.

38. Halsted, C.H. and Tamura, T., in C.S. Davidson (ed.), *Problems In Liver Diseases*. New York: Stratton, 1979, 91–100.

39. Lindenbaum, J., chapter 8, in C.S. Lieber, *Medical Disorders of Alcoholism*. New York: Saunders, in press.

40. Sullivan, L.W. and Herbert, V. Suppression of hematopoiesis by ethanol. *J. Clin. Invest.*, 43: 2048, 1964.

41. Klipstein, F.A. and Lindenbaum, J. Folate deficiency in chronic liver disease. *Blood*, 25:443, 1965.

42. Kobrinsky, N.L. and Ramsay, N.K.C. Acute megaloblastic amemia induced by high-dose trimethoprim-sulfamethoxazole. *Ann. Intern. Med.*, 94: 780, 1981.

43. Seelig, M.S. Magnesium requirements in human nutrition. *Contemporary Nutrition*, 7, 1982.

44. Grimm, R.H. Jr., Leon, A.S., Hunninghake, D.B., et al. Effects of thiazide diuretics on plasma lipids and lipoproteins in mildly hypertensive patients. A double-blind control trial. *Ann. Intern. Med.* 94: 7–11, 1981.

45. Joos, C., Kewitz, H. and Reinhold-Kouniati, D. Effects of diuretics on plasma lipoproteins in healthy men. *Eur. J. Clin. Pharmacol.* 17: 251–257, 1980.

46. Leonards, J.R. and Levy, G. Gastrointestinal blood loss during prolonged aspirin administration. *N. E. J. Med.*, 289: 1020–1022, 1973.

47. Bordman, P.L., and Hart, E.D. Side effects of indomethacin. *Ann. Rheum. Dis.*, 26: 127–132, 1967.

48. Chien, C.P., Townsend, E.J. and Townsend, A. Substance use and abuse among the community elderly: The medical aspect. *Addict Dis.*, 3:357–372, 1978.

49. Guttman, P. Patterns of legal drug use by older Americans. *Addict Dis.*, 3 337–356. 1978.

50. Roe, D.A., *Drug-induced Nutritional Deficiencies*. Westport, Conn.: AVI, 1976, 130–132.

18

·············NUTRITION, ALCOHOLISM····························· AND DRUG ABUSE

ALCOHOL affects virtually every tissue in the body. The fact that alcohol can cause malnutrition has been known for over thirty years. But the prevalence and degree of clinical malnutrition among alcoholics varies with socioeconomic status, pattern of drinking, dietary intake and degree of liver impairment.[1] Interestingly, there has been a decrease in *clinical* nutritional deficiencies (such as scurvy, beriberi, pellagra) among alcoholics since World War II.[2,3,4] This is probably due to the improved economic situation of the total population and the fortification of cereals. But when clinical nutritional deficiencies are identified, the nutrients involved are the same nutrients that act as co-factors in neurochemical physiology associated with alcoholic behavior. This suggests that alcoholics may have an increased need for these nutrients or perhaps that they have some degree of sub-clinical malnutrition that is being overlooked. Some of the behavioral effects that can occur in sub-clinical malnutrition, as discussed earlier in Chapter 17 (Tables 25 and 26), are common among alcoholics and drug addicts.

It is interesting to note that the nutrients investigated and listed in these tables are three of the nutrients at risk for adequacy in alcoholics.[5–9] In addition to these three nutrients, there are at least seven other essential nutrients and amino acids that can be depleted in alcoholism. The box lists four basic ways in which alcohol can cause malnutrition. The box on p. 210 lists the nutrients that have been proven to be at risk or depleted in alcoholism.

The hypothesis that malnutrition might promote or perpetuate alcoholism has been explored. But because the relationship between alcohol and malnutrition is so

---

FACTORS CONTRIBUTING TO MALNUTRITION IN ALCOHOLISM

1) Inadequate food intake
   Anorexia
   Psychoses
   Altered appetite
   Lack of money
   Intoxication
2) Alcohol-induced nutrient losses
   Maldigestion
   Malabsorption
   Increased urinary volume
   Kidney damage
3) Decreased cellular uptake of nutrients
4) Metabolic impairment
   Liver disease
   Other glandular damage

---

complex, simplistic treatment approaches using nutritional supplements have not been very successful. The idea that malnutrition might promote or perpetuate alcoholism has therefore not been widely accepted.

Tipton and others recently reviewed the complexity of the metabolic and nutritional effects of alcohol.[10] Such a complex physiological process demands a physiological approach to alcoholism that is beyond a simple nutrient-replacement program. The alcohol-induced injury and adaptation seen in body membranes may be beyond repair in some individuals. And the complexity of the problem increases substantially when brain neurophysiology is considered. But when the nine nutrients at risk in alcoholism are considered in their role as co-factors for brain neurochemical transmitters and hormone-like substances that can affect behavior, intriguing interrelationships appear. These interrelationships suggest therapeutic roles for vitamins, minerals and other nutrients, combined with a specific dietary program, that may bring about a major advance in the prevention and treatment of alcoholism as well as other drug addictions.

NEUROPSYCHOLOGY OF DEPENDENCE

Recent research in the neurosciences has demonstrated that the concept of "psychic dependence" has physiological correlates that are separate from, but not unrelated to, the withdrawal syndrome generally associated with physical dependence. The failure of clinicians to understand and address the physiological nature of so-called "psychic dependence" may be the single most important missing element contributing to the failure of therapeutic models for alcoholism and other drug addictions.

In order to grasp the physiological nature of "psychic dependence," it may be helpful to look briefly at the motivations for using alcohol and other substances that have psychostimulant action. A review of the controversy regarding motivations to use drugs has been presented elsewhere.[11,12] For the sake of brevity, three of these hypotheses are discussed in order to establish a relationship between neurophysiology and "psychic dependence."

The following oversimplified views of motivational factors for substance abuse should not be construed as support for a particular psychological profile of the chemically dependent person. Carroll and others have pointed out that the diversity of psychological profiles within chemically dependent populations is similar to that of the general population.[13] Miller humorously emphasized this fact when he profiled the average alcoholic as "a passive, overactive, inhibited, acting out, withdrawn, gregarious psychopath with a conscience, defending against poor defenses as a result of excessive and insufficient mothering."[14]

The lack of similarity in psychological profiles of alcoholics and other substance abusers should suggest that perhaps there is an underlying physiological aberration that is not being adequately investigated. The physiological correlates of certain motivational factors for substance abuse support this view.

MOTIVATION TO COUNTERACT PSYCHIC STRESS

Individuals who, for social, relational or physical reasons, are in a state of depression or feel that they might encounter depression, may consciously compensate for this fear by using alcohol or other stimulating substances.[15] One classic example of this type of motivation to use a drug can be seen in the North American Indian's use of peyote. Traditionally, this mescaline-containing cactus was used to counteract a state of collective depression caused by defeat at the hands of the white man.[16] Today, depression from living in a society continually portrayed as being on the brink of nuclear annihilation, "lover's depression," boredom and alienation are examples of this type of motivation to use drugs.

"DEEP-SEATED" MOTIVATION

In 1962, Rado called this type of motivation "prodromal depression."[17] Hartman called it the "basic depressive character."[18] Today it is commonly referred to as endogenous or "vital" depression.[19] The etiology of this type of depression is not universally agreed upon, but current research in the neurosciences is offering provocative findings.

Inwang and others have demonstrated that endogenous depression can be present from early childhood and may involve a congenital incapacity for synthesis, storage and utilization of certain brain neurotransmitters.[20] Individuals with this type of depression may utilize euphoric substances as necessary substitutes for long-standing neurochemical deficiencies.

MOTIVATIONS FOR CONTINUAL ALCOHOL AND DRUG USAGE

Two motivational urges are associated with the difficulty encountered in attempts to break the alcohol- and drug-abuse habit. The state of "wellbeing" and its counterpart, the state of "malaise," have well established neurophysiological correlates commonly called the "reward" and "punishment" or "pleasure" and "pain" centers. In the relatively early days of modern neuroscience studies, Murphy demonstrated that drugs can act as false neurotransmitters, stimulating receptors in the so-called "pleasure" center, resulting in a state of "wellbeing."[21] During withdrawal, reduced amounts of neurotransmitters and thus reduced stimulation of the "pleasure" center, or the ability of another neurochemical system to take over, results in a state of "malaise" or a lowering of the threshold of pain and therefore an increased urge for the drug.

When these three motivational concepts—the motivation to counteract certain psychic states, endogenous motivation, and motivation for drug continuance—are viewed in light of their physiological correlates, the dualistic concept of "psychic dependence" as being something unique and distinct from the concept of "physiological dependence" appears somewhat outdated. This is not to say that social motivations as well as exploratory instincts are unimportant factors in the etiology of alcoholism and other drug addictions. But in order to enhance the alcoholic recovery process, as well as the recovery process in other drug addictions, the neurophysiological correlates of motivations for substance abuse have important therapeutic implications. Thus, it has been suggested that the term "psychic dependence" be replaced with a term such as "neuropsychological dependence."[12]

NEUROTRANSMITTERS, ALCOHOLISM AND OTHER DRUG ADDICTIONS

The common theme running through all of the three motivational concepts discussed is that alcoholics and drug addicts have a drive to overcome depression and achieve a sense of "wellbeing." Early surveys by Woodruff and others in 1973 demonstrated the widespread occurrence of these feelings among alcoholics.[22] In 1969 and 1970 Rosenbaum and others demonstrated similar findings among drug addicts.[23,24] The antidepressive feature of alcohol and other drugs has been substantiated in additional surveys conducted in the early 70s.[25,26]

Studies that have led to our present knowledge of neurotransmitters and depression began in the 1940s. In an attempt to identify a substance in blood responsible for hypertension, 5-hydroxytryptamine, commonly known as 5-HT or serotonin, was identified. In 1957 it was discovered that the antihypertensive drug reserpine depleted serotonin from brain and other tissues. Interestingly, reserpine can create a drug-induced depression that may persist for several months after drug withdrawal and may be severe enough to result in suicide. The relationship between reserpine, serotonin and depression led to extensive research on abnormal serotonin metabolism and behavioral states in man.

In 1957 and in 1966, Brodie and others demonstrated that mood and affect are modulated by a group of brain chemicals known as biogenic amines, which include the chemical serotonin.[27,28] (The biogenic amine theory of affective disorders has recently been reviewed by Van Praag.[29]) In the 1970s, a number of scientists established that alcohol, as well as narcotic drugs, can modulate these biogenic amines.[30–32] Then, in 1974, Takahashi and others demonstrated that alocholics metabolize one of these mood chemicals, serotonin, abnormally.[33] The interrelationship between alcoholism and depression, depression and serotonin, serotonin and alcoholism was thus established. Additional support for this interrelationship was recently published by the Alcohol Research and Treatment Center, Bronx Veterans Administration Medical Center and Mount Sinai School of Medicine. This study showed that alcohol impairs the transport into the brain of an amino acid that is necessary for the synthesis of serotonin.[34]

The precursor for serotonin synthesis is a nutrient generally obtained in the diet, an amino acid called tryptophan. But food sources are generally not effective in altering behavior because of the competitive inhibition of other amino acids that accompany tryptophan in the diet. Studies comparing the antidepressant effects of tryptophan supplements versus therapeutic drugs such as imipramine and amitriptyline have demonstrated that tryptophan is equally effective and has fewer side effects.[35–38]

Dietary factors that can increase serotonin synthesis in the brain include sucrose and excessive fat consumption. Badawy and others demonstrated in 1980 that chronic sucrose ingestion increases serotonin levels.[39] Badawy also showed in 1984 that high-fat diets increase tryptophan availability to the brain.[40] Therefore, in the alcoholic recovery process, cravings for sugar-laden "junk" food, normally high in fat content, are not uncommon. When alcohol is removed from the diet, the alcoholic might unconsciously attempt to compensate for this loss by ingesting foods that enhance serotonin synthesis. Mandating that alcoholics avoid sugar and fatty foods during the recovery process will probably meet with little success unless alternative means of enhancing serotonin synthesis are initiated.

It is interesting to note that many of the nutrients listed on p. 210 as being at risk for adequacy in alcoholics are also necessary cofactors for the synthesis and metabolism of serotonin. Figure 18, p. 214, shows two different metabolic pathways for the amino acid L-tryptophan. There is a significant relationship between metabolic pathways, vitamin B6, depression and alcoholism. As can be seen from this figure, vitamin B6 (PLP) is necessary to convert 5-OH tryptophan to serotonin. Therefore, the vitamin B6 deficiency induced by alcohol may contribute to the alcoholic's depression by decreasing serotonin synthesis. In this case of a drug-induced nutrient deficiency, the drug may actually be a contributing factor to alcoholic depression and play a role in the perpetuation of this disease. In addition to the alcohol-induced B6 deficiency, the alcoholic's diet may be deficient in all the other nutrients listed on page 210. A nutrient-poor diet may therefore also contribute to the depression associated with alcoholism and other drug addictions.

It should be emphasized here that serotonin is only one of the neurotransmitters involved in behavior. Because of the complexity of the role vitamins, minerals, amino acids, fats and carbohydrates play in the metabolism of serotonin and other neurochemical transmitters, a complete discussion is beyond the scope of this chapter. But to the extent that depression is related to the cause and perpetuation of alcoholism and other drug addictions, there is now a sound rationale for including a dietary component with a specially designed set of nutritional supplements that offers exciting potential for improving treatment and prevention programs.

ALCOHOL, OPIATES AND ADDICTION

In the early 1970s various studies demonstrated that the analgesic action of the opiates was the result of an interaction between the opiates and certain receptors in the brain.[41-44] The discovery of these receptors suggested that there may be some naturally occurring substance within the brain that exerts its activity by acting upon these receptors.

Soon after the discovery of these receptors, a number of researchers demonstrated that opiate-like substances did exist in the brain naturally.[45-47] The opiate-like substances, which consisted of five amino acids, were termed enkephalins, meaning "in the head." Other compounds with opiate-like activity were subsequently identified and called endorphins. These opioid peptides can produce a variety of effects. Some of these effects are listed in the box.

During this same period, a theory was developing that would eventually link alcoholism with the physiology of opiate addiction. It was demonstrated that the alcohol metabolite acetaldehyde could combine with a brain chemical and form a compound that belongs to the family of chemicals known as isoquinolines. These substances have opiate-like properties and can interact with the opiate receptors. If alcoholics have an in-

---

SOME OF THE EFFECTS OF THE ENDOGENOUS OPIOID PEPTIDES IN RATS

Analgesia
Catoplexy/epilepsy
Sedation
Meiosis
Respiratory depression
Hypo-/hyperthermia
Memory: Facilitation of passive avoidance and inhibition of extinction of active avoidance.
Blood pressure: Hypotension
Enhance stress ulceration
Sexual behavior: Decreases copulatory behavior
Hormonal effects: growth hormone and prolactin
   ACTH
   TSH
   LH and FSH
   oxytocin
   glucose
Appetite regulation: Enhances feeding

Source: Morley, J. E., Levine, A. S., Yim, G. K., et al., Opioid modulation of appetite, *Neuroscience and Biobehavioral Reviews*, 7:282, 1983.

---

creased need, whether genetically or environmentally induced, for stimulation of certain opiate receptor sites, then the opiate-like substance formed in the metabolism of alcohol would satisfy this need. If this theory is proven, then removal of alcohol from the alcoholic's diet must be accompanied by an acceptable—and, ideally—non-drug replacement to stimulate certain opiate receptors.

It has been demonstrated that alcohol consumption is increased following opiate withdrawal.[48] In recent experiments, attempts have been made to reduce alcohol consumption by using substances that mimic the action of opiates. Ho and Rossi at the Peoria School of Medicine, University of Illinois, have presented preliminary data showing that in rats an endogenous opioid called met-enkephalin can significantly suppress the the consumption of alcohol.[49] If a natural method such as nutritional manipulation could enhance the availability of met-enkephalin to certain opiate receptor sites, it is hypothesized that the drive for alcohol might be suppressed in alcoholics. This is not quite as simple as enhancing neurotransmission by providing dietary precursors, as discussed earlier in the case of dietary supplements of the amino acid tryptophan and serotonin synthesis. If a method existed whereby the met-enkephalin that is naturally produced in the brain, but perhaps in insufficient amounts in the alcoholic and other addicts, could be allowed to accumulate at opiate receptor sites, essentially the same effect of administering met-enkephalin could be achieved.

Normally, enkephalins do not accumulate at receptor sites because they are inactivated by a naturally occurring enzyme called enkephalinase. If enkephalinase is inhibited or inactivated, increased interaction between enkephalins and their respective receptor sites should occur. There are a number of enkephalinase inhibitors that have now been demonstrated to increase enkephalin interaction with opiate receptor sites. Specifically, it was demonstrated in 1981 by French researchers that met-enkephalin is protected by enkephalinase inhibition.[50] This is the enkephalin that Ho and Rossi found able to suppress alcohol consumption in rats.

Currently, there is a non-drug nutritional supplement available that contains an amino acid in a form which has enkephalinase-inhibiting properties.[51,52] This naturally occurring amino acid is called phenylalanine. It is available as a nutritional supplement in both the l and dl forms. Only the "d" form of this amino acid exerts enkephalinase-inhibiting properties. The racemic mixture of these two isomers (dl phenylalanine)is the only legal OTC source of d-phenylalanine. When combined with other nutrients and a special dietary program designed to influence the blood brain barrier, dl phenylalanine offers exciting potential as an adjunct neurochemical modulator for improving the alcoholic and opiate addict recovery process. (*Caution: This nutrient cannot be tolerated by individuals with the inborn error of metabolism known as phenylketonuria.*)

It is now known that a complex interrelationship exists between opiates, whether ingested or occurring naturally in the brain, and monoamines, another type of neurotransmitter associated with behavior. It cannot be overemphasized that single nutrients offer little hope for improving this complex alcoholic recovery process unless integrated into a well-planned dietary program designed with the goal of improving the entire body as well as improving brain neurochemistry. Likewise, a dietary program without an exercise component is less likely to succeed for many of the same reasons as an alcoholic recovery program without a nutritional component. There is now evidence that certain forms of exercise can have a positive influence on opiate receptor sites in the brain which could result in a decreased desire for alcohol. Sacks and Sachs have recently prepared an excellent reference manual on the psychological and some of the physiological benefits of running.[53] Numerous bibliographic citations are included demonstrating the positive effects running can have on the prevention and treatment of alcoholism and other addictions.

There is another opiate-alcohol-nutrition interrelationship that is beginning to surface. A few years ago, Hemmings proposed that psychiatric manifestations occurred in individuals with gluten intolerance, a sensitivity to wheat protein that results from the leakage of incomplete protein metabolites across the gut into the bloodstream. These substances could then influence the immune system and brain chemistry and cause behavioral abnormalities. Recently, it has been proven that digestion of some dietary proteins, such as casein from dairy products and gluten from wheat, can result in the production of substances that have opiate-like activity.[54] These opiate-like substances may produce little or no effect in the so-called "normal" population. Generally, these substances would not be expected to pass from the gut into the bloodstream. Research from the Medical Research Council Clinical Research Centre, Middlesex, England, has shown that alcoholics have increased intestinal permeability, or a "leaky" gut.[55] These findings, are provocative, to say the least. They suggest that perhaps certain protein-like substances in the diet of the alcoholic, and perhaps other addicts, may be intimately involved with behavior and the perpetuation of these disorders.

SUMMARY

The etiology of alcoholism and other drug addictions appears to have some direct interrelationships with current research in neurochemistry and endocrinology. Through nutritional intervention it may now be possible to modulate some of the physiological aberrations that are known to occur in these addictions. But this is not a simple process. Careful dietary planning, accompanied by a delicate balance of nutritional supplements, is necessary to maximize the success of this approach.

In addition to nutrition, an exercise component must be introduced into alcohol and drug addiction treatment models in such a way that even those who have avoided traditional forms of exercise will find it easy to participate. A model utilizing a specific dietary and exercise program to enhance the alcoholic and drug addict recovery process is currently being developed in San Diego. For additional information write Health Media of America, P.O. Box 2173, Del Mar, CA 92014.

REFERENCES

1. Vitale, J.J., and Coffey, J. *Alcohol and Vitamin Metabolism*, in *The Biology of Alcoholism, Vol 1. Biochemistry*, B. Kissin and H. Beglerter (Eds.). New York and London: Plenum Press, 1971.

2. Bean, W. B. Vilter, R.W. and Blankenhorn, M.A. Incidence of pellagra. *J.A.M.A.* 140: 872–873, 1949.

3. Figueroa, W. Sargent, G., Inperiale, F., et al. Lack of vitaminosis among alcoholics. Its relation to fortification of cereal products and the general nutrition of the population. *J. Clin. Nutr.*, 1: 179–199, 1953.

4. Neville, J. N., Eagles, J. A., Samson, G., et al. Nutritional status of alcoholics. *Am. J. Clin. Nutr.*, 21: 1329–1340, 1968.

5. Rosenthal, W.S., Adham, N. F., Lopez, R., et al. Riboflavin deficiency in complicated chronic alcoholism. *Am. J. Clin. Nutr.* 26: 858–860, 1973.

6. Roe, D.A. *A Plague of Corn: The Social History of Pellagra.* Ithaca, N.Y.: Cornell Univ. Press, 1973.

7. Lester, D., Buccino, R. and Bizzocco, D. The vitamin C status of alcoholics. *J. Nutr.* 70: 278–282, 1960.

8. Tomasulo, P. A., Kater, R.M.H. and Iber, F.L. Impairment of thiamine absorption in alcoholism. *Am. J. Clin. Nutr.*, 21: 1340–1344, 1968.

9. Thomson, A., Baker, H. and Leevy, C. M. Thiamine absorption in alcoholism. *Am. J. Clin. Nutr.*, 21: 537–538, 1968.

10. Tipton, K. F., Henehan, G.T.M., and McCrodden, J.M. Metabolic and nutritional aspects of the effects of ethanol. *Bioch Soc Tran* 11: 59–61, 1983.

11. Cocchi, R. and Segala, F. Considerazioni sull'alcolismo, sulle tossicomanie e sulle relative possibilita terapeutiche. *Igiene ment,* 80: 815–825, 1976.

12. Cocchi, R. and Tornati, A. Psychic dependence? A different formulation of the problem with a view to the reorientation of therapy for chronic drug addiction. *ACTA,* 56: 337–346, 1977.

13. Carroll, J.F.X. Personality and psychopathylogy: a comparison of alcohol and drug dependent persons, in Solomon, J. and Keeley, K., *Alcohol and Drugs: Similarities and Differences.* Littleton, Mass.: PSG Publishing, 1981.

14. Miller, W.R. Alcoholism scales and objective assessment methods: A review. *Psychological Bulletin,* 83: 657, 1976.

15. Cocchi, R. Perceptive system, sensitiveness and their relationship to the mind-body problem, some hypotheses. *Proceedings of the 3rd Congress of I.C.P.M.* Rome, 1975, 628–634.

16. Lanternari, V. *Movimenti religiosi di liberta e salvezza dei popoli oppressh Feltrinelli,* Milano, 1974, 67–111.

17. Rado, S. Narcotic bondage, in *Psychoanalysis of Behavior,* Vol 2. New York: Grune & Stratton, 1962.

18. Hartman, H. *Ego Psychology and the Problem of Adaptation.* New York: International Universities Press, 1958.

19. Albert, N., and Beck, A.T. Incidence of depression in early adolescence: A preliminary study. *J. Youth Adoles.,* 4: 301–307, 1975.

20. Inwang, E.E., Primm, B.J. and Jones, F. Metabolic disposition of 2 phenylethylamine and the role of depression in methadone dependent and detoxified patients. *Drug Alcohol Depend* 1: 295–303, 1976.

21. Murphy, D.L. Amine precursors, amines and false neurotransmitters in depressed patients. *Amer. J. Psychiat.* 129: 141–148, 1972.

22. Woodruff, R.A., Guze, S. B., Clayton, P. J. et al. Alcoholism and depression. *Arch Gen Psychiat.* 28: 97–100, 1973.

23. Rosenberg, G. M. Young drug addicts. Background and personality. *J. Nerv. Ment. Dis.* 148: 65–73, 1969.

24. Delteil, P. and Lassere, P. La personnalité des toxicomanes et leur traitement. *Ann Med.-Psychol.* 128: 107–112, 1970.

25. Tart, C.T. *On Being Stoned.* Science and Behavior Books, Palo Alto, 1971.

26. Goode, E. *On Being Stoned.* New York: Knopf, 1972.

27. Brodie, B.B. and Shore, P.A. Biogenic amines and serotonin. *Ann. N.Y. Acad. Sci.* 66: 631, 1957.

28. Brodie, B.B., Comer, M.S., Costa, E. et al. The role of brain serotonin in the mechanism of the central action of reserpine. *J. Pharmacol.* 152: 340, 1966.

29. Van Praag, H.M. Central metabolism in depressions. *Compr. Psychiat.* 21: 30–43, 1980.

30. Shen, F.H., Log, H.H. and Way, E.L. *J. Pharmacol. Exptl. Therap.,* 175: 427, 1970.

31. Rethy, C.R., Smith, C.B. and Villarreal, J. E. *J. Pharmacol. Exptl. Therap.,* 472, 1971.

32. Ho, I. K., Loh, H.H. and Leon-Way, E. *Proc. 36th Ann. Sci. Meeting Natl. Acad. Sci.* (U.S. Comm. Problems Drug Dependence), 474, 1974.

33. Takahashi, St. Yamne, H. Kondo., et al. CSF monoamine metabolites in alcoholism: A comparative study with depression. *Fol. Psych. et Neur. Jap.* 28: 475, 1974.

34. Branchey, L. Shaw, S. and Lieber, C. S. Ethanol impairs tryptophan transport into the brain and depresses serotonin. *Life Sciences,* 29: 2751–2755, 1981.

35. Jensen, K., Fruensgaard, K., Ahlfors, U.D., et al. The effects of tryptophan on depression. *Lancet* II: 920, 1975.

36. Broadhurst, A. D. and Arenillas, L. Pre-trial discussion on antidepressant effects of L-tryptophan. *Curr. Med. Res. Opinion* 3: 413, 1975.

37. Chouinard, G., Young, G. N., Annable, L., et al. Tryptophan dosage critical for its antidepressant effect. *Br. Med. J.* I: 1422, 1978.

38. Herrington, R. N., Bruce, A. Johnstone, E. C., et al. Comparative trial of L-tryptophan and amitriptyline in depressive illness. *Psychol. Med. J.* 6: 673-678, 1976.

39. Abdulla, A., et al. Unsuitability of control sucrose or glucose in studies of the effects of chronic ethanol administration on brain 5-hydroxytryptamine metabolism. *J. Pharm. Meth.* 3: 167–171, 1980.

40. Badawy, A., Morgan, C. J., Davis, N. R., et al. High-fat diets increase tryptophan availability to the brain: Importance of choice of the control diet. *Bioch. J. Letter,* 217: 863–864, 1984.

41. Goldstein, A. L., Lowney, I. and Pal, B. K. Stereospecific and non-specific interactions of the morphone congener levorphanol in subcellular fractions of mouse brain. *Proc. Nat. Acad. Sci.,* 68: 1742–1747, 1971.

42. Pert, C. B. and Snyder, S. H. Opiate receptor: Demonstration in nervous tissue. *Science* 179: 1011–1014, 1973.

43. Simon, E. J., Hiller, J. M. and Edelman, I. Stereospecific binding of the potent narcotic analgesic H-Etorphine to rat brain homogenate. *Proc. Nat. Acad. Sci.* 70: 1947–1949, 1973.

44. Terenius, L. Stereospecific interaction between narcotic analgesics and a synaptic plasma membrane fraction of rat cerebral cortex. *Acta Pharmacol Toxicol* 32: 317–320, 1973.

45. Terenius, L. and Wahlstrom, A. Inhibitors of narcotic receptor binding in brain extracts and cerebrospinal fluid. *Acta Pharmacol. Scand.* 35: 55, 1974.

46. Terenius, L. and Wahlstrom, A. Search for an endogenous ligand for the opiate receptor. *Acta Physiol. Scand.* 94: 74–81, 1975.

47. Hughes, J. Isolation of an endogenous compound from the brain with pharmacological properties similar to morphine. *Brain Res.* 80: 295–308, 1975.

48. Ho, A.K.S. in Messiha, F. and Tyner, G. (eds.), *Alcoholism: A Perspective.* New York: J.D.P. Publications, 1980, 309–327.

49. Ho, A.K.S., and Rossi, N. Suppression of ethanol consumption by met-enkephalin in rats. *J. Pharm.* 34: 118–119, 1982.

50. Patey, G., de la Baume, S. Schwartz, J.C. et al. Selective protection of methionine enkephalin released from brain slices by enkephalinase inhibition. *Science,* 212: 1153–1154, 1981.

51. Ehrenpreis, S. D-Phenylalanine and other enkephalinase inhibitors as pharmacological agents: Implications for some important therapeutic application. *Sub. Alc. Act. Misuse,* 3: 231–239, 1982.

52. Ehrenpreis, S., Balagot, R. C., Mosnaim, A.D., et al. Analgesis in mice and humans by D-Phenylalanine (DPA): Relation to inhibition of enkephalin (ENK) degradation and brain uptake. *The Pharmacologist,* 22: 302, 1980.

53. Sacks, M.H. and Sachs, M.L. *The Psychology of Running,* Chicago: Human Kinetics Publishers, Inc., 1981.

54. Zioudrou, C., Streaty, R. A. and Klee, W. A. Opioid peptides derived from food proteins: The exorphins. *J. Biol. Chem.* 254: 2379–2380, 1979.

55. Bjarnason, I., Ward, K. and Peters, T. The leaky gut of alcoholism: Possible route of entry for toxic compounds. *Lancet,* II: 544, 1984.

GLOSSARY

·······························GLOSSARY·······························

Achlorhydria: the absence of hydrocholic acid in gastric juice.

Acetylcholine: a chemical transmitter for nerve impulses. It is released upon stimulation of the nerve cell and in the presence of calcium.

Achylia: The absence of chyle.

Active transport: The transport of a solute across a cellular membrane against a concentration gradient.

Adenocarcinoma: a malignant tumor or carcinoma in which the cells form a gland.

Adenoma: A benign tumor of which the cells are similar to those from which they arise.

Aerobic: Occurring in the presence of oxygen. An aerobic activity is one in which the intensity allows adequate oxygen intake to meet tissue demands.

Agglutinin: An antibody found in serum that causes the antigen elements to stick together, forming clumps.

Agglutinogen: An antigen which, when introduced into the body, stimulates the formation of specific agglutinin.

Albumin: A water-soluble protein found in tissues and fluids. It is the principle protein in blood and is responsible for osmotic pressure.

Aldehyde: An organic compound containing the group -CHO.

Aldosterone: A steroid hormone produced by the adrenal cortex. It is responsible for the regulation of electrolyte balance by increasing the kidney's reabsorption of sodium and excretion of potassium.

Alopecia: Loss of hair.

Alveolar: Pertaining to the jaw area containing the tooth sockets, or to the air cells of the lungs.

Amenorrhea: The absence or abnormal discontinuation of the menses.

Amine group: A compound formed by replacing one or more hydrogens of ammonia with one or more hydrocarbons or nonacidic organic radicals such as RNH-2 or RNHR-2.

Amino acid: An organic acid containing an amino (NH-2) group. The small building blocks of protein.

Amphoteric: A substance with both acidic and basic properties.

Amylase: A pancreatic or salivary enzyme that breaks down starch into smaller molecules for absorption.

Anabolism: The phase of metabolism in which new molecules are synthesized. Any building process where small substances are combined to form complex compounds.

Anemia: A condition characterized by a deficiency of hemoglobin in red blood cells (and sometimes a concomitant reduction in red blood cell numbers), or red blood cells that are abnormal in size, or both.

Anion: An ion that contains a negative charge of electricity and is attracted to a positively charged anode.

Anorexia: The lack or loss of appetite for food.

Antiaggregatory: To have an inhibitory effect on the clumping of substances; for example, discouraging the normal clumping of certain antibodies and their homologous antigens.

Antiarachitic: An agent that prevents the development of rickets.

Antigen: Any foreign substance, usually a protein, that produces an immune response in animal tissues.

Antioxidant: A substance that prevents or impedes oxidation.

Aromatic: Any organic compound derived from benzene, C-6H-6, or containing at least one unsaturated heterocyclic ring.

Arrhythmia: An irregular heartbeat.

Arteriosclerosis: A variety of conditions in which the artery walls thicken and lose their elasticity. Commonly referred to as "hardening of the arteries."

Ataxia: Irregular muscle action or failure of muscle coordination.

Atherogenic: Anything that has the ability to encourage the development of atherosclerosis.

Atherosclerosis: A form of arterosclerosis. The depositing of fatty plaques along the intima of the artery wall, narrowing the channel and reducing blood supply.

Atony: A lack of normal tone or strength.

ATP: Adenosine triphosphate. A compound consisting of one molecule each of adenine and ribose and three phosphoric acids. The energy currency in the body. When the third phosphate group is cleaved from the compound, energy is released.

Bacteriocidal: A substance that destroys bacteria.

Bacteriostatic: Halting or interfering with the growth of bacteria.

Basal metabolic rate: The energy required for internal or cellular work when the body is at rest; expressed per unit of time and usually per square meter of body surface area.

Bile: A fluid produced by the liver and stored in the gallbladder. When the gall bladder contracts, the bile and its salts are secreted into the intestines to emulsify fats during digestion.

Biliary: Of or pertaining to bile.

Bitot's spots: Small, triangular, silvery spots of epithelial degradation, often accompanied by a foamy surface, on the conjunctiva.

Bolus: The partially digested mass of food prepared by the mouth for swallowing.

Bradycardia: Reduced beating of the heart below 60 beats per minute in the adult and 120 beats per minute in the fetus.

Buerger's disease: Thrombosis and inflammation of the arteries found in young and middle-aged cigarette smokers. Fibrosis develops in the blood vessels of the extremities. The condition is complicated by ischemic changes in the tissues supplied by the damaged blood vessels.

Buffer: A substance that maintains the body's normal acid-base balance.

Calcitonin: A hormone secreted by the thyroid gland that curtails the release of calcium from the bone.

Capillaries: Small blood vessel connecting the smallest arteries with the smallest veins.

Carbohydrase: An enzyme that splits complex carbohydrates into smaller sugars.

Carboxyl group: The group COOH characteristic of organic acids.

Carboxypeptidase: An intestinal enzyme responsible for splitting peptides.

Carcinogen: A cancer-causing substance.

Cardiovascular disease: The combination of heart and blood vessel disorders that include heart attack, stroke, atherosclerosis and congestive heart failure.

Casein: A protein found in milk.

Catabolism: That part of metabolism in which substances are broken down into their component parts and energy is released.

Catecholamine: Any of a family of structurally and functionally similar compounds including norepinephrine, epinephrine and dopamine.

Catatonia: A condition in which the person lacks the will to talk or move and stands or sits motionless.

Cation: An ion that has a positive charge and is attracted to a negatively charged pole.

Celiac disease: A malabsorption syndrome characterized by malnutrition, edema, skeletal disorders, abnormal stools, anemia and peripheral neuropathy. Abnormalities in the intestinal lining require a gluten-free diet.

Ceroid: Yellow to brown pigments insoluble in lipids and representing end metabolites of peroxidation of unsaturated fatty acids.

Cheilosis: A condition characterized by dry scaling of the lips and cracks at the corners of the mouth, commonly found in a riboflavin deficiency.

Cholecalciferol: Vitamin D3 formed from 7-hydrocholesterol.

Cholesterol: A fatty substance or sterol found in all animal fats, bile, skin, blood and brain tissues. The precursor for vitamin D and the sex hormones and important in the formation and maintenance of myelin. At elevated levels in the blood, cholesterol is a primary risk factor in cardiovascular disease.

Chyle: The contents of the intestinal lymph vessels.

Chylomicron: A type of lipoprotein comprised primarily of lipids coated with a thin layer of protein. The initial carrier of fat in the blood after digestion and absorption into the body.

Chyme: A mixture of partially digested food and stomach secretions.

Citric acid: An organic compound comprised of three carboxyl groups.

Coenzyme: The prosthetic group, usually a vitamin, of an enzyme; the binding of a coenzyme to its enzyme activates the complex.

Collagen: A protein substance that forms the primary constituent of connective tissue and the organic matrix in bones and teeth.

Congestive heart failure: A condition in which blood backs up in the veins; accompanied by the accumulation of fluids in various parts of the body; due to insufficient pumping of the heart.

Coronary occlusion: A narrowing or obstruction of one or more of the coronary arteries; blood flow to the receiving tissue is hindered.

Coumadin: The trademark for waffarin, an anticoagulant.

Creatine: A nitrogen-containing end product of muscle metabolism; a phosphorylated form is necessary for muscle contraction.

Creatinine: A nitrogen-containing compound formed from creatine in the presence of urine.

Creatinuria: The occurrence of creatine in the urine.

Cyanosis: A condition in which the skin turns blue because of an insufficient oxygen supply.

Cystic fibrosis: A disorder of unknown etiology, characterized by exocrine and endocrine gland dysfunction, which results in elevated electrolyte concentration, absence of pancreatic enzymes, celiac disease and chronic lung disease.

Deamination: A process of metabolism whereby the nitrogen portion of amino acids is removed.

Deglutition: Swallowing.

Dehydrogenation: The removal of hydrogen.

Dermis: The layer of skin below the epidermis, composed of collagen, elastin, fibroblasts, nerves and blood vessels.

Diglyceride: A fat containing two fatty acids and a glycerol molecule.

Disaccharide: Any sugar—sucrose, lactose or maltose—that yields two monosaccharides when hydrolyzed.

Distal: Away from a point of reference; remote.

Diverticulitis: Inflammation of tiny sacs (diverticula) in the intestines, causing abdominal pain and fever.

Diverticulosis: The development of tiny sacs in weakened areas of the intestines.

Dopaminergic: Characteristics and activities of dopamine and dopamine-like substances.

Duodenum: The upper portion of the small intestine.

Dysplasia: The abnormal development or growth of cells.

Dyspnea: Hard or labored breathing.

Eclampsia: Convulsions occurring during pregnancy; usually associated with edema, hypertension and proteinuria.

Edema: The presence of abnormal quantities of fluid in intercellular tissue spaces in the body.

Elastin: Yellowish elastic protein in connective tissue.

Electrolyte: The ionized form of an ion. Common electrolytes include sodium, potassium and chloride.

Embolism: Spontaneous blocking of an artery by a clot or free-floating obstruction.

Emulsion: A combination of two emiscible liquids in which one is finely divided and held in suspension by the other.

Encephalomalacia: The softening of the brain due to infarction.

Endochondral: Residing within cartilage.

Endothelium: The epithelial lining around the heart, blood vessels and lymphatics

Enriched: The description of processed food that has four nutrients (thiamin, riboflavin, niacin and iron) added back to replace partially those lost in refining.

Enzyme: A biological catalyst that initiates and accelerates chemical reactions.

Epiphysis: The portion of bone that calcifies before uniting with the major part of the bone.

Epithelial: Associated with or composed of the internal and external surfaces of the body, including the lining of blood and lymph vessels, all body cavities and the skin.

Ergocalciferol: Vitamin D2, formed from ergosterol.

Erythrocyte: A mature red blood cell.

Erythropoiesis: The formation of red blood cells.

Essential amino acid: An amino acid that can not be synthesized by the body and must be supplied by the diet.

Essential fatty acid: A fatty acid, such as linoleic acid, that cannot be made by the body and hence must be supplied regularly from the diet.

Ester: The product that results from combining an acid with an alcohol.

Eustachian tube: The tube connecting the middle ear with the pharynx.

Euthroid: A mixture of thyroid hormone salts.

Fatty acid: Open-chained monocarboxylic acid comprised of carbon, hydrogen and oxygen.

Fibrillation: The incoordinate contraction of muscle fibers, often pertaining to the heart muscle.

Fibrinogen: A soluble protein in blood that is converted to fibrin during blood clotting

Fibroblast: A large cell with one or two large, oval and pale-staining nuclei; found often in newly formed tissue or tissue in the process of being repaired.

Fibrosis: The formation of fibrous tissue during the repair process.

Fortification: The addition of one or more nutrients to a food in greater amounts than naturally found.

Free radical: A highly reactive compound with at least one unpaired electron. The central atom is linked to an abnormal number of atoms or groups of atoms.

Fructose: A monosaccharide composed of 6-carbon sugar; found in fruits and honey and obtained by hydrolysis of sucrose or table sugar. Also called fruit sugar or levulose.

Galactose: A monosaccharide resulting from the hydrolysis of lactose.

Gastric juice: The clear, colorless secretion of the glands of the stomach; the pH is about 2.0; contains hydrochloric acid, pepsin, mucin and, in infants, renin.

Glomerulus: A structure in the kidneys composed of a tuft of small blood vessels in Bowman's Capsule.

Glossitis: Inflammation of the tongue.

Glucose: The monosaccharide found in fruits and sugars that forms starch when linked in long strands; the storage sugar in the body; the sugar found in blood, grape sugar and dextrose.

Glucogenic: Glucose forming.

Gluconeogenesis: The formation of glucose from noncarbohydrate substances, such as amino acids.

Glycerol: A three carbon alcohol that forms the backbone of mono-, di- and triglycerides.

Glycogen: The storage form of glucose in the body.

Glycogenolysis: The formation of glycogen from glucose in the liver and muscles.

Glycolysis: The anaerobic conversion of glucose to lactic acid that produces some energy in the form of ATP.

Half-life: The time it takes for half of a substance or characteristic to disappear from a mathematically or physically determined space.

Hematocrit: The volume percentage of red blood cells when centrifuged.

Hemicellulose: An indigestible complex carbohydrate found in the cell walls of plants.

Hemochromatosis: Excessive iron deposition in tissues.

Hemoglobin: A chromoprotein in red blood cells. The incorporated iron has a great affinity for oxygen.

Hemoglobinuria: The presence of hemoglobin in the urine.

Hemolytic: The separation of hemoglobin from red blood cells.

Heparin: A mucopolysaccharide that prevents the clotting of blood.

Hepatic: Of or pertaining to the liver.

Hepatotoxin: Any substance that causes injury or death to the cells of the liver.

Hexose: A monosaccharide containing six carbon atoms.

Histology: The science and study of the minute structure of the body.

Homeostasis: The body's regulatory mechanism that tries to maintain stability and consistency in the various systems, such as body temperature, fluid volume and concentration of electrolytes.

Humoral: Of or pertaining to the humors (fluids or semifluids) of the body.

Hydrocarbons: A compound composed of hydrogen and carbon, such as methane (CH_4).

Hydrocephalus: Distension of the cerebral ventricles from cerebrospinal fluid due to obstruction of fluid flow and absorption.

Hydrolysis: A chemical reaction in which breakdown of a substance into two new compounds is due to the addition of one or more molecules of water.

Hypercholesterolemia: An excess of cholesterol in the blood.

Hyperkalemia: An abnormally high percentage of potassium in the blood.

Hyperplasia: A normal increase in the number of cells within a given tissue.

Hypertrophy: An increase in the size of cells resulting in enlargement of the specific organ or tissue.

Hypokalemia: An abnormally low percentage of potassium in the blood.

Hypovolemia: Reduced blood volume.

Ideopathic: A disease of unknown origin.

Ileitis: Inflammation of the ileum.

Ileum: The lower part of the small intestine between the jejunum and the cecum.

Infarction: The development of dead tissue resulting from the obstruction of blood flow, and subsequent oxygen flow, to the tissue and the inability to remove waste products from the area.

Inositol: A six-carbon alcohol that combines with phosphate to form phytic acid; found in grains and once considered to be a B vitamin.

Intima: The innermost of the three layers comprising a blood vessel.

In vitro: A process or reaction carried out in a petri dish or test tube.

In vivo: A process or reaction carried out in a living organism.

Ion: An atom or a group of atoms that have a positive or negative electrical charge.

Ischemia: A deficiency of blood to a tissue due to constriction or obstruction of the blood vessel.

Islets of Langerhans: An isolated group of cells in the pancreas responsible for the production of the hormones insulin and glucagon.

Isomers: One of two or more compounds having the same type and number of atoms but differing in the molecule's atomic arrangement.

Jaundice: The appearance of bile in the blood.

Jejunum: The middle part of the small intestine between the duodunum and the ileum.

Keratin: An insoluble, sulfur-containing protein found in the skin, hair and nails.

Keratinization: The condition in which epithelial cells, lacking sufficient vitamin A, deposit keratin rather than mucus, resulting in thickened, hardened and scaly tissue.

Ketone: Any one of a number of compounds containing a ketone group (CO), including acetone and acetoacetic acid.

Ketosis: A condition characterized by abnormal accumulation of ketones, resulting from incomplete catabolism of fatty acids.

Korsakoff's disease: A syndrome characterized by confusion, amnesia and apathy; observed in alcoholics and other B-vitamin-deficient individuals.

Kwashiorkor: A protein deficiency disease seen in malnourished children and characterized by growth failure, edema, tissue wasting, decreased resistance to illness and pigment changes in the skin.

Lactose: A disaccharide found in milk and composed of galactose and glucose.

Legume: The seed or fruit of a pod-bearing plant, including dried peas and beans, lentils and chickpeas.

Leukocyte: A white blood cell comprised of a colorless granular mass of protoplasm and varying in size between 0.005 and 0.015 mm in diameter.

Leukopenia: An abnormal reduction of leukocytes.

Ligand: A substance that binds with a metal ion.

Lipase: An enzyme that hydrolyzes fats to fatty acids and glycerol.

Lipid: A term for the family of fats including triglycerides, cholesterol and phospholipids.

Lipogenesis: The formation of fats.

Lipolysis: The splitting of fats into their component parts.

Lipoprotein: A complex of lipid and protein found in blood and responsible for the transportation of fats within the watery medium.

Lipotrophic: Of or pertaining to substances that prevent or curtail the accumulation of fat in the liver.

Lymph: Interstitial fluid within and transported by the lymphatic system; composed of water, salts, proteins and other constituents from blood plasma and containing lymphocytes and other cells.

Lymphatic system: A system of lymph vessels and nodes, ancillary to the blood vessels, that transports lymph.

Lysosomes: Organelles in the cell's cytoplasm that contain digestive enzymes.

Macronutrients: The nutrients that the body requires in relatively large amounts, including protein, carbohydrate, fats and water.

Macrophage: A phagocytotic cell; histocyte.

Maltose: A dissaccharide composed of two glucose units.

Marasmus: A disease of extreme protein-calorie malnutrition characterized by emaciation; found primarily in starving children.

Megaloblast: A large immature red blood cell with an enlarged nucleus.

Megaloblastic anemia: A condition of the blood in which the red blood cells develop improperly to form large and fragile cells with a reduced oxygen-carrying capacity.

Metabolism: The sum total of all anabolic and catabolic chemical reactions within the body.

Methylation: The chemical process of adding a methyl group to a compound.

Micronutrients: The nutrients required by the body in relatively small amounts, including vitamins and minerals.

Microsome: An organelle within the cell comprised of fragments of endoplasmic reticulum and ribosomes.

Micelle: A microscopic particle of fats and bile salts.

Miscible: Capable of mixing in all proportions.

Mitochondria: Rod-shaped organelles within the cell that manufacture and trap ATP; called the cell's "power house."

Monocyte: A large leukocyte with an indented nucleus; precursor to macrophages.

Monoglyceride: An ester of glycerol and one fatty acid.

Monosaccharide: A single sugar, such as glucose, fructose and galactose.

Morphology: The science of structure and form, including anatomy and histology.

Mucopolysaccharide: Any of a group of polysaccharides that are complexed with other molecules, such as protein.

Mucosa: The membrane lining the gastrointestinal, respiratory and genitourinary tracts.

Mutagenesis: The initiation of a genetic mutation.

Mutagen: Any substance causing a genetic mutation.

Myelin: The inner sheath or covering of the medulled nerve fiber.

Myocoardial infarction: Damage or death of a portion of the heart resulting from a reduced blood supply to the region.

Myocardium: The heart muscle.

Myoglobin: A form of hemoglobin found in muscle.

Neoplasm: A new and abnormal growth of tissue that grows at the expense of surrounding tissue and serves no useful purpose.

Neurotransmitter: A chemical that serves as a communication link between neurons.

Neutrophil: A classification of granular leukocyte; the most numerous, constituting 65 to 75 percent of all leukocytes.

Nonessential amino acids: Amino acids that are necessary for growth and maintenance but that can be synthesized by the body from exogenous and endogenous amino acids and other molecules.

Norepinephrine: The primary chemical transmitter at adrenergic nerve terminals; derived from the amino acid tyrosine.

Nucleic acids: Complex molecular substances, such as dioxyribonucleic acid (DNA), that are found in all cells and that carry the cell's genetic code or are responsible for protein synthesis.

Nucleoside: A glycoside formed by the removal of phosphate from a nucleotide; contains a sugar (pentose) with a purine or pyrimidine base.

Nucleotide: A hydrolytic product of nucleic acid containing one purine or pyrimidine base and a sugar phosphate.

Nutrient density: The ratio of nutrients to calories supplied by a food. Foods that provide a substantial amount of nutrients and few calories are considered nutrient dense.

Nyactalopia: Night blindness.

Obstetrics: The branch of medicine concerned with the care of pregnant and lactating women.

Organelle: The various structures within the cell, including lysomes and mitochondria.

Osmolarity: The concentration of a solute in a solution per unit of total volume of the solution.

Osseous: Composed of or pertaining to bone.

Osteoblast: A specialized cell that secretes a collagenous meshwork for new bone formation.

Osteoclast: A specialized cell responsible for bone erosion and resorption.

Oxalic acid: A dicarboxylic acid that forms insoluble salts with calcium; found in spinach, chard and rhubarb.

Oxidation: The chemical reaction in which a substance combines with oxygen.

Parakeratosis: The normal condition of incomplete keratinazation of the topmost epithelial cells of mucous membranes.

Parathyroid hormone: A hormone produced and secreted by the parathyroid gland; responsible for the regulation of blood calcium levels.

Parenteral: Proceeding through the body via channels other than the intestines.

Parietal: Of or pertaining to the walls of a cavity.

Passive transport: Transport of a substance across a membrane by simple diffusion.

Pellagra: A deficiency disease of niacin characterized by skin, gastrointestinal tract and nervous system disorders.

Peptone: An intermediate product of protein digestion.

Peristalsis: The rhythmic, mechanical action of the gastrointestinal tract that churns and pushes food downward.

Peroxide: The oxide of any base that contains the most oxygen.

Phagocyte: A cell capable of ingesting bacteria or other foreign substances.

Phenylketonuria: A congenital deficiency of the enzyme necessary for conversion of the amino acid phenylalanine to tyrosine; characterized by mental retardation.

Phospholipid: A fatty substance containing glycerol, fatty acids, phosphate and a nitrogen base.

Photosynthesis: The process in green plants whereby chlorophyll converts the sun's energy, carbon dioxide and water into carbohydrate.

Plasma: The liquid portion of blood or lymph devoid of cells.

Plaque: A deposit of fatty substances in the intima of the artery wall seen in atherosclerosis; also called atheroma.

Platelets: Cell fragments found in blood.

Polycythemia: An abnormal excess of red blood cells.

Polyhydric: A compound containing more than one hydroxyl group; polyhydroxy.

Polyneuritis: Simultaneous inflammation of numerous nerves.

Polypeptide: A compound of no fewer than three amino acids; an intermediate step in protein digestion.

Polysaccharide: Complex carbohydrates or starches; formed from strings of glucose units.

Portal vein: The vein carrying blood from the small and large intestines, spleen, and stomach to the liver.

Precursor: A substance used as a building block for another.

Prostaglandins: A group of hormone-like substances from linoleic acid and linolenic acid that have wide reaching effects on the body, including contraction of smooth muscle and dilation of blood vessels.

Proteose: A derivative of protein digestion.

Prothrombin: A protein in blood necessary for normal blood clotting.

Purine: A nonprotein heterocyclic nitrogenous base.

Purkinji system: A group of modified cardiac muscle fibers that form the terminal part of the conducting system of the heart.

Ptyalin: A starch-digesting enzyme in saliva.

Purpura: A condition in which hemorrhages occur in the skin, mucous membranes and serous membranes.

Pyrimidine: A cyclic compound containing four carbon and two nitrogen atoms in the ring.

Raynaud's disease: Intermittant pallor, cyanosis or loss of heat from the fingers, toes or both.

Reduction: The decrease of a positive charge of an atom or molecule through the gain of an electron.

Renal: Of or pertaining to the kidneys.

Resorption: The loss of a substance as in the removal of mineral salts from bone.

Rhodopsin: A substance necessary for scoptic vision; produced in the rods of the retina from the protein opsin and vitamin A; visual purple.

Saponin: A glycoside with emulsifying properties widely distributed in nature.

Satiety: A feeling of satisfaction following eating.

Saturated fat: A fat or fatty acid containing the maximum number of hydrogen atoms.

Serotonin: A neurotransmitter formed from the amino acid tryptophan.

Serum: The fluid portion of blood that is left after clotting.

Sprue: A malabsorption syndrome characterized by poor absorption of foods and water; symptoms are associated with nutrient deficiencies.

Steatorrhea: An abnormal excess of fat in the stool.

Stereoisomerism: A state in which two or more compounds are related because they have the same number and kind of atoms in a similar structure, but the compounds have a different arrangement in space.

Steroid: A group of compounds structurally similar to cholesterol, including bile acids, sterols and the sex hormones.

Stomatitis: Inflammation of the mucous membranes in the mouth.

Striated muscle: Muscle characterized by a banding pattern of cross-striped muscle fibers; found in skeletal and cardiac muscle.

Subcutaneous: Below the skin.

Substrate: A substance acted upon by an enzyme.

Synapse: The junction between two neurons where a nervous impulse is transmitted from one neuron to the next.

Sulfonamide: Any of a group of compounds formed from sulfanilamide and used in treating bacterial infections.

Tachycardia: Abnormally fast heart beat (above 100 beats per minute).

Tetany: A condition characterized by intermittent muscle contractions, fibrillations and pain.

Thrombin: A molecule necessary in the coagulation of blood.

Thrombocytopenia: An abnormal decrease in the number of platelets.

Thrombophlebitis: Inflammation of a vein associated with thrombosis.

Thrombosis: The formation of a thrombus.

Thrombus: A stationary blood clot that forms within an artery wall or cavity of the heart.

Triglycerides: Fatty compounds composed of one glycerol and three fatty acid molecules.

Tropocollagen: The fundamental unit of collagen fibrils.

Unsaturated fat: A fat that has one or more double bonds and could accept additional hydrogens.

Urea: The major nitrogen-containing product of protein catabolism.

Uric acid: The end product in the metabolism of purines; excreted in the urine; excess blood levels found in gout.

Vascular: Of or pertaining to blood vessels.

Ventricle: One of the two lower chambers of the heart.

Visual purple: Rhodopsin.

Wernick's encephalopathy: A disease of the nervous system characterized by ataxia, mental confusion and amnesia; seen in alcholics and due to a thiamin deficiency.

Xerophthalmia: A condition in which the eye becomes dry and lusterless; it is followed by inflammation, infection, ulceration, softening and blindness. Caused by a vitamin A deficiency.

INDEX

·····························I N D E X ·····························

About the Authors

Robert H. Garrison, Jr., M.A., R.Ph. is a health and nutrition education specialist for broadcast and print media. He is the publisher of *The Nutrition Report*, a monthly publication summarizing research from over 6,000 scientific sources, and president of Health Media of America, Inc., an educational corporation active in implementing health enhancement and disease prevention programs. Mr. Garrison has lectured extensively throughout the U.S. and has taught numerous courses in nutrition and pharmacology. He is continuing his doctoral studies in health communications and conducting research on the role of nutrition in the alcohol and drug addiction recovery process. He lives in Del Mar, California.

Elizabeth Somer, M.A. is a consulting nutritionist, speaker and writer specializing in health promotion. She has taught university graduate and undergraduate nutrition and health courses and has conducted nutrition seminars, workshops, classes and guest lectures for high school, college, professional and community audiences. She has developed nutrition education programs and counseled patients on controlling health problems through diet and lifestyle modification. Ms. Somer has published numerous articles in the field of nutrition and is currently working with Mr. Garrison on the development of video and films for nutrition programs. She lives in San Diego.